Biomedical Signal Processing for Healthcare Applications

Emerging Trends in Biomedical Technologies and Health Informatics

Series Editors

Subhendu Kumar Pani

Orissa Engineering College, Bhubaneswar, Orissa, India

Sujata Dash

North Orissa University, Baripada, India

Sunil Vadera

University of Salford, Salford, UK

Everyday Technologies in Healthcare
Chhabi Rani Panigrahi, Bibudhendu Pati, Mamata Rath, and Rajkumar Buyya

Biomedical Signal Processing for Healthcare Applications
Varun Bajaj, G. R. Sinha, and Chinmay Chakraborty

Deep Learning in Biomedical and Health Informatics
M. Jabbar, Ajith Abraham, Onur Dogan, Ana Madureira, and Sanju Tiwar

For more information about this series, please visit: https://www.routledge.com/Emerging-Trends-in-Biomedical-Technologies-and-Health-informatics-series/book-series/ETBTHI

Biomedical Signal Processing for Healthcare Applications

Edited by

Varun Bajaj, G. R. Sinha, and
Chinmay Chakraborty

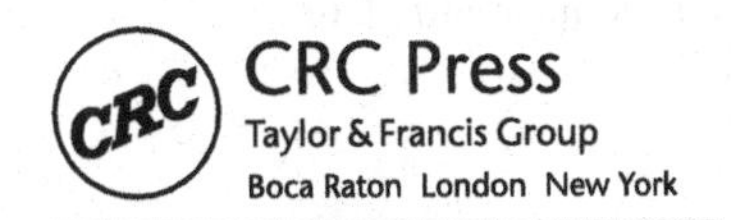

CRC Press is an imprint of the
Taylor & Francis Group, an informa business

First edition published 2022
by CRC Press
6000 Broken Sound Parkway NW, Suite 300, Boca Raton, FL 33487-2742

and by CRC Press
2 Park Square, Milton Park, Abingdon, Oxon, OX14 4RN

CRC Press is an imprint of Taylor & Francis Group, LLC

Library of Congress Cataloging-in-Publication Data
Names: Bajaj, Varun, editor. | Sinha, G. R., 1975- editor. | Chakraborty, Chinmay, 1984- editor.
Title: Biomedical signal processing for healthcare applications / edited by Varun Bajaj, G. R. Sinha and Chinmay Chakraborty.
Description: First edition. | Boca Raton: CRC Press, 2021. | Series: Emerging trends in biomedical technologies and health informatics | Includes bibliographical references and index. | Summary: "This book examines biomedical signal processing in which biomedical signals such as EEG, EMG, ECG are used to analyze and diagnosis various medical conditions. In combination with machine learning tools and other optimization methods, the analysis of biomedical signals will subsequently benefit the healthcare sector"—Provided by publisher.
Identifiers: LCCN 2021005666 (print) | LCCN 2021005667 (ebook) |
ISBN 9780367705879 (hardback) | ISBN 9780367707545 (paperback) |
ISBN 9781003147817 (ebook)
Subjects: LCSH: Biomedical engineering. | Signal processing.
Classification: LCC R856 .B522 2021 (print) | LCC R856 (ebook) |
DDC 610.28—dc23
LC record available at https://lccn.loc.gov/2021005666
LC ebook record available at https://lccn.loc.gov/2021005667

ISBN: 978-0-367-70587-9 (hbk)
ISBN: 978-0-367-70754-5 (pbk)
ISBN: 978-1-003-14781-7 (ebk)

Typeset in Times
by codeMantra

Contents

Preface

The advances of medical image processing and soft computing techniques have made automatic diagnosis of various diseases using different medical image modalities. The area of automatic diagnosis and analysis of medical images is referred to as Computer-Aided-Diagnosis (CAD), which has become an integral part of modern diagnostics and healthcare sector. One of the important research avenues of medical image processing is Biomedical Signal Processing in which biomedical signals such as EEG, EMG, and ECG are used and analyzed, and appropriate classification-based diagnosis is suggested. The analysis of biomedical signals becomes much relevant especially due to Covid-19 issues and challenges. It has been reported that physicians all the world over are interactively using modern CAD-based diagnosis systems so as to provide utmost care to the patients. Also, the fear of job loss, stress and other factors have been causing mental difficulties in youth as well as all sections of society. Biomedical signal processing and analysis has the capability of addressing a number of health issues as a consequence of corona virus, in particular, or other diseases and disorders due to other factors, in general. Despite the availability of globally competent experts, the healthcare is not easily approachable to common masses and in rural areas. Sometimes the physicians also fail to provide the most appropriate diagnosis due to improper understanding and analysis of images. Therefore, the proposed book becomes pertinent in addressing various challenges in healthcare. The use of suitable signal processing methods, machine learning tools, optimization methods and many others would result in a great impact in the analysis of biomedical signals that subsequently benefit the healthcare sector. The proposed book would include all important modalities of biomedical signals, such as EEG, EMG, MEG, ECG, and PCG, which are used in the diagnosis of dangerous illness related to the heart and brain of human beings. The discussion of these modalities will help in better understating, analysis and application of the biomedical signal processing for specific diseases.

The chapter-wise description of the book is as follows: In Chapter 1, sleep is studied of paramount importance to us, and it aids in healing mental as well as physical health of humans. Lack of sleep builds up the risk of serious diseases such as diabetes and cancer. The proficient technique of scoring the sleep stages in electroencephalogram (EEG) is an indispensable tool for medical practitioners to diagnose sleep disorders at an early stage. In this regard, correlation graphs are employed to classify the sleep stage EEG signals. The EEG segments are split to sub-segments, and then by using the statistical methods, the dimensions of the sub-segments are scaled down. Subsequently, each segment is mapped to a graph by taking particular sub-segments as vertices of the graph. In Chapter 2, the authors have constructed a distress phase emotion model using the inherent properties of the arousal, valence, dominance and liking dimensions of emotion representation. Furthermore, a shifted tanh-based normalization scheme is introduced, and the inverse Fisher transformation algorithm is applied to the Database for Emotion Analysis using Physiological Signal (DEAP) dataset. The Radial Basis Function Artificial Neural Networks (RBF-ANN) pattern recognizer was consequently utilized to conduct various experiments and compared the performances of digital image-based feature extraction techniques of Histogram of Oriented Gradient (HOG), Local Binary Pattern (LBP) and Histogram of Images (HIM). Chapter 3 deals with an introduction and background information of heart anatomy and physiology including the biomechanics and electrophysiology. A detailed introduction of ECG signals and complete information required for working with ECG signals including the basics of ECG such as limb and chest leads, electrode placements, components of a tracing rhythm setup, strip analysis and more are presented. During the content review in Chapter 4, a versatile range of feature selection and classification techniques based on deep learning approaches have been compared to differentiate between a healthy human and one who is afflicted by Parkinson's disease. Various classification algorithms are used to achieve better results in terms of efficiency and time. In this chapter, classifiers like Deep Neural Network (DNN), Convolutional Neural Network (CNN), and Deep Belief Network (DBN) are compared on different types of data corpus. In this context, we discuss some possible research directions throwing light on the advantages that deep learning can have for PD detection. This chapter ends with an analysis of the challenges, issues, and opportunities of deep learning models with respect to detection of neurodegenerative disease (ND).

The objective of the study in Chapter 5 is to classify the imagined words and phonological categories and evaluate the feasibility of this task based on the accuracy arising from them. In this regard, EEG data are pre-processed to minimize the effect of artefacts and noise. EEG signal is further decomposed by wavelet transform and empirical mode decomposition to extract meaningful information and evaluate statistical features. The Kruskal-Wallis test is performed to select the highly discriminative features. Different classification algorithms, k-nearest neighbors, decision tree, support vector machine, and ensemble bagged tree are employed for the classification. Chapter 6 aims to investigate the relationship between blood pressure (BP) and two easy-access bio-signals (electrocardiogram (ECG) and photoplethysmogram (PPG)), and use them to measure BP continuously and noninvasively. Since ECG reveals the electrical excitation of the heart, it provides an effective and practicable approach to analyze the heart condition. Furthermore, photoplethysmography that reveals blood volume fluctuations in the peripheral circulation system carries vital diagnostic information about the cardiovascular system. Here, these relationships and the main aspects of proposed models to deal with the issue are discussed. In Chapter 7, four subjects suffering from muscle impairment at different parts of their bodies were treated using acupuncture. The EMG signals at the injured parts were taken before and after the treatment. The results showed that the treatment did not produce any immediate conceivable effect on the patients, i.e. the levels of muscle contraction before and immediately after the treatment were similar. Signs of muscle relief were, nevertheless, observed when the EMG signals were measured 30 minutes after the treatment. This suggests that acupuncture does provide effective medication to the patients, albeit rather slowly. Chapter 8 proposes a method using sign language conversion techniques for recognizing hand gestures and thereby, controlling the appliances. Reducing the physical barriers due to some physical disability is considered the most important objective. These shortcomings may be faced by speaking-impaired people when communicating with others. These can be solved by implementing an electronic device to translate sign language. There are several methods available to recognize the hand gesture. The first method uses the flex sensor to determine the hand gesture to provide the analog output. This analog output of the flex sensor is used to determine the hand gesture made using the sign language. A microcontroller is used to determine the hand gesture made and to transmit the signal using a ZigBee module to the receiver unit which displays the symbol of the hand gesture using an LCD screen. A microcontroller is provided in the receiver circuit which receives the signal from the transmitter using the ZigBee module. In the second method, instead of data glove, the camera is utilized to capture the gesture. The captured images are compared with prestored database. The main objective of the computer-aided drug designing (CADD) in Chapter 9 is to identify the structure of chemical compound that is able to be inserted to a specific binding region of a protein or ligand target both structurally and chemically. Molecular property diagnostic suite (MPDS) is a free-source chemoinformatics portal and a web tool for drug identification and development platform. MPDS tools are planned for identification of enormous diseases that include diabetes mellitus, tuberculosis and metabolic disorder; the main aim is to assess and approximate the drug-likeness of a target molecule. In Chapter 10, with a large number of diagnostic examinations performed every year, chest X-rays are a significant and available clinical imaging instrument for the location of numerous diseases. Out of 1 billion X-rays taken every year, around 40 million X-rays are misdiagnosed leading to high fatality. Notwithstanding, their helpfulness can be restricted by difficulties in translation, which requires fast and intensive assessment of a two-dimensional picture portraying complex, three-dimensional organs and disease measures.

Chapter 11 focuses on providing efficient disease detection with the highest efficiency and the lowest error rate. A comparative study among well-known machine learning classifier models such as Support Vector Machine, Multi-layer perceptron, k-Nearest Neighbor, Decision Tree, Naïve Bayes, Gradient Boost, AdaBoost, and Random Forest is shown in this research. For each of the considered diseases, the most appropriate model is chosen in terms of their prediction efficiency. In Chapter 12, an erudite systematic framework of theoretical and topical efficacious research is done towards the development of real-time smart wearables to monitor and analyze blood sugar level by integrating noninvasive photoacoustic method. An intelligent diagnostic system helps to analyze the level of blood glucose and BP monitoring data by mapping of low and high blood pressures, with several permutation of diabetes insipidus and mellitus, hence serving towards the prime objective. In Chapter 13, the retinal fundus images were fed into the convolutional neural network with pooling and parameter sharing. There is no need for human intervention in executing this architecture. The execution will be user-friendly, accurate, and attractive. The performance of this is comparatively higher than other algorithms. The darkness that can occur in the life of humans through eye diseases can be avoided by diagnosing the diseases using this method at their earlier stages.

The major highlights of the book include biomedical signals, acquisition of the signals, pre-processing and analysis, post-processing and classification of the signals, and application of analysis and classification for diagnosis of brain- and heart-related diseases. The emphasis is given to the brain and heart signals because these lead to major complications and poorer interpretations by the physicians in quite a number of situations. Thus, the book would be an excellent research-oriented reading material and manual that can be used by a wide range of readers such as students, research scholars, faculty, and practitioners in the field of biomedical image analysis and diagnosis.

Acknowledgements

For this important book on Advances in Biomedical Signal Processing for Healthcare, we express our deepest gratitude to our family members, teachers, friends, and well-wishers for their support.

We would like to thank all those who keep us motivated in doing more and more; better and better. We sincerely thank all contributors for providing relevant theoretical background and information about real-time applications of Biomedical Signal Processing for healthcare.

We express our humble thanks to the entire editorial team of CRC Press for their great support, necessary help, appreciation, and quick responses. We also thank CRC Press for their support and the publishing house for giving us this opportunity to contribute on some relevant topic with the reputed publisher. Finally, we want to thank everyone, in one way or another, who helped us in editing this book.

Editors

Varun Bajaj, PhD, (MIEEE 16 SMIEEE20) is working as a faculty in the discipline of Electronics and Communication Engineering at Indian Institute of Information Technology, Design and Manufacturing (IIITDM) Jabalpur, India since 2014. He worked as a visiting faculty in IIITDM Jabalpur from September 2013 to March 2014. He worked as an Assistant Professor at the Department of Electronics and Instrumentation, Shri Vaishnav Institute of Technology and Science, Indore, India during 2009–2010. He earned a BE in electronics and communication engineering at Rajiv Gandhi Technological University, Bhopal, India in 2006, an MTech with honors in microelectronics and VLSI design at Shri Govindram Seksaria Institute of Technology and Science, Indore, India in 2009. He earned a PhD in the discipline of electrical engineering at Indian Institute of Technology Indore, India in 2014.

He is an Associate Editor of *IEEE Sensor Journal* and Subject Editor-in-Chief of *IET Electronics Letters*. He served as a Subject Editor of *IET Electronics Letters* from November 2018 to June 2020. He is a Senior Member of IEEE June 2020, MIEEE 16–20, and an active technical reviewer of leading international journals of IEEE, IET, Elsevier, etc. He has authored more than 100 research papers in various reputed international journals/conferences such as IEEE Transactions, Elsevier, Springer, and IOP. He has edited *Modelling and Analysis of Active Biopotential Signals in Healthcare*, volumes 1 and 2, published by IOP Books. The citation impact of his publications is 2048, h index of 20, and i10 index of 47 (Google Scholar Sep 2020). He has guided six (three completed and three in-process) PhD scholars and six MTech scholars. He is a recipient of various reputed national and international awards. His research interests include biomedical signal processing, image processing, time-frequency analysis and computer-aided medical diagnosis.

G. R. Sinha, PhD, is an Adjunct Professor at International Institute of Information Technology Bangalore (IIITB) and currently deputed as a Professor at Myanmar Institute of Information Technology (MIIT) Mandalay, Myanmar. He earned a BE (electronics engineering) and an MTech (computer technology) with gold medal at the National Institute of Technology Raipur, India. He earned a PhD in electronics and telecommunication engineering at Chhattisgarh Swami Vivekanand Technical University (CSVTU) Bhilai, India. He has been a Visiting Professor (honorary) at the Sri Lanka Technological Campus Colombo for one year, 2019–2020.

He has published 259 research papers, book chapters, and books at the international level, which include *Biometrics* (Wiley India), *Medical Image Processing* (Prentice Hall of India), and seven edited books on cognitive science (Elsevier, 2 vols.), optimization theory (IOP), biometrics (Springer), modelling of bio-potential signals (IOP), and assessment of learning outcomes (IGI). He is currently editing six books on biomedical signals, brain and behavior computing, modern sensors, and data deduplication with Elsevier, IOP, and CRC Press. He is an Associate Editor of three SCI journals: *IET-Electronics Letters*, *IET-Image Processing Journal*, and

IEEE Access-Multidisciplinary Open Access Journal. He has 22 years' teaching and research experience. He has been the Dean of Faculty and Executive Council Member of CSVTU and is currently a member of Senate of MIIT. Dr. Sinha has delivered ACM lectures across the world as an ACM Distinguished Speaker in the field of DSP since 2017. His important assignments include Expert Member for Vocational Training Program by Tata Institute of Social Sciences (TISS) for two years (2017–2019), Chhattisgarh Representative of IEEE MP Sub-Section Executive Council (2016–2019), and Distinguished Speaker in the field of Digital Image Processing by Computer Society of India (2015). He served as a Distinguished IEEE Lecturer at the IEEE India council for the Bombay section.

Dr. Sinha is the recipient of many awards and recognitions, such as TCS Award 2014 for Outstanding Contributions in Campus Commune of TCS, Rajaram Bapu Patil ISTE National Award 2013 for Promising Teacher in Technical Education by ISTE New Delhi, Emerging Chhattisgarh Award 2013, Engineer of the Year Award 2011, Young Engineer Award 2008, Young Scientist Award 2005, IEI Expert Engineer Award 2007, ISCA Young Scientist Award 2006 Nomination, and Deshbandhu Merit Scholarship for five years. He is a Senior Member of IEEE, a Fellow of the Institute of Engineers India, and a Fellow of IETE India.

Dr. Sinha has delivered more than 50 keynote/invited talks and chaired many technical sessions at international conferences in Singapore, Myanmar, Sri Lanka, and India. His special session on "Deep Learning in Biometrics" was included in the IEEE International Conference on Image Processing 2017. He is also a member of many national professional bodies such as ISTE, CSI, ISCA, and IEI. He is a member of various committees of the university and has been the vice president of the Computer Society of India for the Bhilai Chapter for two consecutive years. He is a consultant of various skill development initiatives of NSDC, Government of India. He is regular referee of project grants under the DST-EMR scheme and several other schemes of the Government of India. He has also received several consultancy supports as grants and travel support.

Dr. Sinha has supervised nine PhD scholars and 15 MTech scholars. His research interest includes biometrics, cognitive science, medical image processing, computer vision, outcome-based education (OBE), and ICT tools for developing employability skills.

Chinmay Chakraborty, PhD, is an Assistant Professor (Sr.) in the Department of Electronics and Communication Engineering, Birla Institute of Technology, Mesra, India. He worked at the Faculty of Science and Technology, ICFAI University, Agartala, Tripura, India as a Senior Lecturer. He worked as a Research Consultant in the Coal India project at Industrial Engineering and Management, IIT Kharagpur. He worked as a project coordinator of the Telecommunication Convergence Switch project under the Indo-US joint initiative. He also worked as a Network Engineer in System Administration at MISPL, India. His main research interests include the internet of medical things, wireless body area network, wireless networks, telemedicine, m-health/e-health, and medical imaging. Dr. Chakraborty has published sixty papers at reputed international journals, conferences, book chapters, and books. He is an Editorial Board Member in numerous journals and conferences. He serves as a guest editor of *MDPI-Future Internet Journal, Wiley-Internet Technology Letters, Springer-Annals of Telecommunications, IGI-International Journal of E-Health*, and *Medical Communications*, and he has conducted a session of SoCTA-19, ICICC-2019, Springer CIS 2020, and also a reviewer for international journals including *IEEE,* Elsevier, Springer, Taylor & Francis, IGI, IET, and Wiley publisher. Dr. Chakraborty is co-editing eight books on smart IoMT, healthcare technology, and sensor data analytics with CRC Press, IET, Pan Stanford, and Springer. He has served as a Publicity Chair member at renowned international conferences, including IEEE Healthcom, IEEE SP-DLT. Dr. Chakraborty is a member of the Internet Society, Machine Intelligence Research Labs, and the Institute for Engineering Research and Publication. He has received a Young Research Excellence Award, Global Peer Review Award, Young Faculty Award, and Outstanding Researcher Award.

Contributors

Abdultaofeek Abayomi
ICT and Society Research Group
Durban University of Technology
Durban, South Africa

Balakrishnakumar
Deep Scopy
Coimbatore, India

Samir Kumar Bandyopadhyay
The Bhawanipur Education Society College
Kolkata, India

Veerendra Dakulagi
Department of Electronics and Communication Engineering
Guru Nanak Dev Engineering College
Bidar, India

Shawni Dutta
Department of Computer Science
The Bhawanipur Education Society College
Kolkata, India

Jamal Esmaelpoor
Electrical Engineering Department
Islamic Azad University, Boukan Branch
Boukan, Iran

Pradnya H Ghare
Department of Electronics and Communication
Visvesvaraya National Institute of Technology
Nagpur, India

Subham Ghosh
Department of Electronics and Communication Engineering
JIS College of Engineering
Kalyani, India

Ayesha Heena
KBN College of Engineering
Kalaburagi, India

Delene Heukelman
ICT and Society Research Group
Durban University of Technology
Durban, South Africa

Sudarson Jena
Department of Computer Science and Engineering, SUIIT
Sambalpur University
Burla, India

Ashwin Kamble
Department of Electronics and Communication
Visvesvaraya National Institute of Technology
Nagpur, India

Priyanka Khanna
Department of Information Technology
National Institute of Technology, Raipur
Raipur, India

Vinay Kumar
Department of Electronics and Communication
Motilal Nehru National Institute of Technology
Allahabad, Prayagraj

Jibendu Kumar Mantri
Department of Computer Science and Applications
North Odisha University
Baripada, India

Chinmaya Misra
School of Computer Applications
KIIT Deemed to Be University
Bhubaneswar, India

Mohammad Hassan Moradi
Biomedical Engineering Department
Amirkabir University of Technology
Tehran, Iran

Biswarup Neogi
Department of Electronics and Communication Engineering
JIS College of Engineering
Kalyani, India

Wey Long Ng
Faculty of Engineering and Green Technology
Universiti Tunku Abdul Rahman
Kampar, Malaysia

Humaira Nisar
Faculty of Engineering and Green Technology
Universiti Tunku Abdul Rahman
Kampar, Malaysia

Oludayo O. Olugbara
ICT and Society Research Group
Durban University of Technology
Durban, South Africa

Sudhansu Shekhar Patra
School of Computer Applications
KIIT Deemed to Be University
Bhubaneswar, India

Patrali Pradhan
Department of Computer Science and Engineering
Haldia Institute of Technology
Haldia, India

Reena Raj
SBM
Christ (Deemed to Be University)
Bangalore, India

G Boopathi Raja
Department of Electrical and Computer Engineering
Velalar College of Engineering and Technology
Erode, India

Pugazendi Rajagopal
Department of Computer Science
Government Arts College
Salem, India

Karthikeyan Rajendran
Department of Biotechnology
Mepco Schlenk Engineering College
Sivakasi, India

Sasireka Rajendran
Department of Biotechnology
Mepco Schlenk Engineering College
Sivakasi, India

Shalini Ramesh
Department of Microbiology
Thiagarajar College
Madurai, India

Sneka Ramesh
Department of Biotechnology
Thiagarajar College
Madurai, India

Vinoth Rathinam
Department of Electronics and Communication Engineering
P.S.R. Engineering College
Sivakasi, India

Mridu Sahu
Department of Information Technology
National Institute of Technology, Raipur
Raipur, India

Swati Samantaray
School of Humanities
KIIT Deemed to Be University
Bhubaneswar, India

Zahra Momayez Sanat
Biomedical Engineering Department
Tehran University of Medical Sciences
Tehran, Iran

Padma Selvaraj
Department of Computer Science Technology
Madanapalle Institute of Technology and Science
Madanapalle, India

Bikesh Kumar Singh
Department of Biomedical Engineering
National Institute of Technology, Raipur
Raipur, India

Kamakhya Narain Singh
Department of Computer Science and Applications
North Odisha University
Baripada, India

Sugumari Vallinayagam
Department of Biotechnology
Mepco Schlenk Engineering College
Sivakasi, India

Vignessh B
SBM
Christ (Deemed to Be University)
Bangalore, India

Kim Ho Yeap
Faculty of Engineering and Green Technology
Universiti Tunku Abdul Rahman
Kampar, Malaysia

1 Automatic Sleep EEG Classification with Ensemble Learning Using Graph Modularity

Kamakhya Narain Singh
North Odisha University

Sudhansu Shekhar Patra and Swati Samantaray
KIIT Deemed to Be University

Sudarson Jena
Sambalpur University

Jibendu Kumar Mantri
North Odisha University

Chinmaya Misra
KIIT Deemed to Be University

CONTENTS

1.1 INTRODUCTION

Sleep, as we know, is one of the key activities of the brain. Throughout the sleeping duration, many neurons of the human body are inactive. Any disorderliness in the human sleep cycle may cause lifelong impediments related to the physical performances and mental health of an individual. According to some reputed health organizations of the United States, approximately 60–70 million populace endure sleep distracts like apnea and insomnia. The National Highway Traffic in the United States has reported that many traffic accidents occur due to sleep-related issues.

Sleep (a behavioral state that alternates with waking) has the following characteristics:

- Lying down posture
- Raised threshold to sensory simulation
- Low level of motor output
- Unparalleled behavior dreaming

Sleep scoring is a fundamental procedure in diagnosing sleep distracts, because it can compute the sleep quality in order to support experts in identifying the irregularities in a patient's recording. The study of sleep is called polysomnography (PSG). The major recordings for PSG are as follows:

- Electroencephalography (EEG): Electroencephalogram (EEG) is a test used to evaluate the electrical activity in the brain. Brain cells communicate with each other through electrical impulses. EEG can be used to detect potential problems associated with this activity.
- Electrooculography (EOG): It is a technique for measuring the corneo-retinal standing potential that exists between the front and the back of the human eye. The resulting signal is called the electrooculogram. Primary applications are in ophthalmological diagnosis and in recording eye movements.
- Electromyography (EMG): It is an electrodiagnostic medicine technique for evaluating and recording the electrical activity produced by skeletal muscles. EMG is performed using an instrument called an electromyograph to produce a record called electromyogram.

Besides the above measures, the other recordings are as follows:

- SpO_2: Oxygen saturation (SpO_2) is a measurement of how much oxygen your blood is carrying as a percentage of the maximum it could carry. For a healthy individual, the normal SpO_2 should be between 96% and 99%. High altitudes and other factors may affect what is considered normal for a given individual.
- Electrocardiography (ECG): It records the electrical signal from our heart to check for different heart conditions. Electrodes are placed on our chest to record our heart's electrical signals, which cause our heart to beat. The signals are shown as waves on an attached computer monitor or printer.
- Breathing functions: Breathing provides oxygen to the body parts and eliminates carbon dioxide resulting from cell metabolism. Major physiologic switches in breathing take place during the sleeping period linked to alterations in respiratory drive and musculature.

1.2 RELATED WORK

According to Mora et al. [1], there should be an effective demarcation in the stages of human sleep for treating the sleep disorders including apnea, insomnia and narcolepsy. The sleep process is a physiological activity in recovering from irregularities with the restoration of the energy level in persons and by overruling the exhausting consequences of wakefulness [2]. Currently various biomedical signal analyses such as EEG, EMG, EOG and ECG are functional in clinical setups which are employed for identifying the sleep disorderliness with EEG signal as one of the nearly useful signals in the classification of sleep stages in addition to sleep disorders [3]. Sleep scoring is a process of identifying the sleep disorders and also quantifying the abnormalities in the sleep. A sleep-specialist takes care of the sleep scoring process by following the guidelines of either Rechtschaf-fen and Kales (R&K) or the American Academy of Sleep Medicine (ASMA) [4–7]. Since the data collected are of higher dimension, the dimensionality reduction and feature extraction techniques are used for reducing the dimensionality of the data in the sleep scoring method. There are many sleep scoring methods being developed with one of the following domains: graphs, frequency, time and hybrid domains. Rodríguez-Sotelo et al. [8] suggested to extract entropy metrics from an EEG signal. The feature vector resulted was optimized using Q–α technique, followed by given to a J-means algorithm for clustering. Samiee et al. [9] suggested a Rational Discrete Short Time Fourier Transform (RDSTFT) to discover the various classes of EEG sleep signals. Using RDSTFT, the signals were disintegrated to a collection of frequency bands. From the EEG bands, the desired features are extracted using a basis pursual access method. Random forest classification approach was adopted to classify the evoked features. Aboalayon et al. [10] adopted Butterworth band-pass filters for disintegrating as well as filtering the EEG signal. In this research, distinct frequency characteristics were adopted from the EEG signal with five bands where a SVM classifier was used to distinguish the stages of the sleep state. Though single-channel study in the classification of sleep stages has received much attention, many research studies have been developed based on multi-channel EEG signals. A Multichannel Auto Regressive (MAR) technique was taken for identifying the EEG sleep stages.

In this work, every EEG signal was divided into low blocks. MAR coefficients have been computed by a histogram, and then, it was classified into five different classes. For sleep classification, Zhang et al. [11] proposed a multi-signal technique. In the feature extraction phase, a deep belief neural network was adopted for the classification. For classifying the extracted features, a multiclassifier voting scheme was adopted. A collection of EEG, EOG and EMG signals was used in this study, and the accuracy of the classification was 91%. Amin et al. [12] disintegrated multichannel EEG signals using a discrete wavelet transform. A JPEG2000 technique was employed for the extraction of the required features. The extracted features from the EEGs were fed to an ML classifier.

Recent research suggests that biomedical signals generally show nonlinear deportments as well as irregular practices, as their statistical characteristics alter with the transition of time [13,14]. So many research studies in this field have been formulated with nonlinear techniques [15–17]. Farag et al. [16] proposed a disordered variation analysis to classify sleep stages.

The fast Fourier transform and wavelet transform have [18,19] been used in time domain [20]. Peker [21] proposed a model for sleep classification based on frequency domain in which a dual wavelet transform has been utilized for extracting features for EEG data. Gao et al. [22] suggested a multiclassifier model for classifying the sleep stages which is based on fast Fourier transform using a hamming window length same as the EEG segment length. Czish et al. [23] utilized a normalized wavelet transform to decompose EEG signals to distinct frequency bands. The statistical features were calculated from every decomposed level. The extracted features were then fed into a random forest classifier.

A nonlinear method was applied by Lee et al. [24] for analysis of EEG signals in which fractal scaling exponents were computed depending on a detrended variation analysis and used for classifying the EEG signals. Acharya et al. [25] used a nonlinear feature extraction method for analyzing EEG sleep signals. Diykh et al. [13,15] formulated automatic approaches to discover sleep stages using complex network features and ML methods. Distinct network characteristics were looked and analyzed. This research highlighted that nonlinear features describe the hidden features in the EEG signals. Zhu et al. [26] used visibility graphs for classifying a single-channel EEG signal to six sleep stages. Every EEG segment was mapped to a visibility graph, and then distinct graph features were elicited and then passed through a least square SVM algorithm for further signal processing and modeling.

This chapter makes a modest attempt to develop a trouble-free and prompt technique for sleep-stage identification, based on single-channel EEG signals. The novelty of the work is to classify the single-channel EEG sleep stages into various classifications from the undirected graph. Each segment (after getting divided into subsegments) is mapped to an undirected graph based on the statistical measurements. Ensemble learning with voting technique classifier is used for classifying the undirected graph features. During the training phase, the optimal parameters of the ensemble classifier are tested, and during the training phase, they are determined. The suggested method is compared with the other state-of-the-art methods, and its efficacy is verified with others.

1.3 ELECTROENCEPHALOGRAPHY (EEG)

The cerebral cortex is comprised of six layers. The layer number five has joint pyramidal cells, and the dendrites of this pyramidal cell extend up to the superficial cerebral cortex. Action potential (AP) of the pyramidal neuron is generated at the level of the initial segment. The electrodes in the EEG [27] are placed on the surface of the scalp. Since the electrodes are placed at the surface of the scalp, obviously the electrodes cannot record the electrical activities that occur within the deeper parts of the cerebral cortex. EEG is not the action potential of the brain, though we blindly say that the EEG is the electric activity of the brain. The dendrites are the sites where formation of multiple synapses occurs – there is an excitatory synapse (ES) and also an inhibitory synapse (IS). Whenever excitatory synapse is stimulated, there is a potential generation at the level of dendrites or post-synaptic neuron. This post-synaptic potential generated by the excitatory synapse is excitatory post-synaptic potential (EPSP). Similarly, inhibitory synapses produce the potential inhibitory post-synaptic potential (IPSP), which is again a kind of dendrite potential. It is said that there are trillions of synapses in the cortical region of the brain. All produce some kind of positive or negative voltage; owing to this, there is a flow of current from one part to other part. Due to the flow of the current, there is a shifting electrical dipole. The shifting of electrical dipoles gives rise to waves in EEG. If we place an electrode on the surface of the scalp, it will read certain electrical activities, that is, all the EPSP and IPSP that occur on the dendrites.

We can write this as follows:

$$\text{EEG} = \sum(\text{EPSP} + \text{IPSP}) \tag{1.1}$$

Equation (1.1) shows that EEG is the sum of all the EPSP and IPSP, which occur simultaneously.

But since EPSP + IPSP= Dendritic Potential, Equation (1.1) can be written as

$$\text{EEG} = \sum \text{Dendritic Potential} \tag{1.2}$$

Equation (1.2) shows that EEG is the sum of all the dendritic potential, that is, the local potential and not the action potential (AP). Rather than placing the electrodes on the surface of the scalp, which is done in EEG, if we place them directly above the surface of the cortex just above the pia mater [28], then the same recording will be known as electrocorticogram.

The EEG signals produced spontaneously shows the continuous activity of the brain.

1.3.1 Waves in EEG

EEG waves (or the Berger waves) are the waves created by the brain in all states of the mind [29]. Hans Berger invented the device known as electroencephalogram, which can record the frequencies of the human brain in different states of the mind. The different types of waves produced by the brain are as follows:

- **Beta Brainwaves (β waves)** (13–30 Hz): These waves have the highest frequency amongst all the waves. They are formed at the frontal lobes of the brain and are irregular waves. They normally dominate the usual waking states of consciousness and occur whenever the attention is directed towards cognitive as well as other tasks. These waves are produced when a person is alert, concentrating, attentive, focused and engaged in decision-making or problem-solving. Anxiety and depression have also been linked to beta waves for the reason that they may lead to 'rut-like' thinking patterns. When someone is engaged in a conversation, there is an increase in beta waves.
- **Alpha Brainwaves (α waves)** (8–10 Hz): Alpha waves are very regular and synchronized waves. These waves are generated from parietal lobes or occipital lobes. They are produced when the eyes are closed and during yoga and meditation when the mind is alert, and memory is potentiated. When a painter or musician is doing a creative work, these waves are emitted. These waves are produced in the state of relaxation and aids in improving our memory. Hans Berger was only able to record the alpha waves, and so alpha waves are also known as the Berger waves.
- **Theta Brainwaves (θ waves)** (4–7 Hz): These waves are produced from the hippocampus of the brain. When the mind is disappointed, these waves are generated. In the REM sleep, the theta waves are produced. Just before falling asleep and just after waking up when the mind is not that conscious as in the normal waken state, the theta waves are produced. During deep meditation, these waves are also produced. When we are recollecting the long-forgotten memories, the theta waves are produced by the brain.
- **Delta Brainwaves (δ waves)** (2–4 Hz): These waves are created during the deep sleep state, and they also have several therapeutic effects. They heal the disturbances. Whenever our state of mind is low or we feel sad, and after having a deep sleep when we wake up, we turn out to be energetic, and hence, the delta waves are produced by the brain.

Figure 1.1 shows the different brainwaves. The frequency decreases from Beta towards Delta, and the voltage or the amplitude increases. Frequency depends on the activity of the brain; more the active brain, more will be the frequency, and voltage depends on the synchronicity of different waves. Figure 1.2a shows the synchronous voltages and Figure 1.2b asynchronous voltages. In synchronous, the net voltage will be more, and so amplitude will also be more.

Frequency $\propto$ brain activity

The more active the brain, the more the frequency.

Table 1.1 shows the classification of different brainwaves in terms of frequency (Hz), amplitude (μV), and the recording and location of waves.

In Figure 1.3, the phases of alpha to beta brainwave conversion recordings are shown. During alpha wave, voltage is more, and they are produced when someone is relaxing, eyes are closed and the mind is wandering. If some sensory stimulation

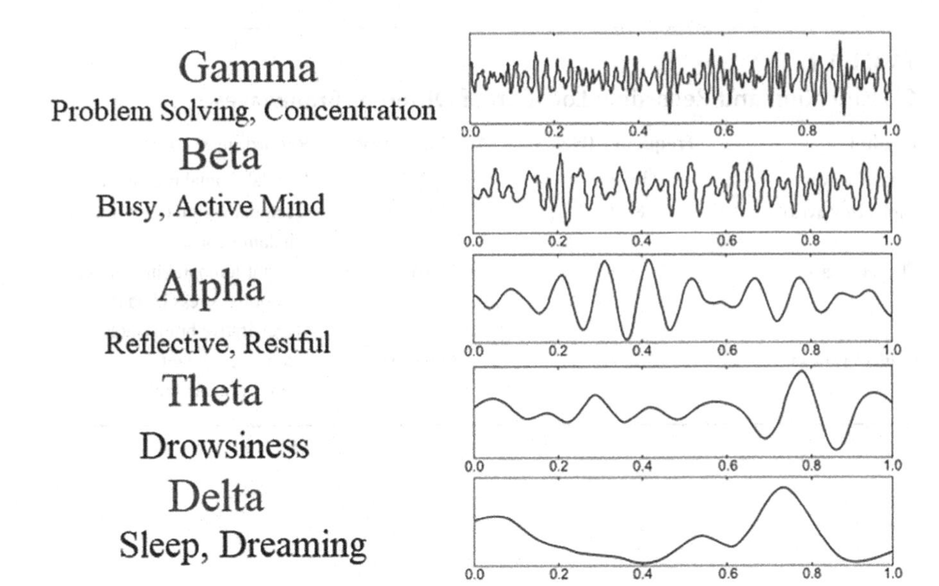

FIGURE 1.1 Different types of brainwaves in EEG.

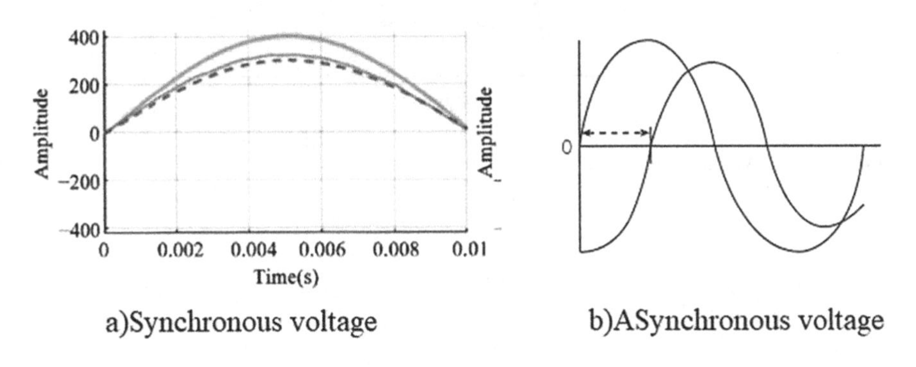

FIGURE 1.2 Types of voltages.

is given, the alpha wave is converted to beta wave. This process is known as alpha block phenomena. When the eyes are open, the beta waves are generated, which are high-frequency active waves. When frequency is high, the voltage is decremented. Since the frequency is so high, it is not even possible to count the picks.

Figure 1.4 reveals where there is a need of clinical attention in a patient. In those waves, the frequency is very high. It can be noted from the figure that within the time scale of 1 second in the delta wave, there is only 3 picks or 3 Hz, and it goes on increasing in theta, alpha and beta waves, respectively. The pathological state where clinical attention is required is the tonic-clonic seizure. There, the frequency is very high. The figure shows that the more the activity in the brain, the more will be the frequency.

TABLE 1.1
Classification and Recording Location of Different Brainwaves

Rhythm	Frequency (Hz)	Amplitude (μV)	Recording & Location
Beta (β waves)	13–30	20	Parietal-frontal region main
Alpha (α waves)	8–10	50–100	Occipital region (more intense), thalamo-cortical
Theta (θ waves)	4–7	Above 50	Parietal-temporal in children Emotional stress in adults Degenerative brain states
Delta (δ waves)	2–4	Above 50	Deep sleep, infant, serious organic brain disease

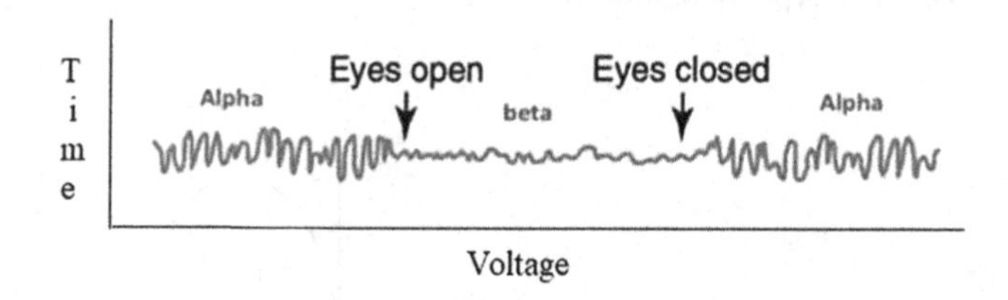

FIGURE 1.3 Alpha block phenomena.

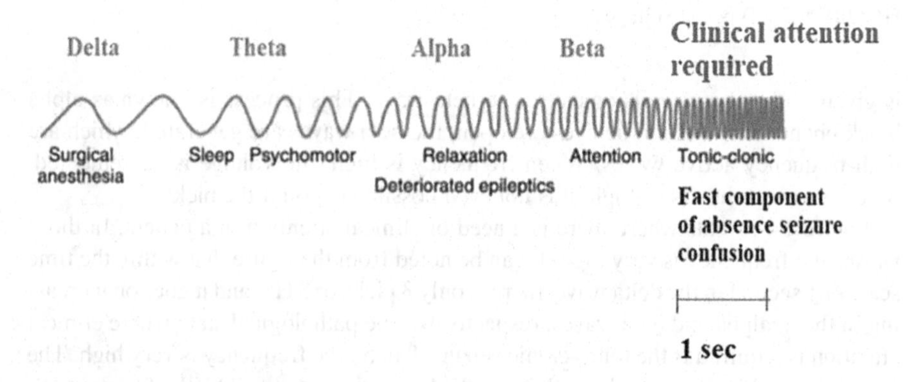

FIGURE 1.4 Different waves in EEG signal.

1.3.2 Types of Sleep

The human brain undergoes quite a number of stable physiological phases during sleep. EEG waves during sleep are divided into three stages:

1. Awake
2. Non-Rapid Eye Movement (Non-REM or NREM)
3. Rapid Eye Movement (REM) sleep [13,30–33]
   - **Awake** stage is divided into two types: the first type of awake stage is 'Eyes Open'. When we go to bed and our eyes are open during that time, beta waves are in higher frequency. The second type of awake stage is 'Eyes Closed', when we are awakened but our eyes are closed, and during that time, alpha waves are produced.
   - **NREM sleep**: Of the entire sleep cycle, 75%–80% of the sleep is of NREM sleep. This is also known as slow-wave sleep. It is a quiet sleep, and during this sleep, all the psychological processes slow down. In this condition, the eyes are usually closed, and many nervous centers become inactive, so rendering the person either partially or completely unconscious and making the brain a less complicated network. No dreams are being registered during this stage. It is broadly categorized into four states: stage 1, stage 2, stage 3 and stage 4. As per AASM, stage 1 is called N1, stage 2 is called N2, and stages 3 and 4 are called N3 [34].
     - During N1 state, the person is in the condition of doziness, and the waves emitted by the brain are the theta waves. Alertness level to the external environment decreases, hypnic jerks may occur, and muscular tone decreases.
     - N2 state is a light sleep stage. 45%–50% of the adults always possess N2 state. The characteristic waves seen during this state in EEG signals are sleep spindles and K complexes. During this state, there is no conscious awareness of external environment, and there is a decrease in muscular activity.
     - N3 state is the deep sleep stage. Delta waves are seen in this stage. The traits featured here are parasomnias, night tremors, night talking and night walking.
   - **REM Sleep.** The new nomenclature is **R stage**. Of the entire sleep cycle, 20%–25% of the sleep is of REM sleep. This is also known as paradoxical sleep. The waves seen during this period are beta waves having the highest frequency with the highest alertness. This is the stage of lucid

TABLE 1.2
Types of NREM Sleep with Features

Recent Stage	%	Features
N1	5	Alpha to theta wave
N2	55	Sleep spindles, K complexes
N3	15	Delta wave

dreaming. Most of the dreams can be registered during this stage, and we can remember them the next morning.

1.3.2.1 Sleep Cycle Stages

Figure 1.5 shows the sleep stages of a person. Every person first enters the N1 stage, followed by N2, N3, REM and again N1. This is known as a sleep cycle. However, this is only for the first cycle of the sleep. After that, the sleep may or may not follow each stage of the sleep. After the first cycle, it may directly enter stage N2 bypassing the stage N1; one may directly enter stage N3 bypassing both N1 and N2 and so on. Only in the first cycle, all the stages are followed; nevertheless, after that, the stages may be irregular. The duration of the first cycle is 70–100 minutes, but the later cycles have 90–120 minutes. So on average, a sleep cycle is considered to be approximately 90 minutes. If someone is sleeping for 6–8 hours, he/she completes around 7–8 sleep cycles depending on the sleep time.

Figure 1.6 shows the stages of a person's sleep with respect to time. When a person enters the sleep, he enters into N1, and then goes to N2, followed by N3; step by step he is moving to N2 again, then N1 and then moving to REM sleep. In Figure 1.6, from 1 to 2, it will be a complete sleep cycle. During this NONREM sleep, there will be theta (θ) and delta (δ) waves. They are the slow-frequency waves, and so it is known as slow-wave sleep. The REM sleep indicates a paradoxical sleep, and we are getting beta-like waves. The beta waves are normally generated when a person is awake or concentrating. In the REM sleep, the person is in sleep, but the signal we are getting is as if the person is awake, so they are contradicting. Recording the eyeball or muscle movements says the person is sleeping, but the EEG recording says the person is awake. Hence, the REM sleep is called 'paradoxical' sleep. From the figure, one can see that when a person moves from the early stage to the late stage of sleep towards the morning, the REM sleep duration increases. Figure 1.7 shows the EOG, EMG and EEG recordings of the REM sleep.

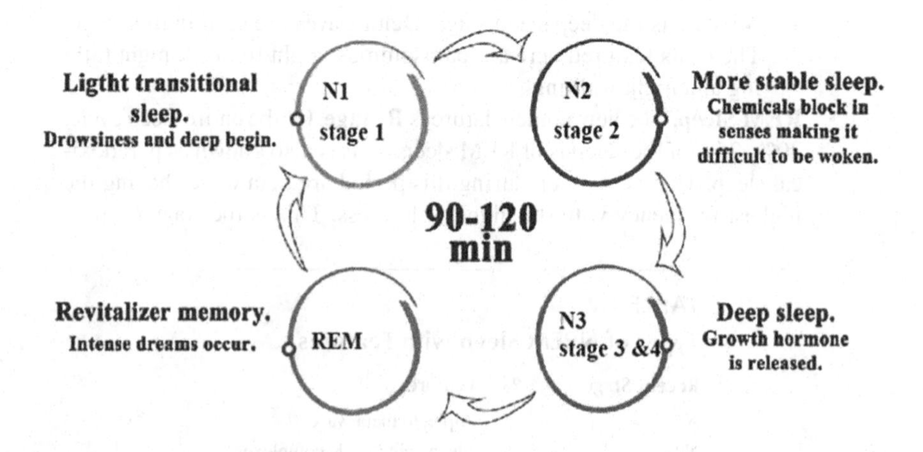

FIGURE 1.5 Sleep cycle stages.

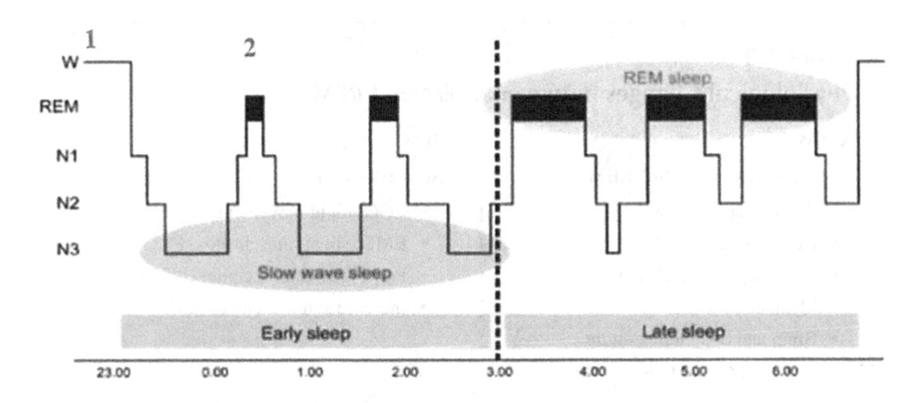

FIGURE 1.6 Stages of the sleep w.r.t time.

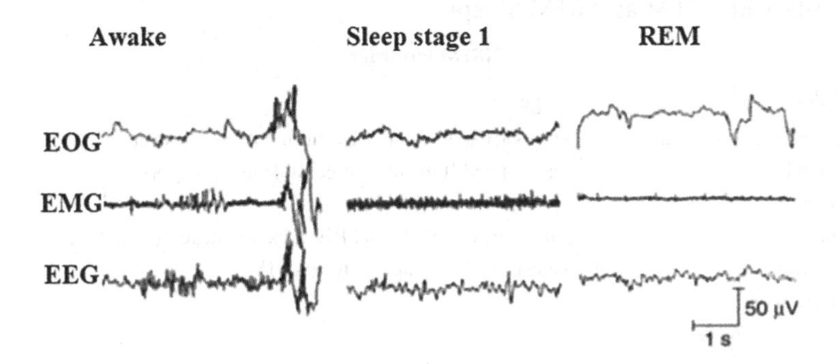

FIGURE 1.7 EOG, EMG and EEG recordings of REM sleep.

1.3.2.2 Physiological Changes between NREM and REM

The physiological changes that can be seen between NREM and REM are shown in Table 1.3.

1.3.2.3 Sleep Period over Life Span

The sleep period changes over the life span of individuals:

- Total sleep time decreases with age.
- All the stages of sleep are reversible except from REM to awake state.
- REM sleep % out of total sleeping time
  - Premature infants = 80% (full-term neonates = 50%)
  - Adult 20–65 years = 25%
  - After 65 years, it decreases (in elderly = 15%)

1.3.2.4 Disorders in NREM and REM Sleep

Table 1.4 shows the sleep disorders during the NREM and REM sleep along with the stages they are generally seen in.

TABLE 1.3
Physiological Changes between NREM and REM

NREM		REM
Resting stage of sleep in NREM.		Active dreaming occurs
• Sympathetic outflow	↓	• EOG: rapid movement
• Heart rate, BP	↓	• EMG: silent, muscle atonia
• Parasympathetic activity	↑	• Ponto-geniculo-occipital (PGO) spikes
• Metabolic rate	↓	• Increase sympathetic outflow
• Brain and body temperature	↓	
• Muscle tone and reflexes intact		

TABLE 1.4
Disorders in NREM and REM Sleeps

NREM Disorder	
Disorder	**Stage**
Sleep walking (somnambulism)	Stages III and IV can occur during the REM sleep
Sleep talking	Stages I and II mainly but possible in all stages
Bruxism	Mainly in stages I and II
Nocturnal enuresis	All stages of NREM and REM, except stage I (max during stage II)
Night terrors	Transition from stage III to stage IV
REM Disorder	
Narcolepsy, nightmare	

1.4 THE EEG DATASET

In this research work, two publicly accessible datasets are used for the classification of the EEG sleep stages. The datasets are gathered from two sources but follow R & K or the AASM rule.

1.4.1 ISRUC-Sleep Database

This dataset is acquired at the Coimbra University Hospital during 2009–2013. It consists of three subgroups. Each subgroup consists of distinct subjects and comprises healthy subjects, subjects having sleep disorders, and subjects with the effects of meditations. The data are recorded from 8, 10 and 100 participants, respectively. The recordings are stored in European Data Format (EDF) files. For the classification, we have considered C3-A2 channel as it gave better classification results [35]. For doing the sleep research, the dataset is publicly available.

The EEG recordings of subjects 1 to 18 are considered in this chapter. 15 males and 4 females in the age group of 22–76 with heights ranging from 68 to 178 cm and weights from 41 to 110 kg are taken.

1.4.2 Sleep-EDF Database

The other set of EEG recordings was collected from PysioNet [36–40]. From two studies, 61 EEG recordings were collected. For simulation, 13 subjects are taken in this chapter. EDF format was used to store all recordings. The signals were sampled at 100Hz. Table 1.5 shows the epochs for EEG sleep stages.

1.5 GRAPH MODULARITY

The modularity in a graph can be denoted as follows:

- Nodes in a real-world graph which aggregates the densely connected subgraphs are known as modules or communities.
- In a module, these nodes are strongly connected with one another as compared to other parts of the network.

Mathematically, graph modularity can be represented as follows:
Let $G=<V,E>$ be a graph. Suppose that $A \subset V$ and $e(A)=\{\{x,y\}\in E : x\in A, y\in A\}$.
Let $M=\{A_1,A_2,\ldots A_k\}$ be a vertex partition of the vertex set V into disjoint subsets.
We can define

$$q(M)=\sum_{i=1}^{k}\left(\frac{e(A_i)}{|E|}-\frac{\left(\sum_{v\in A_i}\deg v\right)^2}{4|E|^2}\right) \tag{1.3}$$

$$q^*(G)=\max_{A} q(M) \tag{1.4}$$

Here in Equation (1.4) $q^*(G)$ is the graph modularity. This is a well-known matric for determining the quality of algorithms for the clustering of complex graph networks.

The modularity is found in the brain network, in the social network where friendship ties tend to be dense within a certain group of people sharing similar social interests. Here we can classify them into different communities or clusters very easily. Figure 1.8a has four modules but (b) has no noticeable modules.

TABLE 1.5
The Number of Epochs of EEG Sleep Stages for Two Different Datasets

Number of Segments from Dataset	AWA	S1	S2	S3	S4	REM	Total
Dataset-1	5900	3500	7170	4320	1900	900	23,690
Dataset-2	1100	900	1050	1160	820	340	5370

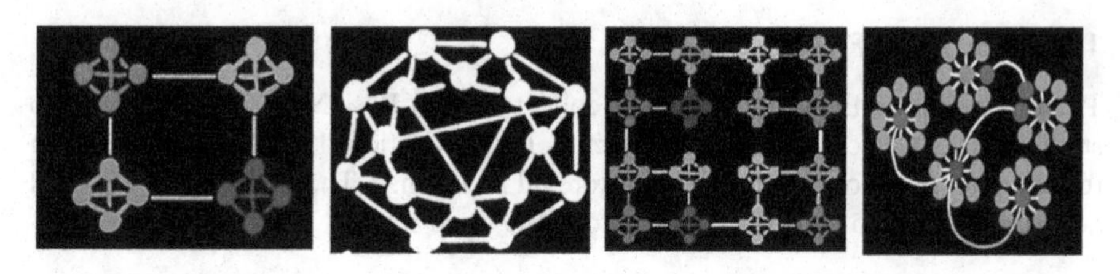

FIGURE 1.8 (a) Modularity, (b) nonmodular graph, (c) hierarchical modularity and (d) modular graphs.

In graph theory, a clustering coefficient is a measurement of the degree to which graph nodes tend to cluster together.

In hierarchical modularity, the real-world graphs are organized hierarchically in their modules such that they contain modules within modules. Figure 1.8c shows hierarchical modularity.

Modular graphs have strong within-module connectivity results and a small number of inter-modular links for maintaining a low characteristic path length in the network [41]. Figure 1.8d shows a modular graph.

The shortest path length L is given in Equation (1.5):

$$L = \frac{1}{N}\sum_{i} l_i = \frac{1}{N(N-1)}\sum_{i\neq j} l_{ij} \tag{1.5}$$

where l_i is the average shortest path from node i to all other nodes.

N is the number of nodes in the graph.

$N(N-1)$ is the number of node pairs excluding self-pairing.

l_{ij} is the shortest path length between nodes i and j.

The benefits of modularity in graph topology argued that modularity and hierarchical organization are essential ingredients for evolvability, adoptability, flexibility and complexity.

1.6 ENSEMBLE TECHNIQUES

The technique of ensemble classifier [42] is the method in which multiple predictors are applied on the same dataset, and based on all the predictions, the final prediction is made by aggregating the predictions resulting from all of them. The problem is a supervised learning prediction problem with multiple inputs, and we have to predict a class. Here the base predictor is the same and we are increasing the accuracy of the classification algorithm by ensemble learning. Figure 1.9 shows the ensemble learning method. Ensemble technique are basically two types

1. Bagging (Bootstrap Aggregation) – One of the techniques in bagging is called Random Forest. Random Forest uses multiple decision trees.
2. Boosting – Boosting is classified into three categories: AdaBoosting, Gradient Boosting (GB) and Extra Gradient boosting (Xgboost).

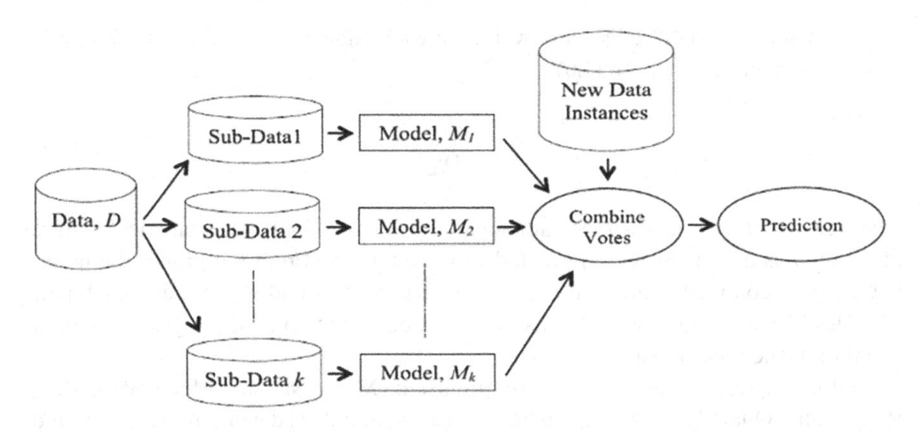

FIGURE 1.9 Ensemble learning model to increase the accuracy of classification model.

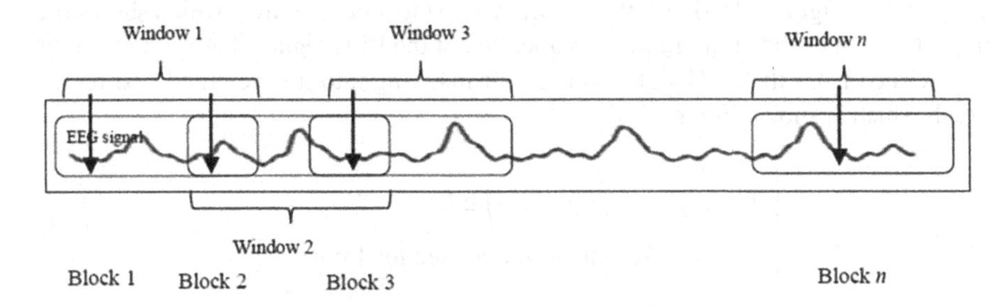

FIGURE 1.10 Using sliding window procedure, the EEG signal is divided into blocks.

1.7 METHODOLOGY

The EEG signal taken for 30 seconds is partitioned into blocks which are of 0.4 seconds each, overlapping to one another using the sliding window method. The dimensionality is reduced as it is the important step in reducing the complexity of the algorithm and the performance improvement. From each block, 12 statistical features are being extracted. The EEG segment of 30 seconds is transferred to weighted undirected graph. Figure 1.10 shows the sliding window procedure for dividing the EEG signal into blocks of window size 1 second each having an overlapping of 0.4 seconds. So the segment of 30 seconds is partitioned into 30/(1−0.4) = 49 blocks which are overlapping. As 12 statistical features are extracted from each block, the extracted feature of 588 features forms a vector to represent each segment of 30 seconds each.

1.7.1 Transforming the Statistical Features to Undirected Weighted Graph

Each vector of statistical features, $T=\{y_1,y_2, \ldots y_m\}$, representing one EEG segment, is transferred to an undirected weighted graph $G=<V, E, W>$ where V, E, and W are the set of vertices, set of edges and weight of each edge, respectively. The weight of an edge is given in Equation (1.6):

$$W_{ij} = \frac{d(ij)}{D_{\max}} \tag{1.6}$$

where $D_{\max}$ is the longest distance among all the points [43,44]. The statistical feature of vector T is a node in the undirected weighted graph. From the graph, the nodes having poor connection are eliminated. For that, a threshold is used, and each pair of nodes is connected only if the distance between any two nodes is greater than or equal to the defined threshold.

In this chapter, 12 statistical features are used: {Mean, Median, Mode, Min, Max, Range, First Quartile, Second Quartile, Variation, Standard deviation, Skewness and Kurtosis}. Out of these 12 statistical features, some are linear, while the others are nonlinear. Skewness and Kurtosis are nonlinear features, whereas the others are linear features. Figure 1.11 shows the accuracy vs. statistical features, which shows the importance of each feature in the classification of the EEG signal. The feature vector T generated from the EEG signal is used for mapping into the weighted undirected graph which is shown in Figure 1.12.

$$\begin{cases} \text{if}\left(v_i, v_j\right) \in E, \text{if } d\left(v_i, v_j\right) \geq \beta \\ \text{else}\left(v_i, v_j\right) \text{eliminate the connection from } G \end{cases} \tag{1.7}$$

where β is a defined threshold.

Figure 1.13 shows the vector using the statistical features mapped to a weighted undirected graph. Let T be the vector given by $\{v_1 = 4.3, v_2 = 4.1, v_3 = 4.2, v_4 = 4.9, v_5 = 4.5, v_6 = 4, v_7 = 3.9, v_8 = 3.8, v_9 = 3.4, v_{10} = 3.6, v_{11} = 3.7, v_{12} = 4.4\}$. For constructing

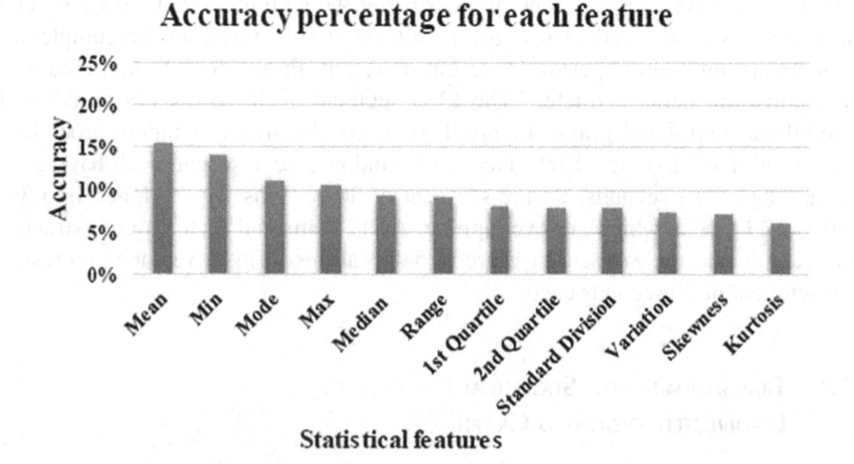

FIGURE 1.11 Classification accuracy depending on the statistical features.

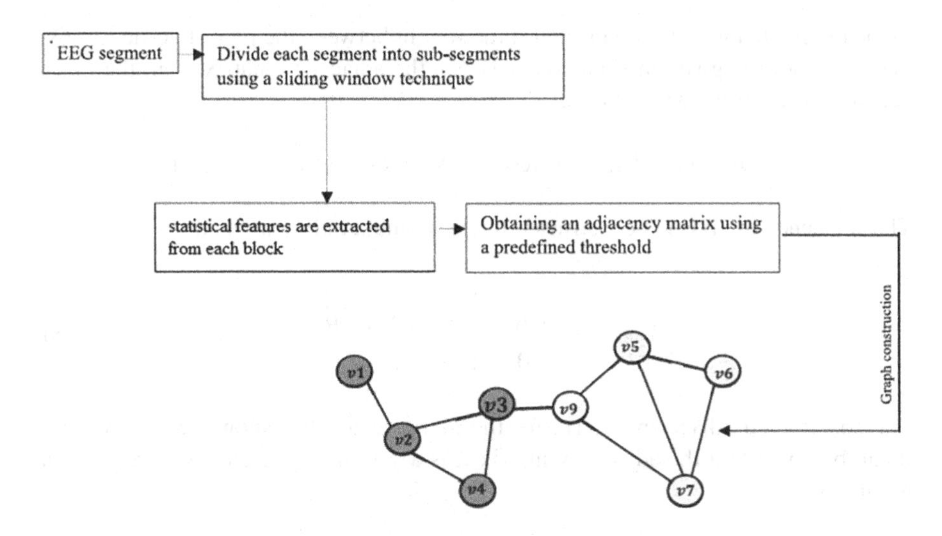

FIGURE 1.12 Undirected graph construction.

0	0	0	0	0	0	0	0	0	0	0	1
0	0	0	1	0	0	0	0	0	0	0	0
0	0	0	0	0	0	0	0	0	0	0	0
0	1	0	0	0	1	1	1	0	1	1	1
0	0	0	0	0	0	0	0	0	1	1	1
0	0	0	1	0	0	0	0	1	0	0	0
0	0	0	1	0	0	0	0	1	0	0	0
0	0	0	1	0	0	0	0	1	0	0	0
0	0	0	0	0	1	1	1	0	1	1	1
0	0	0	1	1	0	0	0	1	0	0	0
0	0	0	1	1	0	0	0	1	0	0	0
1	0	0	1	1	0	0	0	1	0	0	0

FIGURE 1.13 The adjacency matrix (the undirected graph).

the undirected graph, every point of T is taken as a node in the graph. $V_1=4.3$ and $V_2=4.1$ are the first and second nodes of the undirected graph, respectively. The link between A and B is calculated by the Euclidean distance which is 0.2 here. Similarly, for all the edges, it has been calculated. The weighted matrix can be calculated from the distance matrix using Equation (3.6). A threshold is defined. Each pair of vertices in the undirected graph is connected if the weight between the pair of vertices satisfies the condition given in Equation (1.7). So, the adjacency matrix from the given vector T is constructed as follows:

$$T \rightarrow \text{distance Matrix} \rightarrow \text{weighted Matrix} \rightarrow \text{Adjacency Matrix}$$

The adjacency matrix A is constructed by the formula in Equation (1.8):

$$A(v_i, v_j) = \begin{cases} 1, & \text{if } w(v_i, v_j) \geq \beta \\ 0 & \text{elsewhere} \end{cases} \tag{1.8}$$

The constructed adjacency matrix for the given vector T is shown in Figure 1.13. It can be noted that the adjacency matrix A is a symmetric matrix. Vertex V_3 is an isolated vertex.

1.7.2 Transformation of Statistical Features to Undirected Weighted Graph

The proposed model is shown in Figure 1.14 where the undirected weighted graph will be input to the model which is classifying the EEG signal.

1.8 EXPERIMENTAL RESULTS

In the experimental study, six classification techniques are used in the ensemble ML model and used as single classifier: K-means [45], KNN [46], Naive Bayes [47], least square SVM [48], logistic regression [49] and fuzzy C-means [50]. Four individual classifiers are used in identifying the targeted EEG signals [51]. The final decision is based on voting. Here we have used the bagging technique to classify the characteristics of the graph network to sleep stages. Figure 1.15 shows the ensemble classification scheme applied in the experimentation. We have taken the modularity detection or community detection [52,53] for the exploration of the graph. The community detection of the undirected graph is computed as in Equation (1.9):

$$\Delta Q = \left[\frac{\sum_{\text{in}} k_{i,\text{in}}}{2m} - \left(\frac{\sum_{\text{in}} k_{i,\text{in}}}{2m} \right)^2 \right] - \left[\frac{\sum_{\text{in}}}{2m} - \left(\frac{\sum_{\text{tot}}}{2m} \right) \left(\frac{k_i}{2m} \right)^2 \right] \tag{1.9}$$

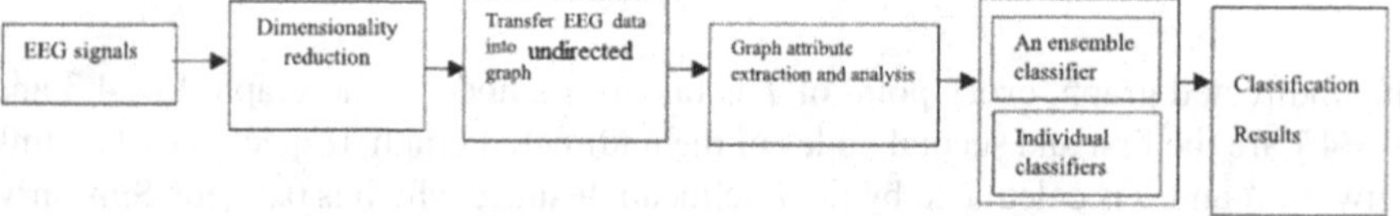

FIGURE 1.14 The proposed method.

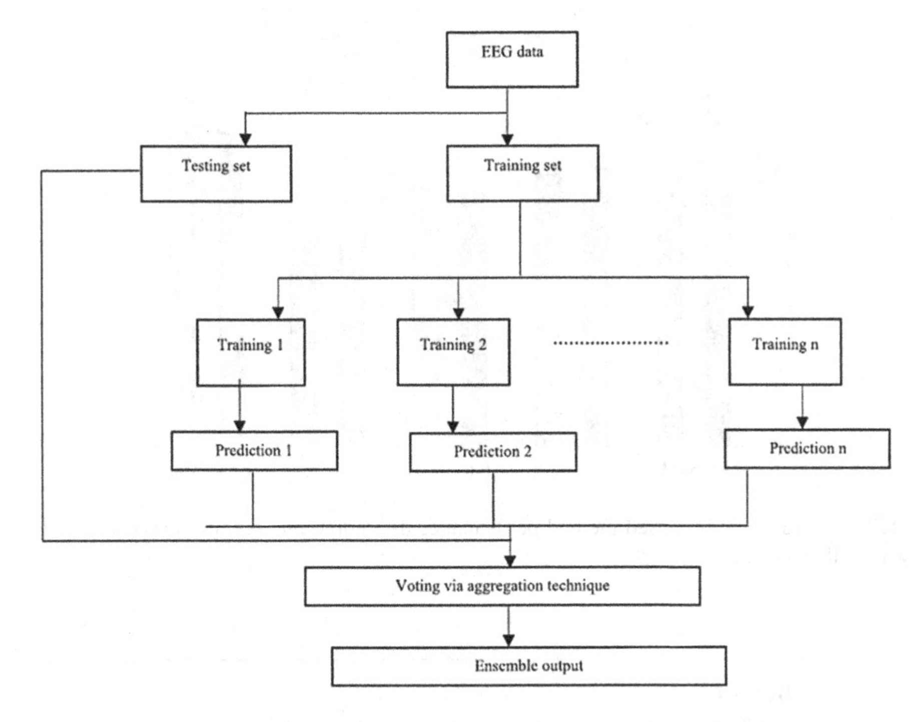

FIGURE 1.15 The ensemble classifier technique in the experimentation.

In community C,

Σ_{in} is the total link weight for all the nodes

Σ_{tot} is the sum total of link weights incident to the nodes

K_i is the total link weights incident to node i

$K_{i,in}$ is the sum of all the weights from node i to other nodes in the whole community

m is the total weight of all the links in the network.

Four community detection algorithms, namely, Walktrap [54], Fast greedy [55], Label Propagation [56,57] and Spinglass, are taken.

Figure 1.16 shows the performance of the ensemble classifier in classifying the EEG signal along with the individual classifiers. The results show that it has an improved result when the ensemble is applied to classify the EEG signal and in turn the undirected graph in comparison to the single classifiers.

Table 1.6 shows the classification results of the suggested method for dataset-1 and dataset-2.

The accuracy, specificity and the kappa coefficients are defined for all types of sleep stages along with the average percentage.

1.9 CONCLUSION

In fine, this chapter discusses an automatic sleep classification procedure on graph modularity in undirected graph assembled by means of an ensemble classifier. The statistical features have been taken for each window, and the vector of every EEG segment

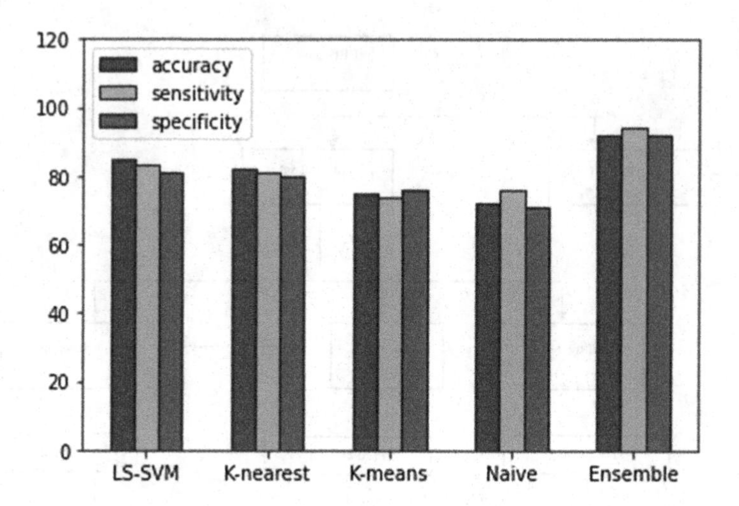

FIGURE 1.16 The proposed method performance depending on ensemble classifier along with individual classifier.

TABLE 1.6
Classification Result Analysis of Dataset-1 and Dataset-2 for the Proposed Method

Sleep Stages	Accuracy (in %)	Specificity (in %)	Kappa Coefficients
	Dataset-1		
AWA	97.9	95.4	0.85
N1	97.3	93.2	0.84
N2	90.5	91.6	0.82
N3	89.8	83.5	0.79
REM	97	96.2	0.88
Average	94.6	92	0.84
	Dataset-2		
AWA	96.3	97.4	0.87
N1	98.2	92.1	0.89
N2	96.1	94.3	0.86
N3	84.5	90.2	0.80
REM	98.2	97.5	0.86
Average	94.7	94.3	0.86

is mapped to a graph. Based on the 12 statistical feature vectors, the undirected graphs are constructed. From the undirected graph using ensemble learning, the sleep is classified. With the aid of data collected from diverse sources, the experiment was conducted with the use of two datasets. The methods put into practice accomplished an approximate average accuracy of 93.3% and 94.5% for dataset-1 and dataset-2, respectively. The suggested approach is a simplified and better method in terms of the feasibility of graph construction; furthermore, hardware devices can be made and implemented in the suggested method to identify the sleep disorders. In comparison to the earlier classification of sleep-stage procedure, the suggested methodology attained a greater classification accuracy. In future, the suggested method can be tested with other EEG data including epilepsy and big data applications may also be enforced to improve the effectualness of the algorithms. The suggested technique can contribute to building a system tool for automatic sleep stage scoring and classification, which will be helpful doctors and neurologists in diagnosing and treating sleep disorderliness and sleep research.

REFERENCES

1. Mora, Antonio Miguel, Carlos M. Fernandes, Luis Javier Herrera, Pedro A. Castillo, Juan Juliàn Merelo, Fernando Rojas, and Agostinho C. Rosa 2010 Sleeping with ants, SVMs, multilayer perceptrons and SOMs. *Proceedings of the 2010 10th International Conference on Intelligent Systems Design and Applications*, IEEE, 1. Cairo, Egypt, pp. 126–131.
2. Estrada, E., Patricia Nava, Homayoun Nazeran, Khosrow Behbehani, J. Burk, and E. Lucas 2006 Itakura distance: A useful similarity measure between EEG and EOG signals in computer-aided classification of sleep stages. *Proceedings of the IEEE Engineering in Medicine and Biology 27th Annual Conference*, IEEE, Shanghai, China, pp. 1189–1192.
3. Ebrahimi, Farideh, Mohammad Mikaeili, Edson Estrada, and Homer Nazeran 2008 Automatic sleep stage classification based on EEG signals by using neural networks and wavelet packet coefficients. *Proceedings of the 30th Annual International Conference of the IEEE Engineering in Medicine and Biology Society*, IEEE, Vancouver, British Columbia, Canada, pp 1151–1154.
4. da Silveira, Thiago L.T., Alice J. Kozakevicius, and Cesar R. Rodrigues 2017 Single-channel EEG sleep stage classification based on a streamlined set of statistical features in wavelet domain, *Medical & Biological Engineering & Computing* 55(2), 343–352.
5. Ebrahimi, Farideh, Mohammad Mikaeili, Edson Estrada, and Homer Nazeran 2008 Automatic sleep stage classification based on EEG signals by using neural networks and wavelet packet coefficients. *Proceedings of the 30th Annual International Conference of the IEEE Engineering in Medicine and Biology Society*, Vancouver, British Columbia, Canada, pp. 1151–1154.
6. Putilov, Arcady A. 2015 Principal component analysis of the EEG spectrum can provide yes-or-no criteria for demarcation of boundaries between NREM sleep stages. *Sleep Science* 8(1), 16–23.
7. Tsinalis, Orestis, Paul M. Matthews, and Yike Guo 2016 Automatic sleep stage scoring using time-frequency analysis and stacked sparse autoencoders. *Annals of Biomedical Engineering* 44 (5), 1587–1597.
8. Rodríguez-Sotelo, Jose Luis, Alejandro Osorio-Forero, Alejandro Jiménez-Rodríguez, David Cuesta-Frau, Eva Cirugeda-Roldán, and Diego Peluffo 2014 Automatic sleep stages classification using EEG entropy features and unsupervised pattern analysis techniques. *Entropy* 16(12), 6573–6589.

9. Samiee, Kaveh, Péter Kovács, Serkan Kiranyaz, Moncef Gabbouj, and Tapio Saramaki 2015 Sleep stage classification using sparse rational decomposition of single channel EEG records. *Proceedings of the 23rd European Signal Processing Conference (EUSIPCO)*, IEEE, Nice, France, pp. 1860–1864.
10. Aboalayon, Khald Ali I., Miad Faezipour, Wafaa S. Almuhammadi, and Saeid Moslehpour 2016 Sleep stage classification using EEG signal analysis: a comprehensive survey and new investigation. *Entropy* 18(9), 272.
11. Zhang, Junming, Yan Wu, Jing Bai, and Fuqiang Chen 2016 Automatic sleep stage classification based on sparse deep belief net and combination of multiple classifiers. *Transactions of the Institute of Measurement and Control* 38(4), 435–451.
12. Amin, Hafeez Ullah, Aamir Saeed Malik, Nidal Kamel, and Muhammad Hussain 2016 A novel approach based on data redundancy for feature extraction of EEG signals. *Brain Topography* 29(2), 207–217.
13. Diykh, Mohammed, and Yan Li. Complex networks approach for EEG signal sleep stages classification. *Expert Systems with Applications* 63, 241–248.
14. Shi, Jun, Xiao Liu, Yan Li, Qi Zhang, Yingjie Li, and Shihui Ying 2015 Multi-channel EEG-based sleep stage classification with joint collaborative representation and multiple kernel learning. *Journal of Neuroscience Methods* 254, 94–101.
15. Diykh, Mohammed, Yan Li, and Peng Wen 2016 EEG sleep stages classification based on time domain features and structural graph similarity. *IEEE Transactions on Neural Systems and Rehabilitation Engineering* 24(11), 1159–1168.
16. Farag, Amr F., Shereen M. El-Metwally, and Ahmed Abdel Aal Morsy 2013 Automated sleep staging using detrended fluctuation analysis of sleep EEG. In: Balas V., Fodor J., Várkonyi-Kóczy A., Dombi J., Jain L. (eds.) *Soft Computing Applications* (Springer, Berlin) pp. 501–510.
17. Lee, Jong-Min, Dae-Jin Kim, In-Young Kim, Kwang Suk Park, and Sun I. Kim 2004 Nonlinear-analysis of human sleep EEG using detrended fluctuation analysis. *Medical Engineering & Physics* 26(9), 773–776.
18. Taran, Sachin, and Varun Bajaj 2019 Sleep apnea detection using artificial bee colony optimize hermite basis functions for EEG signals. *IEEE Transactions on Instrumentation and Measurement* 69(2), 608–616.
19. Taran, S., V. Bajaj, and D. Sharma 2017 Robust Hermite decomposition algorithm for classification of sleep apnea EEG signals. *Electronics Letters*, 53(17), 1182–1184.
20. Hsu, Yu-Liang, Ya-Ting Yang, Jeen-Shing Wang, and Chung-Yao Hsu 2013 Automatic sleep stage recurrent neural classifier using energy features of EEG signals. *Neurocomputing* 104, 105–114.
21. Peker, Musa 2016 An efficient sleep scoring system based on EEG signal using complex-valued machine learning algorithms. *Neurocomputing* 207, 165–177.
22. Gao, Vance, Fred Turek, and Martha Vitaterna 2016 Multiple classifier systems for automatic sleep scoring in mice. *Journal of Neuroscience Methods* 264, 33–39.
23. Czisch, Michael, Victor I. Spoormaker, Katia C. Andrade, Renate Wehrle, and Philipp G. Sämannn 2011 User Research Sleep and functional imaging. *Brain* 41, 5–8.
24. Lee, Jong-Min, Dae-Jin Kim, In-Young Kim, Kwang Suk Park, and Sun I. Kim 2004 Nonlinear-analysis of human sleep EEG using detrended fluctuation analysis. *Medical Engineering & Physics* 26(9), 773–776.
25. Acharya, U. Rajendra, Shreya Bhat, Oliver Faust, Hojjat Adeli, Eric Chern-Pin Chua, Wei Jie Eugene Lim, and Joel En Wei Koh 2015 Nonlinear dynamics measures for automated EEG-based sleep stage detection. *European Neurology* 74(5–6), 268–287.
26. Zhu, Guohun, Yan Li, and Peng Wen 2014 Analysis and classification of sleep stages based on difference visibility graphs from a single-channel EEG signal. *IEEE Journal of Biomedical and Health Informatics* 18(6), 1813–1821.

27. Binnie, C. D., and P. F. Prior 1994 Electroencephalography. *Journal of Neurology, Neurosurgery & Psychiatry*, 57(11), 1308–1319.
28. Hutchings, Margaret, and Roy O. Weller 1986 Anatomical relationships of the pia mater to cerebral blood vessels in man. *Journal of Neurosurgery*, 65(3), 316–325.
29. Kaur, Bhavneet, Meenakshi Sharma, Mamta Mittal, Amit Verma, Lalit Mohan Goyal, and D. Jude Hemanth 2018 An improved salient object detection algorithm combining background and foreground connectivity for brain image analysis. *Computers & Electrical Engineering* 71, 692–703.
30. Amin, Hafeez Ullah, Aamir Saeed Malik, Nidal Kamel, and Muhammad Hussain 2016 A novel approach based on data redundancy for feature extraction of EEG signals. *Brain Topography* 29(2), 207–217.
31. Fraiwan, Luay, Khaldon Lweesy, Natheer Khasawneh, Mohammad Fraiwan, and H. Wenz 2010 Classification of sleep stages using multi-wavelet time frequency entropy and LDA. *Methods of Information in Medicine* 49(3), 230–237.
32. Lajnef, Tarek, Sahbi Chaibi, Perrine Ruby, Pierre-Emmanuel Aguera, Jean-Baptiste Eichenlaub, Mounir Samet, Abdennaceur Kachouri, and Karim Jerbi 2015 Learning machines and sleeping brains: Automatic sleep stage classification using decision-tree multi-class support vector machines. *Journal of Neuroscience Methods*, 250, 94–105.
33. Zhang, Junming, Yan Wu, Jing Bai, and Fuqiang Chen 2016 Automatic sleep stage classification based on sparse deep belief net and combination of multiple classifiers. *Transactions of the Institute of Measurement and Control*, 38(4), 435–451.
34. Berry, Richard B., Rita Brooks, Charlene E. Gamaldo, Susan M. Harding, C. Marcus, and Bradley V. Vaughn 2012 The AASM manual for the scoring of sleep and associated events, Rules, Terminology and Technical Specifications, Version 2.2, Darien, Illinois, American Academy of Sleep Medicine, 176.
35. Khalighi, Sirvan, Teresa Sousa, José Moutinho Santos, and Urbano Nunes 2016 ISRUC-Sleep: A comprehensive public dataset for sleep researchers. *Computer Methods and Programs in Biomedicine* 124, 180–192.
36. Goldberger, Ary L., Luis AN Amaral, Leon Glass, Jeffrey M. Hausdorff, Plamen Ch Ivanov, Roger G. Mark, Joseph E. Mietus, George B. Moody, Chung-Kang Peng, and H. Eugene Stanley 2000 PhysioBank, PhysioToolkit, and PhysioNet: Components of a new research resource for complex physiologic signals. *Circulation* 101(23), 215–220.
37. Kemp, Bob, Aeilko H. Zwinderman, Bert Tuk, Hilbert AC Kamphuisen, and Josefien JL Oberye 2000 Analysis of a sleep-dependent neuronal feedback loop: The slow-wave microcontinuity of the EEG. *IEEE Transactions on Biomedical Engineering*, 47(9), 1185–1194.
38. Mourtazaev, M. S., B. Kemp, A. H. Zwinderman, and H. A. C. Kamphuisen 1995 Age and gender affect different characteristics of slow waves in the sleep EEG. *Sleep* 18(7), 557–564.
39. Kemp, Bob, Alpo Värri, Agostinho C. Rosa, Kim D. Nielsen, and John Gade 1992 A simple format for exchange of digitized polygraphic recordings. *Electroencephalography and Clinical Neurophysiology*, 82(5), 391–393.
40. Van Sweden, B., B. Kemp, H. A. C. Kamphuisen, and E. A. Van der Velde 1990 Alternative electrode placement in (automatic) sleep scoring. *Sleep* 13(3), 279–283.
41. Reichardt, Jörg, and Stefan Bornholdt 2006 When are networks truly modular? *Physica D: Nonlinear Phenomena* 224(1–2), 20–26.
42. Polikar, Robi 2012 Ensemble Learning. In: Zhang C., and Ma Y. (eds.) *Ensemble Machine Learning*, Springer Science & Business Mediapp (Springer, Boston, MA), 1–34.
43. Micheloyannis, Sifis, Ellie Pachou, Cornelis J. Stam, Michael Vourkas, Sophia Erimaki, and Vasso Tsirka 2006 Using graph theoretical analysis of multi channel EEG to evaluate the neural efficiency hypothesis. *Neuroscience Letters*, 402(3), 273–277.

44. Sousa, Teresa, Aniana Cruz, Sirvan Khalighi, Gabriel Pires, and Urbano Nunes 2015 A two-step automatic sleep stage classification method with dubious range detection. *Computers in Biology and Medicine*, 59, 42–53.
45. Liao, T. Warren 2005 Clustering of time series data—A survey. *Pattern Recognition* 38(11), 1857–1874.
46. Wilson, D. Randall, and Tony R. Martinez 2000 Reduction techniques for instance-based learning algorithms. *Machine Learning* 38(3), 257–286.
47. John, G. H., and P. Langley 1995 Estimating Continuous Distributions in Bayesian Classifiers. *Proceedings of the Eleventh Conference on Uncertainty in Artificial Intelligence*, Montreal, Quebec, Canada.
48. Suykens, Johan AK, and Joos Vandewalle 1999 Least squares support vector machine classifiers. *Neural Processing Letters* 9(3), 293–300.
49. Peng, Chao-Ying Joanne, Kuk Lida Lee, and Gary M. Ingersoll 2002 An introduction to logistic regression analysis and reporting. *The Journal of Educational Research*, 96(1), 3–14.
50. Havens, Timothy C., James C. Bezdek, Christopher Leckie, Lawrence O. Hall, and Marimuthu Palaniswami 2012 Fuzzy c-means algorithms for very large data. *IEEE Transactions on Fuzzy Systems*, 20(6), 1130–1146.
51. Taran, Sachin, Prakash Chandra Sharma, and Varun Bajaj 2020 Automatic sleep stages classification using optimize flexible analytic wavelet transform. *Knowledge-Based Systems*, 192, 105367.
52. Zhang, Han, Chang-Dong Wang, Jian-Huang Lai, and S. Yu Philip 2017 Modularity in complex multilayer networks with multiple aspects: A static perspective, *Applied Informatics*, 4(1), 7.
53. Zhang, Xian-Kun, Jing Ren, Chen Song, Jia Jia, and Qian Zhang 2017 Label propagation algorithm for community detection based on node importance and label influence. *Physics Letters A* 381(33), 2691–2698.
54. Pons, Pascal, and Matthieu Latapy 2005 Computing communities in large networks using random walks. *Proceedings of the International Symposium on Computer and Information Sciences*, Springer, Berlin, Heidelberg, pp. 284–293.
55. Newman, Mark EJ 2006 Modularity and community structure in networks. *Proc: National Academy of Sciences*, 103(23), 8577–8582.
56. Raghavan, Usha Nandini, Réka Albert, and Soundar Kumara 2007 Near linear time algorithm to detect community structures in large-scale networks. *Physical Review E*, 76(3), 036106.
57. Zhang, Xian-Kun, Jing Ren, Chen Song, Jia Jia, and Qian Zhang 2017 Label propagation algorithm for community detection based on node importance and label influence. *Physics Letters A* 381(33), 2691–2698.

2 Recognition of Distress Phase Situation in Human Emotion EEG Physiological Signals

Abdultaofeek Abayomi, Oludayo O. Olugbara, and Delene Heukelman
Durban University of Technology

CONTENTS

2.1 INTRODUCTION

The understanding of emotion expressed by people is a big challenge in affective computing, human computer interaction and social communication. Deployed solutions of human emotion recognition tasks could play an important role in various intelligent affective communication systems [1]. Emotion is also very useful in our understanding of human social behaviors and richly embedded in human nonverbal communications. An important part of human-to-human communication is an expected change in the emotional state of a subject [2]. This could indicate emphasizing or clarifying spoken words, expressing agreements or disagreements, comprehending intentions, and interacting with others and environments [3].

Human emotion is related to physiological signals and are influenced by physiological changes, external events and relationship with others, therefore representing a complex and dynamic state of human mind [1]. However, physiological signals originate from the peripheral and the autonomic central nervous system, which is one of the most complex systems of the human body. The nervous system is fundamental in human behaviors because it empowers human with the ability to perceive, understand and react to environmental events such as emotions, desires and thoughts that are transmitted to the nervous system through the neuropeptides. In addition, human brain, which is an essential component of the central nervous system, generates brain waves, which contain electrical signals that are collected using electrodes attached to the scalp. These EEG waveforms from the brain represent the wave pictures of the electrical activity in the brain. They are physiological signals that capture human emotional states and are obtained from the nervous systems using bio-sensors [4]. The peripheral nervous signals that have been collected in the literature include galvanic skin response (GSR), skin temperature (TEMP), electrocardiogram (ECG), electroencephalogram (EEG), electromyogram (EMG), electrooculogram (EOG), respiration (RESP), blood volume pulse (BVP), heart rate (HR) and heart rate variability (HRV) [5]. In the literature, emotion recognition using physiological signals has received relatively less attention in comparison to the audiovisual methods of facial expression and speech [6,7–9]. Meanwhile, the audiovisual methods have some intrinsic drawbacks, they are capable of being easily faked, and the subject needs to be within a perimeter defined by the camera or must always listen to an audio signal. However, physiological signals evolve automatically and spontaneously. They are human reactions over which they have less controls and are less influenced by social, language and cultural differences [4,6,9,10].

In this study, our objectives include the construction of an emotion model by leveraging on the attributes of the arousal, valence, dominance and liking dimensions of emotion representation. In addition, we acquired EEG physiological data from the emotion DEAP corpus and analyzed it while introducing a shifted tanh-based normalization scheme after which the inverse Fisher transformation algorithm was applied. Secondly, we desire to extract distinctive features from the transformed EEG physiological data using the HOG, LBP and HIM techniques which are popular shape, texture and pixel intensity distribution descriptors, respectively, in the digital image processing domain. Thirdly, we aim to utilize the RBF-ANN pattern recognizer to compare the performances of the three different feature descriptors in recognizing human emotional states along the happy, distress and casualty classes of our constructed distress phase emotion model.

The rest of this chapter is structured as follows: the relevant literature and related works are discussed immediately after the Introduction section. This is then followed by the Materials and Methods section wherein the dataset acquisition, emotion representation modeling, data preprocessing steps, physiological signals transformation, feature extraction techniques and the classification algorithm applied are fully described. The proposed experimental models are presented in the next section to validate the performance of the various methods introduced. This is then followed by the Results and Discussion section wherein the results obtained are presented and discussed. Finally, the chapter is concluded by giving a brief discussion about the results obtained and comparing them with the literature, while also giving future directions.

2.2 LITERATURE REVIEW

In comparison with the audiovisual emotion channels consisting of facial expressions, gestures and speech, relatively few research works have been conducted on emotion recognition using physiological signals [1,6,7,8]. While appreciable but varied recognition accuracy results were recorded in these relatively few works, feature extraction and fixing an agreed recognition accuracy remain open issues in pattern recognition and affective computing research [6,11]. There are also wide disparities in the number of emotions to be recognized, the number and types of bio-signals measured, dataset used and its quality, the number of subjects sampled, emotion stimulus, modality considered, emotion models and the pattern recognizer employed [4,6,11].

The subject-independent approach is the focus of many current studies [12–14] as a large number of subjects ensure reliability of results. Consequently, we followed this approach in this current study as it addressed the apparent limitations of the subject-dependent approach such as its low degree of generalization, lack of inter-person variability in emotional feelings and inability of applications based on it to be readily deployed for practical usage [9,11,15]. However, the most critical challenge in developing subject-independent emotion recognition system is the identification of the most discriminatory features among the subjects which obviously impacts recognition results obtained.

It was observed that by using different methods [1,3,6,15–19] various results have been recorded in the literature as the issue of feature extraction which is germane for performance attained in a pattern recognition system that still remains open. In this study, we have used the digital image feature descriptors of HOG, LBP and HIM because of their strong performances in pattern recognition studies [20–28]. We used the subject-independent approach and observed the performances of the RBF-ANN classifier to determine whether we could obtain favorable and reliable results with the various configurations including our data processing and transformation method as well as features employed than those in the literature.

Wang and Shang [29] introduced a Deep Belief Network (DBN)-based system that automatically extracts features from four channels' raw physiological data consisting of two EOG and two EMG channels, respectively, under an unsupervised scheme while building classifiers that predict human emotion along the arousal, valence and liking classes. The classification accuracies obtained were 60.9%, 51.2% and 68.4%, respectively, which compares favorably with the results achieved by the same authors while using the Naïve Bayes classifier.

Li et al. [30] adopted a two hidden-layer DBN architecture configured with visible and hidden nodes as 128-10-10 to classify EEG signals of the DEAP dataset along the binary label scheme for valence, arousal, dominance and liking, respectively, using unsupervised training and future learning. Classification of experiments was done along individual subject as well as across all subjects. A support vector machine

(SVM) classifier was applied on the power spectral density (PSD) as well as the DBN features in order to compare the manually extracted features with the DBN features. Recognition accuracies of 58.2% (valence), 64.3% (arousal), 65.1% (dominance) and 66.3% (liking) were achieved with the PSD features across all subjects, while 58.4%, 64.2%, 65.8% and 66.9% accuracies, respectively, were recorded for the DBN features. There is no significant difference between the results of the two features as the possibility of learning affective features through a deep learning and manually generated feature approaches were explored. This indeed confirms the potency of manually generated features competing favorably with deep learning-based features as also obtained in this present study.

Zhuang et al. [31] utilized the DEAP dataset and applied the empirical mode decomposition (EMD) method to extract the first difference of time series, the first difference of phase and the normalized energy features from EEG signals which were decomposed into intrinsic mode functions (IMFs), and classification was done along the arousal and valence classes using the SVM classifier. Classification accuracies of 71.99% and 69.10%, respectively, was achieved for the arousal and valence classes using 8 EEG channels of Fp1, Fp2, F7, F8, T7, T8, P7 and P8, while classification accuracies of 72.10% and 74.10% were achieved for arousal and valence with 32 EEG channels. These performances are better than the results obtained by the same authors using other methods and features such as the fractal dimension, sample entropy and discrete wavelength transformations.

Furthermore, EEG signals' characteristics such as spatial, frequency domain and temporal were integrated by Li et al. [32] and mapped to a two-dimensional image from which EEG multidimensional feature images (MFI) were built to represent varied emotions in EEG signals. A deep learning approach of CLRNN involving hybriding the convolution neural networks (CNN) and long short-term-memory (LSTM) recurrent neural networks (RNN) was then applied on the EEG MFI obtained from the DEAP dataset. With each subject, an average best emotion classification accuracy of 75.21% was achieved with a 2-second time window frame as against the available 60-second window size containing all the EEG data per sample. In addition, the results of other classification methods such as *k*-NN, random forest and SVM with the features and method proposed by the authors are below the 75.21% recorded. But aside the computationally expensiveness of deep learning techniques, we opted for a shallow machine learning approach because it is believed that the classification accuracy obtained in these deep learning-based studies can be improved upon if the discriminatory strength of features is enhanced through novel feature engineering method proposed by us in this study rather than relying on auto-generation of features as obtained in deep learning approaches.

A multiple-fusion-layer-based ensemble classifier of stacked autoencoder (MESAE) for recognizing human emotions was proposed by [33], which involves the identification of the deep structure based on physiological data-driven approach. Stable feature representations of the physiological signals were obtained as the unwanted noise in the physiological signals' features was filtered by the three hidden layers in each stacked autoencoder. The stacked autoencoder ensembles were achieved by using an additional deep model, and the physiological features are divided into many subsets based on various feature extraction methodologies with each subset separately encoded by a stacked autoencoder. The derived SAE abstractions were merged based on the physiological modality to create six sets of encodings which subsequently served as input to a three-layer, adjacent-graph-based network for feature fusion whose features were used for human emotion recognition along the binary arousal and valence emotion states. Average classification accuracies of 77.19% and 76.17% were achieved for the arousal and valence states, respectively, using the MESAE scheme with deep classifier, while the accuracies reached 84.18% and 83.04% with ensemble classification schemes.

In another study, Alhagry, Fahmy and El-khoribi [34] applied LSTM recurrent deep neural network on the EEG physiological signals in the DEAP dataset. An average recognition accuracy of 85.65% was achieved for the arousal class, while 85.45% and 87.99% average accuracies were recorded for the valence and liking classes, respectively.

In the research study carried out and reported by Menezes et al. [35], features were extracted from EEG signals for affective state modeling using the Russell's circumplex model [36]. The SVM and random forest classifiers were applied on the EEG features of statistical measures, band power as well as higher order crossing extracted from the DEAP dataset to classify human emotion into the valence and arousal classes. The highest classification accuracy obtained with the bandwaves PSD features by the SVM classifier was 69.2% and 88.4% for the bipartite scheme of arousal and valence classes, respectively, while the tripartite scheme recorded 59.5% and 55.9%. However, the random forest classifier recorded its best classification accuracies of 74.0% (arousal) and 88.4% (valence) along the bipartite labeling scheme (high or low) with the statistical bandwaves features and 63.1% (arousal) and 58.8% (valence) with the same features but for the tripartite labeling scheme (high, medium and low). Diverse lower results were, however, recorded for each and combined bandwaves of Delta (δ), Theta (θ), Alpha (α) and Beta (β) by both the SVM and random forest classifiers for the bipartite and tripartite labeling schemes using statistical bandwaves or PSD features.

Lastly, a framework to automatically search for the optimal subset of EEG features using evolutionary computation (EC) algorithms including the particle swam optimization (PSO), ant colony optimization (ACO), genetic algorithm (GA), simulated annealing (SA) and differential evolution (DE) was introduced by Nakisa et al. [37]. This is aimed at removing inefficiency and redundancy resulting from high dimensionality introduced by combining all possible EEG features. The framework used frequency, time and time-frequency domain features of EEG signals from which some discriminatory features were selected using the EC algorithm and the probabilistic neural network pattern classifier was applied to classify human emotions into four classes. The DE algorithm yielded the best recognition accuracies of 96.97% and 67.47% for the MAHNOB and DEAP datasets, respectively. Though the results obtained are promising, the challenge with this framework and method is its computation complexity as it takes about 80 hours to achieve convergence. This is not ideal for a real-time situation where efficient, prompt and accurate classifications are required. We therefore explored our proposed method of the EEG physiological data transformation and feature extraction to determine if we could attain better results above those of the deep learning approaches reported in the literature.

2.3 MATERIALS AND METHODS

2.3.1 Acquisition of Dataset

The DEAP dataset was developed by [8] using video clips stimuli to elicit human emotions from 32 subjects (16 females), and their physiological data such as the EEG, EOG, EMG, GSR, RESP, BVP and TEMP were concurrently collected as they watched 40 one-minute extracts of music videos. These clips are capable of eliciting the target or reported felt emotions of anger, contempt, disgust, elation, envy, fear, guilt, hope, interest, joy, pride, relief, sadness, satisfaction, shame and surprise. The physiological signals comprising the central nervous system, for instance the EEG, and the peripheral nervous system physiological signals consisting of the EOG, EMG, GSR, RESP, BVP and TEMP data were collected, but only the EEG signals were consequently utilized for experimentations in this current study. During each trial, subjects also undertook and reported a self-assessment of their degrees of arousal, valence, dominance and liking on a continuous 9-point scale using a self-assessment manikin (SAM). For each subject, there were 40 trials/samples. Each subject's samples contain down-sampled 63-second EEG physiological signals of average size $40 \times 40 \times 8064$ (video/trial $\times$ channel $\times$ data) which gives a total of 1280 trial samples available for the analysis of all the 32 subjects considered. As also done in other related research studies, we utilized all the available 1280 samples in the DEAP dataset. In order to avoid overfitting of the classifier during training especially when the dataset is not large, utilizing a technique that is robust to outliers in the dataset as well as selecting the most important feature in the dataset have been suggested in the literature, and we applied this in the current study.

2.3.2 Emotion Representation Modeling

In the DEAP dataset, each sample of the EEG physiological signals was labeled by the subjects along the dimensional approach of emotion representation which include arousal, valence, dominance and liking as they quantitatively describe human emotions. The valence scale measures the pleasantness or unpleasantness feelings of an emotion and can include happy, joy, peaceful and cheerful emotions for the pleasant or positive emotions and sad, fear, stress and angry emotions for the unpleasant or negative emotions [3,8]. On the other hand, the arousal scale measures the intensity of emotional feelings and includes both for positive and negative valence emotions. For instance, both pleasure and joy emotions have a positive valence but low and high arousal, respectively, while both sadness and anger have negative valence but low and high arousal, respectively. Dominance scale ranges from a weak and helpless feeling to being in control while liking scale measures the taste and preference of subjects [3,8]. The valence and arousal scales may be represented either way on the vertical or horizontal axis in the valence-arousal representation plane. This is to enable a quadrant categorization of emotion to include low arousal, positive valence (LAHV); high arousal, positive valence (HAHV); low arousal, negative valence (LALV); and high arousal, negative valence (HALV). But in order to map the subjects' ratings in the DEAP dataset with the emotion quadrant, since the quantitative score ranges from 1 to 9 and no negative figures

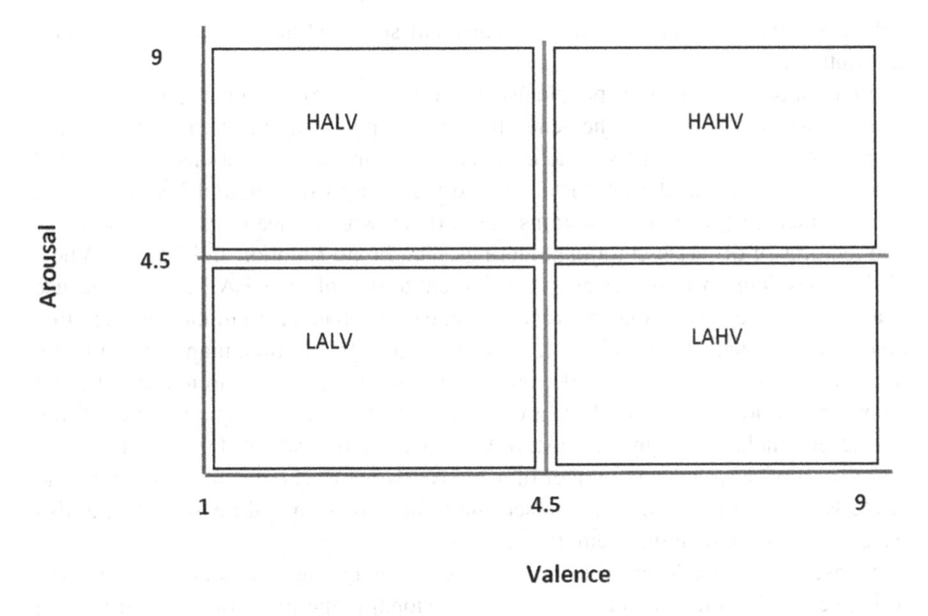

FIGURE 2.1 Participant ratings mapped to HALV, HAPV, LALV and LAHV dimensions.

recorded, the negative valence is therefore represented as low valence, while the positive valence is represented as high valence as shown in Figure 2.1.

Furthermore, the dominance dimension measures the control ability expressed by an individual under a certain emotional state. The dominance and liking emotion representation can occur in any emotion type whether it is a high or low valence or arousal dimensions [8]. For instance, an individual experiencing a joy emotion may have a weak feeling or helpless indicating that he is not in control or has been overpowered by the emotion, while another individual experiencing an anger or sadness emotion may still have a strong feeling and be in control. In addition, the liking scale does not also always connote a positive valence scale because an individual may like a sadness or anger emotion which are both negative valence emotions, as well as any materials capable of eliciting these emotions and vice versa [8]. This subject's liking rating and preference for instance is despite the fact that negative valence emotions are characterized with unpleasantness and displeasure.

Therefore, we model our human emotion recognition in distress phase situation problem along the combined four emotion representations of arousal, valence, dominance and liking. This entails tackling a classification problem involving three emotion classes namely happy, distress and casualty phases which were built from the arousal, valence, dominance and liking ratings in the DEAP physiological signal dataset. In addition, we appropriately map discrete emotions into the identified three classes of happy, distress and casualty phases of our emotion model. We achieved this by drawing inspirations from the target or felt emotion wheel consisting of anger, contempt, disgust, elation, envy, fear, guilt, hope, interest, joy, pride, relief, sadness, satisfaction, shame and surprise emotions in the DEAP dataset. This enables us to appropriately categorize these discrete emotions along the valence-arousal-dominance-liking dimensional space while also utilizing the participants' ratings.

In addition, since various people use different words to mean the same emotional feeling, in order to enhance the generalization capability of our distress phase situation emotion model in terms of definitions and meanings of emotions, we extended the emotion wheel in the DEAP dataset to the Funto Emotion and Feeling Wheel as contained in [38] which contains some other words, meanings, characteristics and features of different emotional feelings. The Funto Emotion and Feeling Wheel [38] is considered over others as a complement to that of the DEAP dataset because it attempts to resolve some inherent challenges in other past emotion wheels that contains more negative emotions than positive ones. In addition, many scientifically identified feelings and emotional words were not on the other emotion wheels, and from real world experience, there are many "emotions" that people are identifying but weren't included in any, or most, of the other emotion wheels [38]. Furthermore, apart from offering a huge number of affective words to choose from, compare and relate with those in the DEAP dataset, the Funto Emotion and Feeling Wheel also have all the six basic human emotions.

Consequently, we leveraged on Russell's [36] mapping of human emotions and affective words to the valence-arousal dimensional plane to enable the constructed distress phase emotion model, after taking cognizance of the participants' ratings, to appropriately map a detected human emotion into the valence-arousal dimensional plane. Having thresholded the ratings of the arousal, valence, dominance and liking scales along two classes namely low or high by placing the threshold in the middle as done in [8] such that all subjects' ratings above 4.5 score are respectively mapped to high arousal, high valence, high dominance and like, while ratings below 4.5 score are mapped to the respective low dimensions and dislike emotion representations. Therefore, the distress phase emotion model phases developed in this study are constructed as follows.

The happy phase in the emotion model as shown in Table 2.1 consists of EEG physiological signals of all positive or high valence emotion scores as rated by the participants in the DEAP dataset. We are guided by the human emotions and hedonism theory that people are motivated to seek pleasure and avoid pain [39] as happy phase involves maximizing the positive effects of the various human sensory systems. Positive valence emotions include elation, joy, glad, delighted, satisfaction, pride, happiness, relief, amusement, love, satisfaction, pleased, satisfied, calm, serene, relaxed, at ease and jubilation, among others, as these are pleasurable and desired by people [39]. Individuals with these positive valence emotions are characterized with humor, self-confidence, optimism, cheerful, gratitude, sense of accomplishment, creativity and a sense of personal control traits. Therefore, we configured that whatever the arousal, dominance and liking scores are for a subject, the most important emotion representation index for the happy phase is the positive or high valence as shown in Table 2.1. This phase indicates pleasure, and it is generally desired with no associated harm and thus wouldn't require any emergency assistance to be prompted and provided in our distress phase situation model.

The other two phases to be considered in our emotion model are the distress and the casualty phases. The aim is to build an affective model that can trigger emergency

TABLE 2.1
Emotion Representation Scores for Distress Phase Emotion Modelling

Phase	Emotion Types	Emotion Representation Scores			
		Valence	**Arousal**	**Dominance**	**Liking**
Happy	Amusement, Joy, Love, Satisfaction, Happiness, etc.	+ (only positive or pleasant valence emotions)	± (both low/high arousal)	± (both low/high dominance)	± (both like/dislike)
Distress	Fear, Anger, Distress, Annoyed, Alarmed, etc.	– (negative or unpleasant valence emotions)	+ (high arousal)	+ (high dominance)	± (both like/dislike)
Casualty	Sadness, Shame, Grief, Sorrow, Depressed, etc.	– (negative or unpleasant valence emotions)	– (low arousal)	– (low dominance)	± (both like/dislike)

assistance once danger is imminent in order to avoid a casualty phase where a loss would be suffered. These two phases will both therefore have a low or negative valence score since humans are motivated to avoid pain [39], thus requiring the prompting of an emergency service whenever there is a threat to pleasure. Negative valence emotions indicate unpleasantness, displeasure and aversive feelings of an emotion. They are characterized with suffering, insecure, pain – which may include physical and mental pain – panic, nervousness and helplessness [38]. Some negative valence discrete emotions include sadness, anger, fear, disgust, distressed, shameful, guilty, depressed, agony, hate, frustrated, distressed and contempt, among others. Since both the distress phase and casualty phase have low or negative valence emotions, we utilized the arousal and dominance ratings to alienate these two phases. This is because the arousal rating quantities heightened physiological activity and provide emotional responses in terms of "fight", "freeze" or "flight" to daily life experiences being confronted, while the dominance ratings denote weak, helpless and in control emotional feelings.

High arousal rating indicates more will and determination to fight or "flight"; it connotes that an individual can still muster strength to face the impending threat. The distress phase is therefore mapped to a high arousal as similarly done by [36] and high dominance ratings because it is exactly at this point that an emergency service is required not when the emotional arousal is very low indicating a helpless situation, freeze, less will and determination to confront the danger, thus possibly leading to a casualty phase. Out of the negative valence emotions listed, relying on Russell [38] as well as the emotion wheel adopted in the DEAP dataset, the discrete emotions and affective words that could be mapped to the distress phase include fear, angry, distress, tense, hope, contempt, disgust, envy, arouse, alarm and annoyance. The distress phase is characterized with hope, acknowledging that there is impending trouble but with a conviction that things can turn out fine and well, though fearing the worst but always expecting the best. It is believed that with prompt emergency assistance and all depths of individual efforts, a positive outcome is expected to be achieved.

The casualty phase, on the other hand, is what the proposed distress phase emotion model wants to avert as it is not desired because a tragedy has already occurred in real-life situations leading to loss of probably life, limb, valuables, successful kidnapping, rape and fire burns among others, thus necessitating the mapping of the casualty phase to low arousal, low dominance and negative valence emotions and affective words. The casualty phase is characterized with helplessness, overpowered, irrevocable loss, dejection, defeat and sorrow. The discreet emotions and affective words that are mapped to this phase include sadness, regret, shame, hurt, disappointed, displeased, suffering, grief, despair, depress, miserable and droopy [36,38]. The respective feature samples that would be extracted from the DEAP dataset EEG physiological signals samples that have been appropriately mapped to the happy phase, distress phase and casualty phase labels in the configured distress phase emotion would consequently be passed as a tripartite scheme for human emotion recognition and performances compared in order to determine the best obtainable result.

2.3.3 Preprocessing and Transformation of the Physiological Signals

In order to process the data using our proposed methodology, firstly, we normalized the raw EEG physiological data channel by channel. There are different normalization schemes available in the literature among which the Min-Max and Z-score are famous. In particular, the Z-score has been used in the study of physiological data [40] because it has capability to dramatically simplify clinical interpretations [41]. However, both Min-Max and Z-score normalizations have received criticisms as they are both sensitive to outliers, and their performances are sometimes poor [42]. The Min-Max normalization scheme also usually scales data to a fixed range of 0–1, thereby giving smaller standard deviations. But the Z-score normalization is often preferred to the Min-Max scheme especially when applied with the principal component analysis (PCA) procedure in order to compare similarities between features as the components that maximize the variance are often the focus [43]. The tanh estimator, suggested as a robust scheme in place of Min-Max and Z-score because of its robustness, efficiency and elegance [42] as a simple normalization scheme based on the tanh function, is hereby introduced. The tanh estimator's robustness to outliers is essential because removing the impact of outliers is required for getting a sensible model and result with a small dataset as overfitting is avoided.

The general tanh function is given as

$$t(u(x)) = \frac{e^{u(x)} - e^{-u(x)}}{e^{u(x)} + e^{-u(x)}} \tag{2.1}$$

where

$$u(x) = \frac{(x - \overline{x})}{\sigma_x} \tag{2.2}$$

is the Z-score that ensures normalization with a mean $(\overline{x})$ of zero and standard deviation (σ_x) of one.

The expression in Equation (2.1) can be further simplified by multiplying the right-hand side by e^x and at the same time divide it by e^x to give

$$f\left(u(x)\right) = \frac{e^{2u(x)} - 1}{e^{2u(x)} + 1} \tag{2.3}$$

The expression in Equation (2.3) corresponds to the inverse Fisher transform that has the advantage that it is compressive and for large absolute values, the output is compressed to one at most while also removing low amplitude variations. The inverse Fisher transform is analogous to edge sharpening in digital image processing. Moreover, it is the exact solution of the standard fractional Riccati differential equation (FRDE) [44] of the form

$$D^{(\alpha)} f(t) + y^2(t) - 1 = 0; t > 0, 0 < \alpha \leq 1 \tag{2.4}$$

where

$$\alpha = 1, f(0) = 0, t = u(x) \tag{2.5}$$

The values of $F\ (u(x))$ lies in the interval [−1, 1] but a normalizer that computes values in the interval $[0, L]$ where L is the maximum grayscale value such as 255 is desired. If 1 is added to both sides of Equation (2.3), it gives

$$1 + f(u(x)) = \frac{2}{1 + e^{-2x}} \tag{2.6}$$

To achieve the desired goal of having a normalizer that computes values in the interval $[0, L]$, we multiply both sides of Equation (2.6) by L and at the same time divide by 2 to have

$$\frac{L\left(1 + f\left(u(x)\right)\right)}{2} = \frac{L}{1 + e^{-2u(x)}} \tag{2.7}$$

By substituting Equation (2.2) into Equation (2.7) and dividing the left-hand side of Equation (2.7) by $f\ (u(x))$, we have

$$f\left(u(x)\right) = \frac{L}{1 + e^{\frac{-k(x - \bar{x})}{\sigma_x}}} \tag{2.8}$$

Equation (2.8) is the desired normalizer, which is a particular form of growth function with L being the modifier, $\bar{x}$ is the data mean, σ_x is the data standard deviation, k=2,3,4,5… is the normalizer and the value of $f(x)$ lies in the interval $[0, L]$. This function corresponds to the inverse Fisher normalizer with k=2.

After the normalization and applying the inverse Fisher transform on the EEG physiological data which involve mapping the transformed data to grayscale image space, channels' images of each channel's data are thereafter formed. This is to enhance the digital image processing techniques which are to be applied for feature extractions. The subjects' quantitative ratings ranging from 1 to 9 were thresholded for each of the valence, arousal, dominance and liking scales along the two classes namely low or high by placing the threshold in the middle as also done in [8] such that all subjects' ratings above 4.5 score are respectively mapped to high arousal, valence, dominance and like, respectively, while ratings below 4.5 score are mapped to the respective low emotion and dislike dimensions. This indicates the labels against each sample of the EEG physiological data.

We proceeded to extract the histogram of oriented gradient (HOG), local binary pattern (LBP) and histogram of the images (HIM) features from the inverse Fisher transformed EEG physiological data. These features are called 'local' features as they were extracted from each channel of each sample. The step-by-step procedure for the data preprocessing and transformation, feature extraction and classification for emotion recognition is itemized in Algorithm 2.1.

Algorithm 2.1

1: Read the raw EEG physiological data from the DEAP dataset
2: Determine EEG physiological data class using emotion representation – arousal, valence, dominance and liking
3: Preprocess the EEG physiological data by applying the inverse Fisher transformation
4: Map the transformed EEG physiological data to hyperspectral images
5: Extract features from the hyperspectral images using different standard algorithms of digital image processing techniques – HOG, LBP and HIM
6: Apply principal component analysis to the extracted features to compute dimensionally reduced Eigen features
7: Select the desired Eigen features using the Kaizer criterion of Eigenvalues greater than one
8: Use pattern recognizer to recognize the selected Eigen features as happy, distress and casualty

This preprocessing, feature extraction and classification procedure in conjunction with the implementation was done using MATLAB 2018a environment.

2.3.4 Feature Extraction Techniques

Feature extraction is an important task in pattern recognition. It involves the use of specific algorithms to acquire discriminating characteristics from the raw data for recognition. We have experimented with the HOG, LBP and HIM techniques to extract discriminatory features from the DEAP physiological signals for human emotion recognition task in this study. The HOG, LBP and HIM feature extraction techniques have recorded great success in digital image processing, speech processing, bioinformatics and other pattern recognition research studies [20–26,45–47], thus informing our decision to utilize them.

2.3.4.1 Histogram of Oriented Gradient

The histogram of oriented gradient (HOG) was developed for human recognition and object detection, considering that local object appearance and shape of an image can be represented by the distribution of intensity gradients or edge orientations [46,47]. Since the digitized physiological data have been presented as images, the intensity gradient of the images can be computed to represent discriminatory features. The implementation of the HOG involves dividing an image into cells and compiling the histogram of gradient directions for the pixels within the cells. The aggregation of these histograms represents the HOG features. To compute the HOG feature from a given image, four essential steps are required which are masking, orientation binning, local normalization and block normalization. The research work reported in [46] contains detailed information regarding the computations and characteristics of the HOG features.

2.3.4.2 Local Binary Pattern

The local binary pattern (LBP) descriptor was originally developed by Ojala, Pietikainen and Harwood [45]. It describes the texture of an image and has been widely applied in diverse applications [45,48–50]. It assigns numeric label for the block of pixels of an image through a thresholding process that uses a 3×3 neighborhood of the center pixel value while treating the result obtained as a binary number. Since the neighborhoods to the center pixel consist of eight pixels, the texture descriptor is derived from the histogram of the $2^8 = 256$ different labels. The LBP value is computed following the steps described in [45]. We chose the LBP descriptor because of its proficiency in appropriately describing the texture of an image [45,51]. In addition, it has a modest theoretical definition which is the foundation of its status as a computationally efficient image texture descriptor [52].

2.3.4.3 Histogram of Images

Digital image processing involves the procedure of obtaining useful information from images by determining an image's pixel properties and variations for the purpose of analysis, classification and recognition or identification. The histogram of an image represents the pixels' intensity values in the image. It is a graphical representation that covers all the various intensity values in the image. Thus, after preprocessing and applying the inverse Fisher transform on the DEAP dataset, the data obtained for each sample is converted and mapped into a grayscale image representation with pixel intensity values ranging from 0 to 255. As an image processing algorithm, the histogram features in the various grayscale images are computed using an automatic binning algorithm that yields bins with a uniform breadth which are selected to cover the range of pixel intensity elements, thus revealing the underlying unique shape and patterns of the distribution. Histogram as features has strong capabilities for identification and differentiation of patterns, and we therefore employ it for human emotion recognition along the happy, distress and casualty class labels. The histogram-based features have been used for image processing and in several pattern classification studies with promising results [27,28], thus necessitating its choice as a third option to the HOG and LBP descriptors employed.

Consequently, for instance, to extract features from the 40 channels of each sample, 81 HOG feature vectors of each channel are concatenated such that each sample of the physiological signal has a vector size of $81 \times 40 = 3240$. For the LBP and HIM descriptors, the feature vector size of 256 elements per channel gives a vector size of $256 \times 40 = 10{,}240$ for each sample after concatenating the 40 channels. A simple dimensionality reduction algorithm based on the PCA with the associated eigenvectors indicating the most dominant elements of the feature vectors, respectively, is thereafter applied to these feature vectors extracted from each channel before concatenation as dimensionally reduced feature vectors can improve classifiers' performance as reported in the literature [53]. The PCA is aimed at standardizing data using inherent relationship existing in the data, which are often linear or almost linear, thus making the data responsive to analysis. It rotates original data to new coordinates by finding a low-dimensional linear subspace such that when the data is projected, information loss is minimized while making the computation of eigenvalues and eigenvectors of the covariance matrix achievable.

In order to compute the PCA, for each feature vector I_i extracted by a pattern descriptor such as the HOG, LBP and HIM from N samples, I is an $m \times n$ matrix of each extracted feature vector where $i = 1, 2, 3, \ldots, N$. The matrices for N samples are averaged and represented as I_{avg}, the covariance matrix C is thus computed [54] as shown in Equation (2.9):

$$C = \sum_{i=1}^{N} (I_i - I_{\text{avg}})' (I_i - I_{\text{avg}}) \tag{2.9}$$

The covariance matrix C is evaluated to obtain the eigenvalues and the corresponding eigenvectors; y eigenvectors are selected based on the principal eigenvalues. The size of matrix D containing the selected y eigenvectors is $n \times y$ such that the extracted feature F_i of each sample is obtained by projecting the feature vector I on matrix D as shown in Equation (2.10):

$$F_i = I_i . D \tag{2.10}$$

Thus, after applying the PCA and obtaining the eigenvectors, the local HOG, LBP and HIM features of each channel for the EEG data, for instance, are reduced from 81, 256 and 256 feature vector sizes, respectively, to 10, 31 and 31 most dominant features, respectively. By this step, for each sample of the physiological signals to be trained by the RBF-ANN pattern recognizer, the feature vector sizes of the HOG, LBP and HIM features are now 320, 992 and 992, respectively, after concatenating features for all the 32 channels available in each sample of the EEG data. With this procedure, the new feature vector size was realized with about 90% dimensionality reduction of the original size thus minimizing computational complexity and also proved useful in avoiding overfitting during classifier's training as only dominant features are selected.

2.4 CLASSIFICATION ALGORITHM FOR EMOTION RECOGNITION

Feature classification involves the cataloguing of the extracted features into appropriate classes or states using a pattern recognition or classification algorithm. Such pattern classifier is always trained to learn the inherent characteristics in the different extracted features and attempt to match features with similar patterns into the same class. The RBF-ANN is the pattern classifier that was utilized for the various experiments conducted in this study.

The RBF-ANN can be described as a particular type of feed forward artificial neural network for solving problems of pattern recognition/classification and function approximation [55,56]. The concepts of RBF are ingrained in earlier pattern recognition techniques such as clustering, spline interpolation, mixture of models and function approximation [56,57]. A typical RBF neural network architecture consists of an input layer, one hidden layer consisting of RBF neurons and an output layer of artificial neuron for each class to be classified [55–58]. Each neuron in the hidden layer implements a radial basis activation function that represent an arbitrary basis for the input vectors, while the network output is a linear combination of radial basis functions of the input and neuron parameters.

According to McCormick [55], classification task performed by a RBFNN measures the input similarity to samples from the training dataset. A "prototype" representing one of the samples in the training dataset is stored in each RBFNN neuron as classification of a new input involves each neuron computing the Euclidean distance between the new input and its prototype. The new input is classified as belonging to class 1 prototype if it more closely resembles class 1 than class 2 prototype. The prototypes are indeed cluster centers computed as the average of all the data points in the cluster.

Each of the n-dimensional feature vectors of the HOG, LBP, HIM for the EEG modality signals is extracted from the DEAP dataset and, respectively, fed into the RBF network through the input layer for classification. This PCA dimensionally reduced n-dimensional feature vector is displayed to each of the RBF neurons in the hidden layer. A "prototype" feature vector obtained from one of the feature vectors in the training dataset is stored in each RBF neuron which compares an input feature vector with its prototype and a measure of similarity with values between 0 and 1 is the output. If the new input matches the prototype, the output of that particular RBF neuron will be 1 otherwise 0. The RBF neuron's response has a bell curve shape as the value of the neuron's response is termed its activation value while the prototype feature vector is otherwise called the neuron's center because it is located at the center of the bell curve.

In computing a measure of similarity between the input feature vector and its prototype vector obtained from the training samples, there are various choices of similarity functions that could be applied. Because of its reputation for good performance, the Gaussian radial function as the most popular similarity function was employed as a one-dimensional input vector in the RBF-ANN classifier configurations for the experiments conducted in this study. A Gaussian with a one-dimensional input is as shown in Equation (2.11):

$$f(x) = \frac{1}{\sigma\sqrt{2\pi}} e^{-\frac{(x-\mu)^2}{2\sigma^2}} \tag{2.11}$$

where x is the input feature vector, σ is the standard deviation and μ is the mean which is the center of the familiar bell curve produced from the Gaussian function. However, the RBF neuron activation function wherein the prototype vector is at the center of the bell curve is similar to Equation (2.11) but as n-dimensional vectors and computed as

$$\varphi(x) = e^{-\beta x - \mu^2} \tag{2.12}$$

As shown in Equation (2.12), both the outer and inner coefficients of Equation (2.11) have been removed as the beta coefficient now controls the width of the bell curve and the output nodes learn the correct coefficient or weight to the neuron's response.

In addition, the RBF network output is made up of a set of nodes consisting of one per each class that is to be classified, and a "score" is computed for each of the related category. Thus, in arriving at a classification decision, the new input feature vector is assigned to the class with the highest score which is computed by obtaining a weighted sum of the activation values from every RBF neuron. A weight value which is associated with each of the RBF neurons by an output node is multiplied by the neuron's activation and then added to the total response to obtain the weighted sum. Each output node in the network computes the weighted score for a category, and thus, every output node has its own set of weights. Typically, a positive weight is given by an output node to the RBF neurons that belong to its category and a negative weight to others in the different categories.

In summary, the RBF-ANN classifier is noted for its ability to approximate continuous function arbitrarily. It has a faster training process because of its local mapping attribute as compared to other neural networks, very robust to noise [59–61] while also capable of yielding at least 10% higher accuracy than can be obtained by the back-propagation ANN algorithm [62]. More details about the RBF-ANN pattern classifier can be obtained in the literature [55,56].

2.5 EXPERIMENTAL MODELS

The generic architecture for the design and implementation of the procedures for the experimental models proposed consisting of the three experiments conducted in this study is shown in Figure 2.2.

The first step in the architecture is the DEAP dataset from which the physiological signals as our experimental data were acquired. This step was followed by data preprocessing procedure which includes data normalization. Thereafter, the inverse Fisher transform algorithm and mapping of the transformed data to image space were conducted. Feature extractions using the signal and digital image processing

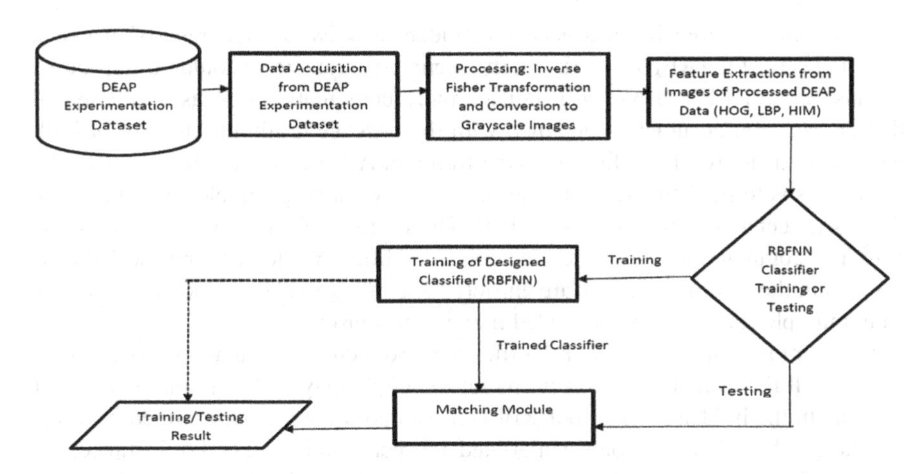

FIGURE 2.2 The generic architecture of the human emotion recognition experimental model.

algorithms such as the HOG, LBP and HIM were subsequently applied, and the dimensionally reduced extracted features were passed to the RBF-ANN pattern classifier for training/testing, and the results of human emotion recognition were obtained.

The experimental models in this study were conducted on the 32 EEG channels of DEAP physiological data. There are 1280 samples in the dataset which was obtained from the 32 subjects' 63s (60-second trial and 3-second pretrial) duration physiological signals of 40 trials per subject. Three experiments were conducted to determine how best the EEG physiological data could accurately recognize human emotions along our developed distress phase emotion model. The inverse Fisher transformed 32 EEG channels of the DEAP dataset were used, and the HOG, LBP and HIM feature descriptors were applied to extract the corresponding features, respectively. In the first experiment conducted, we utilized the HOG features and applied the RBFNN classifier in order to classify the extracted features into the three classes. The HOG features have 320 elements as feature vectors for each of the 1280 training samples fed into the RBF network. The number of neurons in the input layer is thus 320, while the output layer has three neurons for the three emotion classes indicating the happy, distress and casualty tripartite phases for classification.

In order to train an RBFNN network, determining the number of neurons in the hidden layer is very essential as this affects the result that can be obtained. The prototypes as well as the beta coefficient of the RBF neurons and the matrix of output weights between the RBF neurons and the output node are the parameters that must be carefully selected in determining the number of neurons in the hidden layer [55]. There exists no strict rule in the literature for selecting the prototypes for the RBF neurons. One approach is to create an RBF neuron for each training sample [53] such that for the problem at hand, we would have 1280 neurons, while the other is to randomly select *k* prototypes from the training samples [55]. These requirements are slack because with an adequate number of neurons, an RBFNN can outline any random complex decision boundary and recognition accuracy can always be improved upon by adding more RBF neurons in the hidden layer. However, a trade-off between the efficiency of the RBF network and the accuracy parameters should be considered because more RBF neurons will indicate more computation cost as it is essential that an excellent accuracy is obtained with the possible minimum number of RBF neurons so as to avoid overfitting during training. A novel method for selecting the prototypes is to perform *k*-Means clustering on the training sample while selecting the cluster centers as the prototypes [55]. The average of all the data points in the cluster is computed as the cluster centers. In addition, while utilizing the *k*-means algorithm, the training samples are clustered according to classes such that samples from multiple classes are not included in the same cluster.

In order to enhance the network's efficiency and reduce computation costs, instead of using all the available 1280 neurons for the hidden layer, the optimal number of neurons in the hidden layer of our RBFNN configuration was determined by varying the number of clusters between 50 and 150 per emotion class. For instance, the distress phase emotion model has three classes and with 50 clusters per class, this indicates 150 neurons in the hidden layer of the network for the 1280 training samples. We chose 150–450 number of neurons as we leveraged on [53] where the same range of neurons were chosen for each hidden layer in the MLP-ANN configuration consisting of 534 training samples, two hidden layers and 14 classes. The authors also utilized all the available 534 neurons in the hidden layer for the RBF network configuration in their study. Our configured RBF network is therefore much simpler and efficient than the MLP-ANN and RBF configurations reported in [53] as maximum fewer hidden neurons (35.16%) were utilized out of the available 1280 neurons to avoid overfitting. The results obtained with the varied number of neurons for the HOG feature were chronicled.

We extended and concluded this experiment by separately using the LBP and the HIM features of the EEG data. The number of neurons in the input layer is 992 each for both the LBP and the HIM features. This huge number of input neurons is as a result of the higher number of dominant components in these features extracted from the EEG physiological data. However, the output layer still has three neurons consisting of the happy, distress and casualty classes. The features were passed to the RBF-ANN classifier, and performance accuracy was determined as done in the first experiment. Thus, the three sets of experiments yielding three results were performed with the varied features extracted from the EEG data. The general differences in the three experiments conducted lie in the features extracted, the number of input neurons fed to the network and the optimal number of neurons in the hidden layers. The number of output neurons is, however, the same for all the three experimental models as three neurons were utilized to represent the three emotion classes.

2.6 RESULTS AND DISCUSSION

The results of the three experiments conducted in this study are hereby presented. The qualitative results of the inverse Fisher transformation of the emotion physiological data are to ascertain the similarities across subjects' emotional responses despite the variation in individual's emotional experiences [63]. Out of the 40 experimental trials of each subject, 8 trials were randomly selected per subject such that the trials selected for each of the 32 subjects (S1–S32) are unique. This is to enable an appropriate trial mix toward enhancing the generalization and reliability of inferences drawn and results obtained. From the 32 EEG channels, the Fp1, F7, T7, P7, Fp2, F8, T8 and P8 channels were identified and selected having been reported in the literature to be directly related to human emotions [6,35,37,64–67]. The grayscale image plots of the inverse Fisher transformed physiological data of ten subjects for eight random trials against the identified channels are shown in Figure 2.3 indicating the

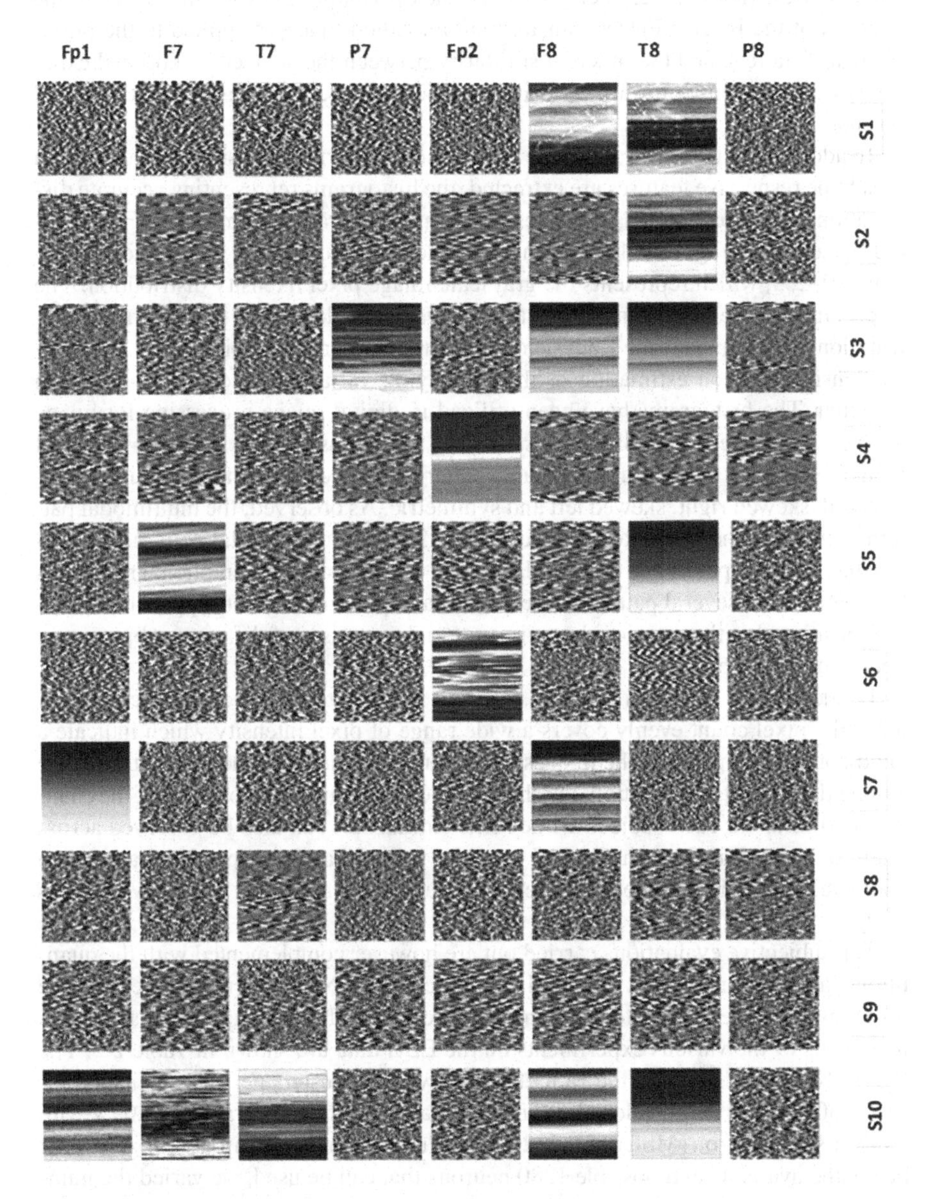

FIGURE 2.3 Images of the inverse Fisher transformed EEG physiological data.

similarities in the patterns of the images across the subjects. As shown in Figure 2.3, there seems to be a similar textural pattern in the majority of the images across the subjects despite the individual variability that do exist in emotional experiences which necessitates the little variations noticed in the patterns of the few images of one or two channels per subject.

The textural similarity in the images across the subjects is observed in the dense and coarse patterns of the images with observed varied brightness or darkness as a result of the different pixel intensity values and distributions in each image. Thus, the strength of the inverse Fisher transformation method that was applied to the physiological data revealed the inherent similarity between the subjects' emotional experiences and responses toward ensuring a subject-independent based inferences and results.

In addition to the grayscale image plot of the transformed physiological data from which the respective features are extracted, the histograms representing accurate distributions of the pixel intensity values for each of the grayscale images in Figure 2.3 are presented in Figure 2.4. The range of pixel intensity values was binned to 256 that is 0–255, which represents the grayscale image pixel intensity distribution. The importance of the histogram data is that it reveals the density of the underlying distribution of the transformed physiological data and can be employed for probability density function estimation of the underlying variable especially by a pattern classifier. The histograms have been utilized in digital image processing for image analysis, brightness, equalization, stretching and thresholding. There is no ideal image' histogram shape, but the notable patterns include the unimodal, multimodal, bimodal, skewed right, skewed left and symmetric. As observed, the multimodal pattern dominates the histogram plots in Figure 2.4. The multimodal pattern distribution has multiple peaks and could indicate that the physiological emotional responses of subjects have several patterns of responses and preferences that support the literature position that the emotional experiences and responses of different subjects may not be the same [63].

In addition, as shown in Figure 2.4, for all the selected channels and across subjects, the pixel count evenly covers a wide range of pixel intensity which indicate a good contrast property of the images as well as a similarity in the contrast property among the subjects. In addition, the shape of the histogram plots for some of the channels is similar for each subject, while some similarities can also be observed across many subjects. It is from these pixel intensity values that the respective features are computed for a subject-independent emotion recognition task that is employed in this study.

The subjective evaluations carried out are however complemented with the quantitative analysis and results obtained using the RBF-ANN pattern classifier and the respective feature descriptors are hereby presented. In our experimental model, the results of the various experiments on the EEG data are shown in Table 2.2. The RBF-ANN classifier using the HOG features with 50 clusters per class which represents 150 neurons in the hidden layer achieved a recognition accuracy of 76.09% with a mean square error (MSE) of 0.6922. Since the number of neurons utilized is far below the available and possible 1280 neurons that can be used, we varied the number of clusters which determines the number of neurons that are used in the hidden

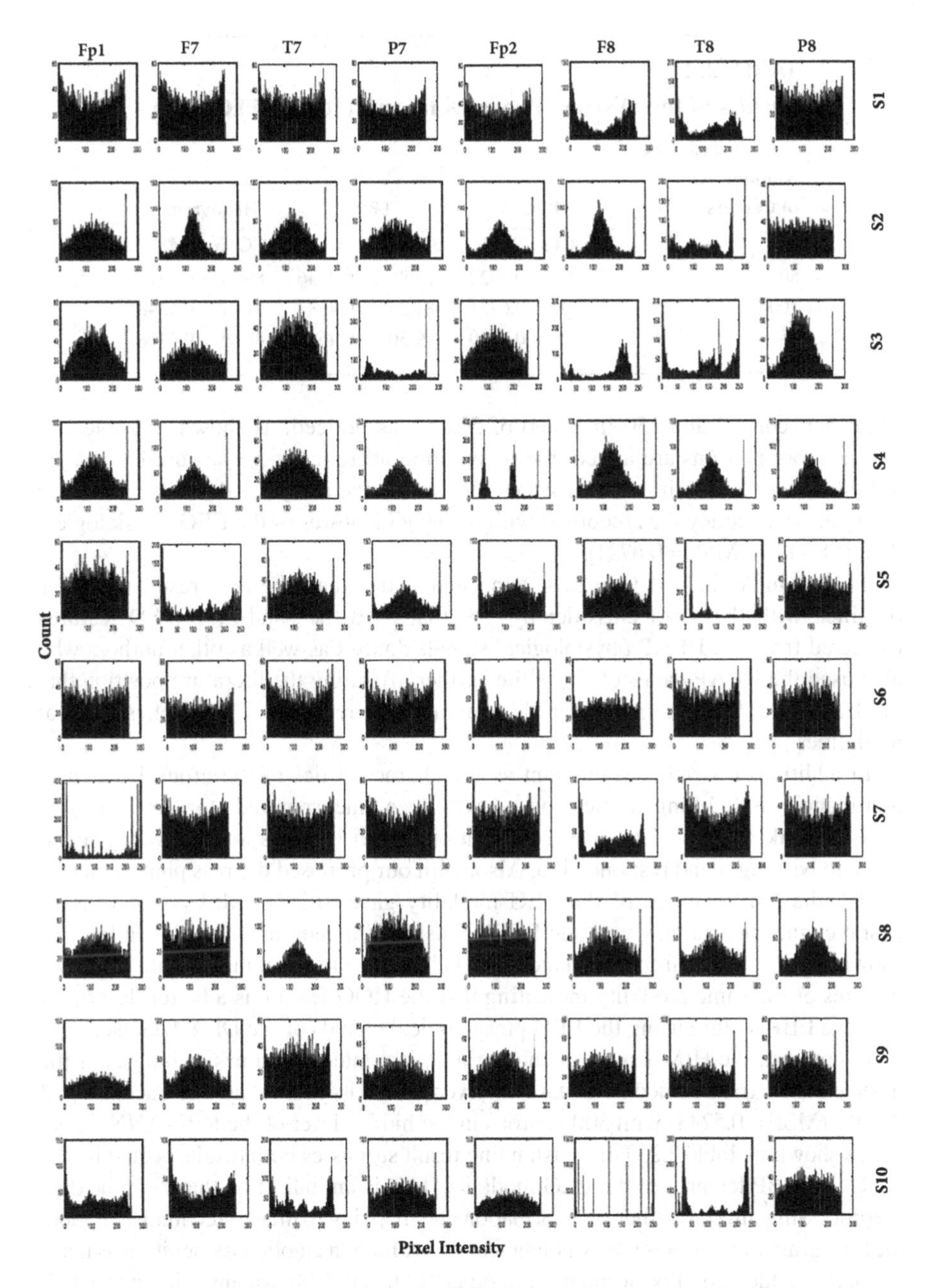

FIGURE 2.4 Histogram plot of the inverse Fisher transformed EEG physiological data.

TABLE 2.2
Results of the Distress Phase Dimension for the EEG Data

Number of Centers \ Features	HOG		LBP		Histogram	
	ACC (%)	MSE	ACC (%)	MSE	ACC (%)	MSE
50	76.09	0.6922	75.86	0.4546	89.77	0.2978
100	84.14	0.6721	81.25	0.4583	91.41	0.5248
150	83.59	0.8660	79.30	0.4688	88.05	0.4408

layer, between 50 and 150 in a step of 50. It was noticed, as shown in Table 2.2, that as more neurons are added, the recognition accuracy increases until it peaked at 84.14% while utilizing 300 neurons after which the accuracy dwindles. The best recognition accuracy thus recorded with the HOG features of the EEG physiological data is 84.14% (MSE = 0.6721).

This result is indeed very promising and better than the best result of 69.2% obtained with the SVM classifier by [35] that used the bandwaves PSD features extracted from the DEAP physiological signals dataset as well as other authors who also used the DEAP dataset [37], while further affirming the literature position that the EEG modality is capable of producing a better result than other physiological modalities [3].

In addition, it is more significant as the characteristics of the arousal, valence, dominance and liking dimensions have been incorporated for an effective decision-making in a distress phase situation which involves an emergency assistance to be sought and responded to. Also, with our proposed distress phase emotion model, the LBP features of the EEG modality gave 81.25% (MSE = 0.583) as its best recognition accuracy with the RBFNN using 300 neurons in its hidden layer as shown in Table 2.2. This performance falls below the 84.14% obtained with the HOG features of the same modality indicating that the HOG feature is a better descriptor than the LBP feature using the EEG physiological signals of the DEAP dataset.

In contrast, the HIM features denoting the pixel intensity values of images of the inverse Fisher transformed EEG data however posted its best recognition accuracy of 91.41% (MSE = 0.5248) with 300 neurons in the hidden layer of the RBF-ANN classifier as shown in Table 2.2. This outstanding result surpasses both results posted by the HOG and LBP features of the EEG modality. This is an indication that with the data preprocessing, inverse Fisher transformation and mapping to images technique applied, the histogram of images is a very potent feature for human emotion recognition as it has similarly yielded good performances in other studies [27,28]. Meanwhile, the 91.41% (MSE = 0.5248) recognition result is better than the results obtained in different recent research studies that have utilized the DEAP dataset [32,33,35,37]. In emotional signal processing including speech signal, an amplitude is otherwise referred to as intensity and can be computed in various ways which are a measure of the maximum change in a quantity that occurs when the signal is being transmitted [68] as a peak amplitude is a measure of emotional intensity. It has also been established in the literature that as a rule, the larger the amplitude, the greater is the intensity of the signal [68] including emotional speech and physiological signals. In addition, an increase in emotional intensity will trigger an increase in performance up to an optimal point [69]. However, human emotions are associated with amplitude fluctuations, and a highly significant effect of amplitude in various emotions does exist [70–72]. Emotions such as fear, sadness, fear, disgust, joy and boredom have been detected with high, medium and low amplitudes expressed by various subjects [72,73].

The images of the histogram features of the three classes catalogued under the distress phase emotion model, which are happy, distress and casualty for six sampled uniformly selected subjects, are investigated to examine some characteristics in these features among the subjects and the classes that necessitated the results obtained. The happy class has the highest amplitude, followed by the distress class and then the casualty class, thus enhancing classification by the pattern recognizer. Among the uniformly selected subjects, these were observed for subjects S4, S12 and S22, while for S8, S18 and S27, the amplitude values of the distress class are the lowest among the three. This confirms that the classes are, however, separable and can be classified accordingly.

The summary of the best results obtained under each feature is shown in Table 2.3. It is noted that these best results outperform those reported in similar research studies [8,29–31,33,35]. In the table, for instance, the overall best recognition result that was achieved in the experiments is 91.41% and was obtained by the HIM features of the EEG data. This is hereby recommended for human emotion recognition in distress phase situations using the DEAP dataset.

To enable replicability of the RBF neural network experimentations in this study, the parameters that were optimized to obtain the recognition results include the number of neurons that was utilized in the hidden layer which was experimentally determined for the HOG, LBP and HIM features, respectively, for the various modalities. There are three neurons in the output layer, which denote the number of emotional states to be classified. The hidden layers and output layer implemented a hyperbolic tangent sigmoid transfer function which is considered simple and suitable above the rectified linear unit (ReLU) of multi-layer deep neural networks, while the linear transfer function was applied in the input layer.

According to the literature, emotional physiological data exhibit significant nonlinearity [74] as most physiological data do not increase linearly even for only a subject while experiencing an emotional state. We leveraged on the peculiar nonlinearity

TABLE 2.3
Summary of Experimental Results across the Different Features

	Features					
	HOG		LBP		HIM	
Emotional Dimension	ACC (%)	MSE	ACC (%)	MSE	ACC (%)	MSE
Distress Phase	84.14	0.6721	81.25	0.4583	91.41	0.5248

of emotional physiological data and the inherent capability of neural network models to perform efficiently when the data distribution is nonlinear to achieve higher emotion recognition accuracies in the study at hand. Thus, the artificial neural network models were able to achieve greater recognition accuracies as a result of their capabilities to approximate arbitrary nonlinear functions [75]. This is in addition to the models' strength of tacitly detecting and extracting intricate nonlinear relationships between independent and dependent variables as well as their capabilities of detecting every probable interaction between predictor variables [76]. Therefore, in order to navigate the computational complexity drawbacks in deep learning approaches and explore the possibilities of getting better results, as a shallow classifier, the RBF-ANN was applied to the extracted HOG, LBP and HIM features in the experiments conducted in this study.

Thus, the three set objectives of this study have been successfully achieved. These objectives are as follows: (i) to construct an emotion model suitable for detecting distress situations that require an emergency assistance and acquire EEG physiological data from the DEAP corpus for the purpose of human emotion state recognition to validate the constructed model; (ii) to extract discriminatory features from the EEG physiological data using the HOG, LBP and HIM feature extraction techniques; and (iii) to compare the performances of the RBF-ANN models using the three different features for the task of human emotion recognition especially in distress phase situations as might be experienced in real life. In summary, based on our findings and results in this study, we recommend a combination of HIM features and EEG physiological data for classification in order to carry out emotion recognition task using physiological signals. This combination gave the best result of 91.41% (MSE = 0.5248) when compared to the other feature sets and configurations. The various results obtained in this current study are also better than the results reported in similar research works that utilized the same DEAP dataset [29–35,37,77–81]. In addition, the 91.41% (MSE = 0.5248) overall result surpasses most of the results reported in [82] and keenly competes with those in [83–85]. This is despite the fact that various deep learning classifiers were applied in some of these studies to recognize only four emotions.

2.7 CONCLUSION

The automatic recognition of human emotion remains very challenging in affective computing as physiological data are continuously being researched to enhance emotion recognition accuracies. In this study, we constructed an emotion model for recognizing human emotions especially in distress situations by using EEG physiological signals, and it becomes handy in prompting emergency services once a distress state is detected. We compared the HOG, LBP and HIM feature extraction techniques adapted from the digital image processing domain to extract discriminative features from the EEG data in the DEAP physiological dataset. Different RBF-ANN classifier configurations were experimentally compared as we explored the intrinsic ability of the neural network models to handle nonlinearity in data to achieve promising results. With the current results, there is a huge prospect of the adoption of an automated emotion recognition paradigm in application domains such as emergency services, call centers, customer services, safe driving, biomedicine and psychiatric disorder research. Future work will include comparing other machine learning methods, merging of audio and physiological signals, the discovery and adoption of other physiological feature extraction algorithms and the practical prototyping for real-time application purpose.

REFERENCES

1. Maaoui C. and Pruski A. 2010 Emotion recognition through physiological signals for human-machine communication. Cutting Edge Robotics, Vedran Kordic (Ed.) pp. 1–18.
2. Zhihong Z., Pantic M., Glenn I. R. and Thomas S. H. 2009 A Survey of affect recognition methods: audio, visual and spontaneous expressions, *IEEE Transactions on Pattern Analysis and Machine Intelligence* **31**(1), 39–58.
3. Soleymani M., Jeroen L., Pun T. and Pantic M. 2012 A multimodal database for affect recognition and implicit tagging, *IEEE Transactions on Affective Computing* **3**(1), 42–55.
4. Heng Y. P., Lili N. A., Alfian A. H. and Puteri S. S. 2013 A study of physiological signals-based emotion recognition systems, *International Journal of Computer and Technology* **11**(1), 2189–2196.
5. Chun-yan N., Hai-xin S. and Wang J. 2013 The relationship between chaotic characteristics of physiological signals and emotion based on approximate entropy. *Proceedings 2nd International Conference on Computer Science and Electronics Engineering (ICCSEE 2013)*, (22–23 March, Hangzhou, China. Atlantic Press), pp. 552–555.
6. Noppadon J., Setha P. and Pasin I. 2013 Real-time EEG based happiness detection system, *The Scientific World Journal* **2013**, 1–13. Article id 618649, Hindawi Publishing Corporation.
7. Wagner J., Jonghwa K. and Andre E. 2005 From physiological signals to emotion: Implementing and comparing selected methods for feature extraction and classification. *Proceedings of the IEEE International Conference on Multimedia and Expo (ICME)*, Amsterdam (July 2005), pp. 940–943. doi: 10.1109/ICME.2005.1521579.
8. Koelstra S., Muhl C., Soleymani M., Jong-Seok L., Yazdani A., Ebrahimi T., Pun T., Nijholt A. and Patras I. 2012 DEAP: A database for emotion analysis using physiological signals, *Affective Computing* **3**(1), 18–31.
9. Chanel G., Kronegg J., Grandjean D. and Pun T. 2006 Emotion assessment: arousal evaluation using EEG's and peripheral physiological signals. *Proceedings of the Multimedia Content Representation, Classification and Security (MRCS 2006)*, eds. B. Gunsel, A. K. Jain, A. M. Tekalp and B. Sankur (Lecture Notes in Computer Science, Springer, Berlin) vol. 4105, pp. 530–537.
10. Eun-Hye J., Byoung-Jun P., Sang-Hyeob K. and Jin-Hun S. 2012 Emotion recognition by machine learning algorithms using psychophysiological signals, *International Journal of Engineering and Industries* **3**(1), 55–66.
11. Jerritta S., Murugappan M., Nagarajan R. and Wan K. 2011 Physiological signals based human emotion recognition: A review. Signal processing and its applications (CSPA). *Proceedings of the IEEE 7th International Colloquium on Signal Processing and Its Applications*, Penang, pp. 410–415. doi: 10.1109/CSPA.2011.5759912.
12. Jing C., Bin H., Yue W., Philip M., Yongqiang D., Lei F. and Zhijie D. 2017 Subject-independent emotion recognition based on physiological signals: A three stage decision method, *BMC Medical Informatics and Decisions Making* **17**(3), 45–66.
13. Xiang L., Dawei S., Peng Z., Yazhou Z., Yuexian H. and Bin H. 2018 Exploring EEG features in cross-subject emotion recognition, *Frontiers in Neuroscience* **12**(162), 1–15.
14. Yuan-Pin L. and Tzyy-Ping J. 2017 Improving EEG-based emotion classification using conditional transfer learning, *Frontiers in Human Neuroscience* **11**(334), 1–11.

15. Rigas G., Katsis C. D., Ganiatsas G. and Fotiadis D. I. 2007 A user independent, biosignal based, emotion recognition method. *Proceedings of the 11th International Conference on User Modeling (2007)*, eds. C. Conati, K. Mccoy and G. Paliouras (Lecture notes in Computer Science, Springer, Berlin), vol. 4511, pp. 314–318.
16. Panagiotis C. P. and Leontios J. H. 2010 Emotion recognition from EEG using higher order crossings, *IEEE Transactions on Information Technology in Biomedicine* **14**(2), 186–197.
17. Vyzas E. and Picard R. W. 1999 Offline and online recognition of emotion expression from physiological data. *Proceedings of the Workshop on Emotion-Based Agent Architectures, 3rd International Conference on Autonomous Agents* (May 1999), (Seattle, Washington, United States), pp. 135–142.
18. Cong Z. and Chetouani M. 2009 Hilbert-Huang transform based physiological signals for emotion recognition. *Proceedings of the IEEE International Symposium on Signal Processing and Information Technology (ISSPIT)*, Ajman, UAE Dec 2009, pp. 334–339. doi:10.1109/ISSPIT.2009.5407547.
19. Mohammad Y and Nishida T 2009 Measuring naturalness during close encounters using physiological signal processing. *Next-Generation Applied Intelligence: Proceedings of the IEA/AIE 2009*, eds. B. C. Chien, T. P. Hong, S. M. Chen and M. Ali (Lecture Notes in Computer Science, Springer, Berlin) vol. 5579 pp. 281–290. doi:10.1007/978-3-642-02568-6_29.
20. Uroš M. and Božidar P. 2015 Automated facial expression recognition based on histograms of oriented gradient feature vector differences, *Journal of Signal Image and Video Processing (SIViP)* **9**(1), 245–253.
21. Wang X., Jin C., Liu W., Hu M., Xu L. and Ren F. 2013. Feature fusion of HOG and WLD for facial expression recognition. *Proceedings of the 2013 IEEE/SICE International Symposium on System Integration (SII)*, Kobe (Dec 2013), pp. 227–232. doi:10.1109/SII.2013.6776664.
22. Manar M. F. D., Aliaa A. A. Y. and Atallah H. 2014 Spontaneous facial expression recognition based on histogram of oriented gradients descriptor, *Computer and Information Science* **7**(3), 31–37.
23. Yunan Z., Yali L. and Shengjin W. 2015 Facial expression recognition using coarse-to-fine classifiers. *Computer Science and Applications*, ed. Hu pp. 127–131. doi:10.1201/b18508-24.
24. Ramchand H., Narendra C. and Sanjay T. 2013 Recognition of facial expressions using local binary patterns of important facial parts, *International Journal of Image Processing (IJIP)* **7**(2), 163–170.
25. Happy S. L. and Aurobinda R. 2015 Automatic facial expression recognition using features of salient facial patches, *IEEE Transactions on Affective Computing* **6**(1), 1–12.
26. Hamed M., Sazzad H. M. and Rafael A. C. 2014 Using remote heart rate measurement for affect detection. *Proceedings of the 27th International Florida Artificial Intelligence Research Society Conference Pensacola Beach*, Florida (May 2014) ed W Eberle and C Boonthum-Denecke (AAAI Press: Palo Alto, California) pp. 118–123.
27. Iman B., Norihide M., Hiroshi M., Hasan D. and Gholamreza A. 2017 Histogram-based feature extraction from individual gray matter similarity-matrix for Alzheimer's disease classification, *Journal of Alzheimer's Disease* **55**(4), 1571–1582.
28. Thamizhvani T. R., Hemalatha R. J., Babu B., Dhivya A. J. A., Joseph J. E. and Chandrasekaran R. 2018 Identification of skin tumours using statistical and histogram based features, *Journal of Clinical and Diagnostic Research* **12**(9), 11–15.
29. Wang D. and Shang Y. 2013 Modeling physiological data with deep belief networks, *International Journal of Information and Education Technology* **3**(5), 505–511.

30. Li X., Zhang P., Song D., Yu G., Hou Y. and Hu B. 2015 EEG based emotion identification using unsupervised deep feature learning. *Proceedings of the SIGIR2015 Workshop on Neuro-Physiological Methods in IR Research*, Santiago, Chile. NeuroIR'15 (Aug 2015) pp. 1–3.
31. Zhuang N., Zeng Y., Tong L., Zhang C., Zhang H. and Yan B. 2017 Emotion recognition from EEG signals using multidimensional information in EMD domain, *BioMed Research International* **2017**(1), 1–9. Article ID 8317357.
32. Li Y., Huang J., Zhou H. and Zhong N. 2017 Human emotion recognition with electroencephalographic multidimensional features by hybrid deep neural networks, *Applied Sciences* **7**(1060), 1–20.
33. Yin Z., Zhao M., Wang Y., Yang J. and Zhang J. 2017 Recognition of emotions using multimodal physiological signals and an ensemble deep learning, *Computer Methods and Programs in Biomedicine* **140**, 93–110.
34. Alhagry S., Fahmy A. A. and El-Khoribi R. A. 2017 Emotion recognition based on EEG using LSTM recurrent neural network, *International Journal of Advanced Computer Science and Applications* **8**(10), 355–358.
35. Menezes M. L. R., Samara A., Galway L., Sant'Anna A., Verikas A., Fernandez A. F., Wang H. and Bond R. 2017 Towards emotion recognition for virtual environments: an evaluation of EEG features on benchmark dataset, *Personal and Ubiquitous Computing* **21**(6), 1003–1013.
36. Russell J. A. 1980 A circumplex model of affect, *Journal of Personality and Social Psychology* **39**(6), 1161–1178.
37. Nakisa B., Rastgoo N. M., Tjondronegoro D. and Chandra V. 2018 Evolutionary computation algorithms for feature selection of EEG-based emotion recognition using mobile sensors, *Expert Systems with Applications* **93**, 143–155.
38. Chadha R. 2016. The Junto emotion wheel: Why and how we use it. Funto Institute of Entrepreneurial Leadership. Chicago. U.S.A. http://blog.thejuntoinstitute.com/the-junto-emotion-wheel-why-and-how-we-use-it.
39. Franken R. E. 1994 *Human Motivation*, 3rd ed. (Brooks/Cole Publishing Company, Belmont, CA).
40. Chubb H. and Simpson J. M. 2012 The use of Z-scores in paediatric cardiology, *Journal of Annals of Pediatric Cardiology* **5**(2), 179–184.
41. Colan S. D. 2013 The why and how of Z scores, *Journal of the American Society of Echocardiography* **26**(1), 38–40.
42. Singh Y. N. and Gupta P. 2007 Quantitative evaluation of normalization techniques of matching scores in multimodal biometric systems. *Advances in Biometrics*, eds. S.-W. Lee and S. Z. Li. ICB Lecture Note in Computer Science, (Springer, Berlin) vol. 4642, pp. 574–583.
43. Raschka S. 2014 About feature scaling and normalization - and the effect of standardization for machine learning algorithms, https://sebastianraschka.com/Articles/2014_about_feature_scaling.html.
44. Salehi Y. and Darvishi M. T. 2016 An investigation of fractional Riccati differential equations, *Optik* **127**, 11505–11521.
45. Ojala T., Pietikainen M. and Harwood D. 1996 A comparative study of texture measures with classification based on feature distributions, *Pattern Recognition* **29**(1), 51–59.
46. Dalal N. and Triggs B. 2005 Histograms of oriented gradients for human detection: Pro. *IEEE Computer Society, International Conference on Computer Vision and Pattern Recognition CVPR'05* (San Diego, United States) 1 pp. 886–893.
47. Dipankar D. 2014 Activity recognition using histogram of oriented gradient pattern history, *International Journal of Computer Science, Engineering and Information Technology* **4**(4), 23–31.

48. Ojala T. and Pietikäinen M. 1999 Unsupervised texture segmentation using feature distributions, *Pattern Recognition* **32**(3), 477–486.
49. Ojala T., Valkealahti K., Oja E. and Pietikäinen M. 2001 Texture discrimination with multidimensional distributions of signed gray-level differences, *Pattern Recognition* **34**(3), 727–739.
50. Ojala T., Pietikäinen M. and Mäenpää T. 2002 Multi resolution gray-scale and rotation invariant texture classification with local binary patterns, *IEEE Transaction on Pattern Analysis and Machine Intelligence* **24**(7), 971–987.
51. Garcia-Olalla O., Alegre E., Fernandez-Robles L., Garcia-Ordas M. T., and D. Garcıa-Ordas. 2013. Adaptive local binary pattern with oriented standard deviation (ALBPS) for texture classification. *EURASIP Journal on Image and Video Processing* 1(31): 1–11.
52. Rahim M. A., Hossain M. N., Wahid T. and Azam M. S. 2013 Face recognition using Local Binary Patterns (LBP), *Global Journal of Computer Science and Technology Graphics & Vision* **13**(4), 1–9.
53. Adetiba E. and Olugbara O. O. 2015 Improved classification of lung cancer using radial basis function neural network with affine transforms of Voss representation, *PLoS One* **10**(12), e0143542. doi:10.1371/journal.pone.0143542.
54. Abdelrahman S. A. and Abdelwahab M. M. 2018 Accumulated grey-level image representation for classification of lung cancer genetic mutations employing 2D principle component analysis, *Electronics Letters* **54**(4), 194–196.
55. McCormick C. 2013 Computer vision and machine learning projects and tutorials, Radial Basis Function Network (RBFN) Tutorial.
56. Bors A. G. 2001 Introduction of the radial basis functions (RBF) networks, The York Research database, Online Symposium of Electronics Engineers.
57. Ugur H. 2004 Artificial neural networks EE543 Lecture Notes Ch 9.
58. Xianhai G. 2011 Study of emotion recognition based on electrocardiogram and RBF neural network, *Procedia Engineering* **15**, 2408–2412.
59. Leonard J. A. and Kramer M. A. 1991 Radial basis function networks for classifying process faults, *IEEE Control Systems Magazine* **11**(3), 31–8.
60. Cha I. and Kassam S. A. 1995 Channel equalization using adaptive complex radial basis function network, *IEEE Journal on Selected Areas in Communications* **13**(1), 122–31.
61. Andina D. and Pham D. C. 2007 *Computational intelligence for Engineering and Mathematics*, (Springer Science & Business Media, Berlin) pp. 120–121.
62. Chapman R. A., Norman D. M., Zahirniak D. R., Rogers S. K. and Oxley M. E. 1991 Classification of correlation signatures of spread spectrum signals using neural networks. *Proceedings IEEE National Aerospace and Electronics Conference* (NAECON 1991, Dayton, OH, USA) vol. 1 pp. 485–491. doi:10.1109/NAECON.1991.165794.
63. Siemer M., Mauss I. and Gross J. J. 2007 Same situation—different emotions: How appraisals shape our emotions, *Emotion* **7**(3), 592–600.
64. Davidson R. J., Jackson D. C. and Kalin, N. H. 2000 Emotion, plasticity, context and regulation: Perspectives from affective neuroscience, *Psychological Bulletin* **126**(6), 890–909.
65. Niemic C. P. 2002 Studies of emotion: A theoretical and empirical review of psychophysiological studies of emotion, *Journal of Undergraduate Research* **1**, 15–18.
66. Noppadon J., Setha P. and Pasin I. 2013 Emotion classification using minimal EEG channels and frequency bands. *Proceedings of the 10th International Joint Conference on Computer Science and Software Engineering JCSSE 2013* (Maha Sarakham, Thailand 2013) pp. 21–24. doi:10.1109/JCSSE.2013.6567313.
67. Petrantonakis P. C. and Hadjileontiadis L. J. 2010 Emotion recognition from EEG using higher order crossings, *IEEE Transactions on Information Technology in Biomedicine* **14**(2), 186–197.

68. Glenn E. 2010 *The physics hypertextbook: Intensity vs amplitude*, Physics info https://physics.info/intensity/summary.shtml.
69. Nasoz F., Alvarez K., Lisetti C. and Finkelstein N. 2004 Emotion recognition from physiological signals using wireless sensors for presence technologies, *Cognition, Technology & Work* **6**(1), 4–14.
70. Burkhardt F. 2005 Emofilt: The simulation of emotional speech by prosody-transformation. *Proceedings of the Interspeech '05- Eurospeech, 9th European Conference on Speech Communication and Technology* (Lisbon, Portugal September 2005) pp. 509–512.
71. Hammerschmidt K. and Jurgens U. 2007 Acoustical correlates of affective prosody, *Journal of Voice* **21**(5), 531–540.
72. Hartmut R. P. and Christian K. 2008 Amplitude and amplitude variation of emotional speech. *Proceedings of the Annual conference of the Interspeech '08* (Brisbane, Australia Sep 2008) pp. 1036–1039.
73. Lech M., Stolar M., Bolia R. and Skinner M. 2018 Amplitude-frequency analysis of emotional speech using transfer learning and classification of spectrogram images, *Advances in Science, Technology and Engineering Systems Journal* **3**(4), 363–371.
74. Healey J. 2014 Physiological sensing of emotion. *The Oxford Handbook of Affective Computing*, eds. R. Calvo, S. D'Mello, J. Gratch and A. Kappas (Oxford University Press, Oxford).
75. Cybenko G. 1989 Approximation by superpositions of a sigmoidal function, *Mathematics of Control, Signals and Systems* **2**, 303–314.
76. Jack V. T. 1996 Advantages and disadvantages of using artificial neural networks versus logistic regression for predicting medical outcomes, *Journal of Clinical Epidemiology* **49**(11), 1225–1231.
77. Chen J., Hu B., Wang Y., Moore P., Dai Y., Feng L. and Ding Z. 2017 Subject-independent emotion recognition based on physiological signals: A three-stage decision method, *BMC Medical Informatics and Decision Making* **17**(3) 167, 45–66.
78. Arnau-González P., Arevalillo-Herráez M. and Ramzan N. 2017 Fusing highly dimensional energy and connectivity features to identify affective states from EEG signals, *Neurocomputing* **244**, 81–89.
79. Qiu J. L., Li X. Y. and Hu K. 2018 Correlated attention networks for multimodal emotion recognition. *Proceedings of the IEEE International Conference on Bioinformatics and Biomedicine (BIBM)* (Madrid Spain, Dec. 2018) pp. 2656–2660.
80. Choi E. J. and Kim D. K. 2018 Arousal and valence classification model based on long short-term memory and DEAP data for mental healthcare management, *Healthcare Informatics Research* **24**(4), 309–316.
81. Liu J., Meng H., Li M., Zhang F., Qin R. and Nandi A. K. 2018 Emotion detection from EEG recordings based on supervised and unsupervised dimension reduction, *Concurrency and Computation Practice Experience* **30**, 1–13.
82. Khare S. K. and Bajaj V. 2020 An evolutionary optimized variational mode decomposition for emotion recognition, *IEEE Sensors Journal*, 1–8 doi: 10.1109/JSEN.2020.3020915.
83. Khare S. K., Nishad A., Upadhyay A. and Bajaj V. 2020 Classification of emotions from EEG signals using time-order representation based on the S-transform and convolutional neural network, *Electronics Letters* **56**(25), 1359–1361.
84. Khare S. K. and Bajaj V. 2020 Time-frequency representation and convolutional neural network-based emotion recognition, *IEEE Transactions on Neural Networks and Learning Systems* 1–9. doi: 10.1109/TNNLS.2020.3008938.
85. Khare S. K., Bajaj V. and Sinha G. R. 2020 Adaptive tunable Q wavelet transform-based emotion identification, *IEEE Transactions on Instrumentation and Measurement* **69**(12), 9609–9617.

3 Analysis and Classification of Heart Abnormalities

Ayesha Heena
KBN College of Engineering

CONTENTS

3.1 INTRODUCTION AND BACKGROUND INFORMATION

The heart is an extremely sophisticated and most significant organ of the human body. Interestingly, our heart starts beating before the brain is formed in the mother's womb. The fact is the nervous system does not initiate the heartbeat. It is actually self-initiated by our creator. Hence, we can say the heart is the center of human beings and not the brain. Recently, we have learned there are over 40,000 neurons in the heart that are communicating. There is a two-way communication between our brain and our heart. Our heart needs nourishment just like we need oxygen to breathe since cells need life, and if we stop breathing, cells die, and exactly our heart also needs to breathe for its nourishment for the heart to be healthy. Like any other disease, prevention is the key to avoid heart diseases and optimize treatment. Heart abnormalities are very common in India and all over the world, but with better understanding of different signs and symptoms of heart problems, proper diagnosis and prognosis are possible, so that early treatment is initiated. Heart diseases are seen as a common cause with multiple symptoms.

3.2 ANATOMY AND PHYSIOLOGY, BIOMECHANICS AND ELECTROPHYSIOLOGY OF THE HEART

Our heart is a fist-sized muscular organ located over the diaphragm. The biomechanics refers to the mechanical events generated within our heart because of the action potentials which in turn results from circulation of blood through our body; when heart beats in rhythm, as a result, a sequence of electrical events are generated. The electrical activity activated by the muscle tissues of the heart constitutes current flow throughout our body that results in potential differences in millivolts. The current is constituted because of movement of ions resulting due to muscle contraction and muscle relaxation in the heart. The heart is comprised of four chambers, two atria and two ventricles with some unique structural and electrical properties. Mainly blood flow in heart begins from right atrium, which receives blood from superior and inferior venae cavae; from here, blood passes into right atrium, across the tricuspid valve to the right ventricle as shown in Figure 3.1 in anatomy and physiology of heart figure. From the right ventricle, further blood is pumped across pulmonary valve into pulmonary artery, which distributes blood to the lungs. The heart receives pure oxygenated blood from left atrium through veins and enters left ventricle through mitral valve, where it enters the aortic valve and then the peripheral circulation proceeds through aorta as shown in Figure 3.1.

The process of pumping of blood and its circulation through the chambers of the heart is referred to as cardiac cycle. The phase of cardiac cycle which results in contraction is called systole referring to ventricular contraction v/s atrial contraction, and the relaxation phase of the cardiac cycle is called diastole; it is this phase in which the ventricles are filling, and the diastolic phase is always much longer than systole. Myocardial fibers possess specialized electrical properties; examples are pacemaker cells, excitability and conductivity. Pacemaker cells are unique cells with the ability to generate an electrical impulse independently. The

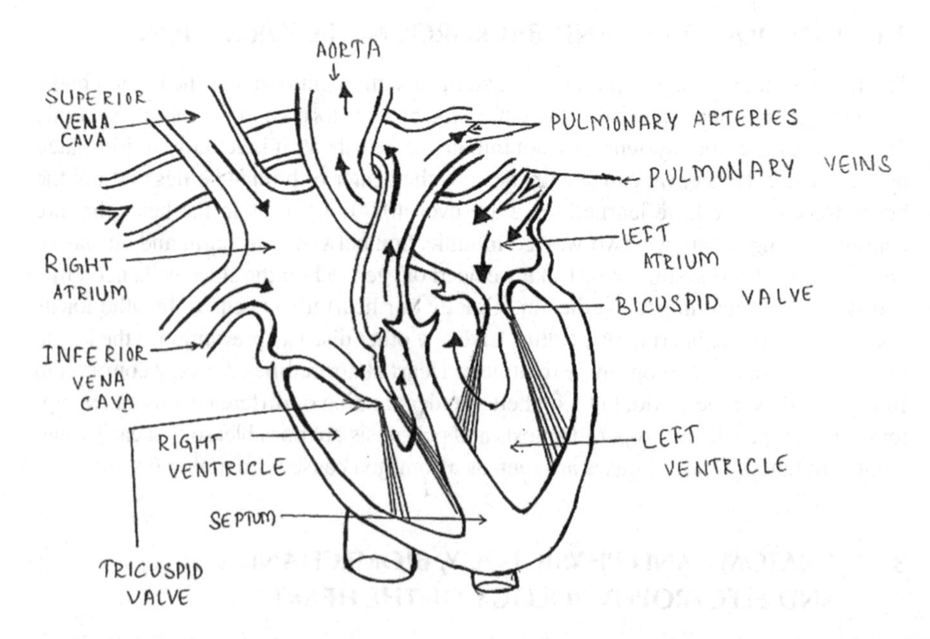

FIGURE 3.1 Anatomy and physiology of the human heart depicting circulation of blood through various parts within the structure of the heart.

ability of cells to respond to electrical stimulation is referred to as excitability. The ability of passing or propagating electrical impulses from one cell to another is defined as conductivity in the heart. The electrical conduction system of the heart comprises these three properties. This entire system is a network of structures in which the electrical impulses spread through the heart at much faster rate than they spread along muscle cells alone. The process of generation of electrical impulses through electrical conduction system is called depolarization. This is a process in which the electrolyte concentration shifts on either side of the cell membrane due to change in electrical charge of a cell. The contraction of muscle fiber is due to the stimulation of the electrical charge. A resting cell is referred to as a polarized cell, a condition wherein the inside of the cell is electrically more negative than the outside of the cell. When the permeability of the cell wall changes due to change in electrical stimulation, it allows positively charged ions, particularly sodium (Na^+), to move into the cell. With the influx of calcium (Ca^+) which is slow, sodium rushes inside the cell changing the inside of the cell from negative to positive. This activity of the cell is depolarization, resulting in contraction of muscle as a response to electrical charge. It is the conductivity due to which the rapid movement of depolarization takes place from cell to cell and then throughout the muscles of the heart. Myocardial cells are supposed to return to resting state of internal negativity after depolarization. The re-establishment of negative charge internally inside the cell is referred to as repolarization which is achieved through entry of potassium (K^+) into the cell and pumping of Na^+ out of the cell. After the understanding of movements of electrolytes, now it's time to see this process of depolarization and repolarization using electrocardiogram or ECG, which shows the electrical activity and not the mechanical health of the heart. Human body is a great conductor of electrical current. ECG is used for detecting the electrical activity that originates in the heart from the surface of the body [1].

3.3 INTRODUCTION OF ECG SIGNALS

An ECG is a signal that measures the electrical activity of the heart. An ECG records the potential differences in the heart. This measurement involves use of electrodes; these electrodes are attached to the surface of the skin over a fixed amount of time. Because of very low magnitude of the measured signals, the impact of noise on the measurements is very significant. The analysis of ECG so obtained is performed using processing of the signals. Signal processing encompasses a wide range of concepts that deal with different types of processing. For further analysis and extracting more details of information, the use of modification and processing is a common practice. Depending upon the various computing platforms available, various operations such as reading of ECG, decoding and recording data can be performed by using software for implementation of ECG. ECG waveforms can be used to find the various parameters and any disease that affect the heart. For identification and analysis of irregularities or abnormalities related to the heart and diseases of the heart, ECG signals are extensively helpful. Each portion of heartbeat is representation of electrical activity of the heart and produces a totally different deflection.

The study of ECG signal is generally used to characterize whether ECG is normal or not and discussing the various types of abnormalities and various parameters of consideration to effectively analyze and classify heart defects.

The application of electrodes to the skin is for measuring voltage changes in the cells, which are amplified and visually displayed on oscilloscope and graph paper. ECG analysis involves a step-wise procedure as follows:

Step 1: ECG corresponds to series of waves and deflections that records the activity of the heart from a view.

Step 2: Lead monitors the change in voltage between electrodes by placing them in different positions on the body.

Step 3: Leads as mentioned earlier from V1 to V6 are unipolar, are single positive electrodes with a negative reference point found at electrical center of the heart.

Step 4: Voltage changes so obtained are amplified and visually displayed on an oscilloscope and graph paper.

However, an ECG tracing looks different in each lead because of the recorded angle of electrical activity changes with each lead. Care must be taken during placement of electrodes, otherwise a normal ECG may turn out into an abnormal one. Normally a cable attached to the patient which is divided into different colored wires is used. Most preferred are 10- or 12-lead ECG. Recording of ECG involves paper tracing of patterns from the monitoring lead, rhythm strips are inscribed on graph paper which highlights various electrical components of an ECG and plays a significant role in ECG analysis. The vertical lines on graph paper measure time and horizontal lines on graph measure voltage. Say for example, one small box equals 0.04 seconds, and one large box equals 0.20 seconds. These boxes help us in measuring the duration of events. The voltage measurement is only relevant to calibrated tracings such as 12- or 15-lead ECG.

The various components of an ECG tracing include wave, complex, segment, interval, P wave, PR interval, QRS complex; ST segment, T wave, QT interval and U wave as shown in Figure 3.2. A single cardiac cycle inscribes various deflections on graph paper which are electrical activities described as below:

- **Wave**: A deflection, away from baseline of the ECG tracing either positive or negative.
- **Complex**: Involves more than one wave.
- **Segment**: Is a line between waves and complexes.
- **Interval**: Comprises a segment and a wave.

The electrical components are described as follows:

- **P wave**: The first wave that appears slightly rounded and upright positive represents atrial depolarization.
- **PR interval**: Distance between beginning of P wave and beginning of QPRS complex; measures the time duration in which depolarization wave travels from atria to ventricles.

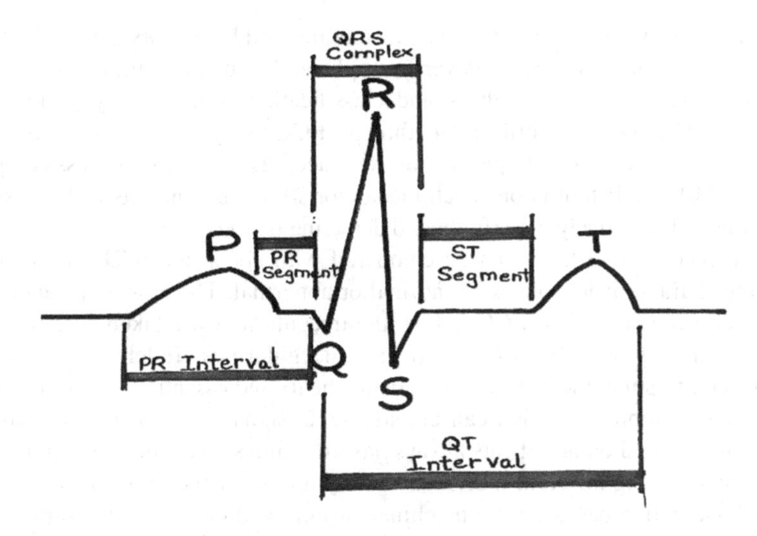

FIGURE 3.2 Various electrical components of an ECG.

- **QRS complex**: Three deflections following P wave indicates ventricular depolarization.
- **Q wave**: The first negative deflection.
- **R wave**: The first positive deflection.
- **S wave**: The first negative deflection after R wave.
- **ST segment**: Distance between the end of S wave and the beginning of T wave measures time between ventricular depolarization and beginning of repolarization.
- **T wave**: Round upright positive wave following the QRS complex in the ST segment indicates ventricular repolarization.

ECG has many uses. It is used to reflect anatomic, hemodynamic, molecular, ionic and drug-induced cardiac abnormalities. ECG may be very helpful for proper diagnosis and therapy provides significant information required for many heart-related problems. In fact, ECG is extensively applied in clinical diagnosis of heart diseases and can be reliably used as a measure to monitor the overall functionality of the cardiovascular system. ECG signals are simple and noninvasive and hence widely used for detection and analysis of heart diseases. The most important factor for analysis and diagnosis of heart diseases is feature extraction and classification. The performance of ECG pattern classification strongly depends on the characterization power of the features extracted from ECG signal and the design of classifier.

3.4 VARIOUS HEART-RELATED ABNORMALITIES

Heart abnormalities are very dangerous and can result in death. It is always the need of the hour to come up with improvements in diagnosis and treatment and are always appreciated by the medical fraternity. For heart patients, one of the most useful diagnostic tools would be the ECG. The technique used by doctors/physicians traditionally for the analysis of ECG is very complicated, time consuming and requires expertise. Computer-based analysis and classification is immensely preferred in diagnostics. The need of an efficient method for ECG analysis and classification is to develop a method which is simple yet has good accuracy and requires less computation time. MATLAB tool is one such means for study and analysis of ECG signal processing and effectively classifying and detecting heart defects.

A reference normal ECG can be compared with abnormal ECG for classification using characteristics to classify normal or abnormal. The most important challenge in classification of an ECG is how the irregularities are taken care of which are characteristics of an ECG signal. If these irregularities are left unnoticed, it is very difficult to study the status of a, patient's heart and essentially, there is a need of an efficient approach which can classify ECG signals with a higher accuracy. Classification based on heartbeats always has difficulties since these waveforms are not the same among different individuals. They are discussed by some unique features. Classification based on the machine learning approach has in several recent research studies proven to be more accurate using the unique features as input to machine learning algorithms. These are again discussed later in the chapter.

Any emergency situation genuinely will have only minutes or less for to interpret ECG correctly and ensure the possible right treatment for the patient. An increase in size of the heart is always abnormal; however, in case of athletes, the slow heart rates even from normal heart can reflect mild cardiomegaly because of higher-than-average cardiac output. However, pathophysiology of heart failure is uniquely portrayed due to specific chamber enlargement. An increase pulmonary lucent area due to the chronic setting decreased flow is the hallmark of right heart failure. The characterization of acute left sided heart failure by bat wing appearance is most common, usually seen in case of acute MI or acute MR due to chordal rupture; B-Lines characterizes the chronic left sided heart failure. The acute right-sided heart failure is mostly a result of massive pulmonary embolism. In patients with the problem of right-sided heart failure, lucent lungs flow pattern is found. The more the severity of tricuspid regurgitation (reverse flow of blood), the more the enlargement of the right-sided chamber. Consequently, severe left heart failure results in right heart failure. Also, in patients suffering from mitral stenosis leading to severe tricuspid regurgitation, the situation is exemplified.

Scientifically, now heart diseases refer to conditions involving the heart, its vessels, muscles, valves or internal electric pathways responsible for muscular contraction. So together, the common heart diseases include the following:

- Coronary artery disease
- Heart failure
- Cardiomyopathy
- Heart valve diseases.

Ischemia is commonly detected using diverse electrocardiography. Myocardial ischemia is a condition wherein there is a mismatch between supply and demand of oxygen within the cardiac cells. When supply of oxygen doesn't meet the demand, it leads to shift in metabolism from aerobic toward anaerobic substrates. This in turn results in accumulation of metabolic end products such as lactate which is followed by impaired mechanical function. Ischemia results due to reduced coronary blood flow from fixed stenosis. Depletion of high-energy phosphate stores is also a result of the anaerobic metabolism. The purpose of stress testing is to provoke myocardial Ischemia. By the help of surface ECG, myocardial ischemia may be documented by proper examining of perfusion of myocardia or wall motion of the left ventricle. The parameters used for defining the test accuracy is obtained by calculating diagnostic sensitivity and specificity. The highest accuracy corresponds to the tests with values of the sensitivity and specificity greater than 80%. The accuracy of exercise ECG during routine work up of patients varies with those of abnormal studies. Catheterization is required for patients having negative stress results. It is significant to use these measures (sensitivity and specificity) in clinical practices to know whether these tests can be applied as a gatekeeper to angiography (sensitivity of 100% and specificity of 0% is a right choice for gatekeeping). Methods are available to correct verification bias. Exercise ECG needs to be analyzed and interpreted very carefully. The factors that are confound to the interpretation of exercise ECG include medications, hormonal status, resting ST wave changes of ECG, prior myocardial infarction and more importantly functional capacity. In case of certain subsets of patients, it is evident that the exercise ECG will be of diminished value. A low QRS voltage can also lead to false positive results. In ECG abnormalities such as left ventricular hypertrophy, left bundle branch block and Wolff-Parkinson-White syndrome, patients need to be referred to cardiac imaging. In patients heart rate of 75 beats per minute is resting heart rate or above and vary with subjects during exercise and after exercise. Evaluation of functional capacity should be included in test suggested for the patient that also includes information about ventricular ectopy, heart rate recovery, hemodynamic and chrono topic responses to stress. For a proper timing of inducible ischemia, patients are suggested exercise in order to gain insight about patient's capabilities. For a growing segment of population, including obese or diabetic patients, the correct choice of exercise protocol is paramount so as to overcome stress. The symptoms of arrhythmia often include dizziness, and hence often such patients are referred to electrophysiologists for confirming that the symptoms are caused by arrhythmia or not. It is possible to positively determine an arrhythmic cause only if ECG is recorded when exactly the event occurs. Actually, a correct direction of diagnosis is to have a detailed patient history. The ECG may help in revealing factors leading to cause of dizziness including myocardial infarction, cardiac hypertrophy, sinus node dysfunction, conduction abnormality, white syndrome, etc. Evaluation of ECG may lead to a variety of cardiac diagnosis. For patients who present with dizziness, it is worth knowing the cause of dizziness whether it is vertigo or true light headedness, or if the patient feels like the room is spinning or has a sensation that everywhere there is darkness or feeling like unconsciousness, since cardiovascular dizziness does not actually produce vertigo. Palpitations are occurring with different outcomes, including skipped beats, a sudden thump, hard beating, fluttering in the chest, a jittery sensation, or a rapid pulse. It has been found that many patients feel a strong heartbeat that is palpitation and hence irregular heartbeats and this must be properly differentiated. Palpitations are often more prominent at night, especially observed in patients who lie on their left side. It is also preferable to always sleep on your right-side during night. For proper diagnosis and therapeutic reasons an electrophysiologic study is required. For infrequent arrhythmias noninvasive monitoring is often futile. A definitive analysis for proper diagnosis is required using implantable recorders for electrophysiologic studies.

It has been doctor's experience that in certain patient's alcohol and caffeine are arrhythmogenic although its effect on arrhythmia patients is very less, sustained ventricular tachycardia its effect is high. Patients may present with symptoms such as fatigue, chest pain or dizziness that are unrelated to arrhythmia. Many patients do not suffer palpitations but present with either fatigue, shortness of breath or episodic weakness. Although such symptoms often direct the clinician to a different road but actually may cause arrhythmia since there are also cases of patients with no palpitations but present symptoms of heart failure.

Heart rate variability (HRV) is used to assess cardiac status, wherein variations in sinus cycle length is used as a basis of analysis. The standard deviation of normal to normal (SDNN) beats or all of RR intervals is a commonly used method. To develop a power spectral density frequency domain method applies frequency domain representation of the signal. This represents the distribution of variance of the signal (i.e., power) as a function of frequency. The post-myocardial risk stratification uses HRV. There is an increased rate of sudden death when HRV is decreased. Also, post-myocardial infarction increases in HRV with treatment results in protective effects [2].

Some of the common cardiac arrhythmias are atrial fibrillation (AF), tachycardia and atrial flutter. The most common sustained cardiac arrhythmia is indeed atrial fibrillation in clinical practice. Also, this arrhythmia is most prevalent and is often associated with deterioration of hemodynamic and results in a wide spectrum of symptoms and significant morbidity, mortality and medical costs. Perhaps no single therapy will prove to be the best for all, and there are a variety of treatment strategies applied to different arrhythmias. These treatments include no therapy at all, rhythm control and rate control with both pharmacologic and nonpharmacologic options. Due to uncoordinated atrial contraction and disorganized atrial electrical activation, atrial fibrillation results. Although disorganized atrial activation may reveal further analysis, ECG has the characteristic appearance of a regular rapid atrial rhythm. Careful measurement will disclose variability in PP interval, and this is often misinterpreted as atrial flutter. At the initial stage of detection of AF, however, the subsequent pattern of recurrences may be difficult to ascertain. Only after two or more episodes, AF is classified as recurrent. Episodes that generally last less than 7 days (and most less than 24 hours) are self-terminating; they can be classified as persistent only after the termination of an episode, whereas those lasting for more than 7 days often require electrical or pharmacologic cardioversion. When cardioversion fails, AF is classified as permanent, and no further treatment works. Although this classification method is generally useful, AF pattern is treatment-dependent. Thus, even persistent AF sometime may change to paroxysmal (only when lasting for less than 7 days) during pharmacologic therapy with antiarrhythmic medications. It has been demonstrated from studies that AF patients further have risk of stroke, and also, it is age-dependent. Stroke is the most feared consequence of AF, and prevention would be the only focus of managing such patients [3]. There is general consensus that AF that has been present for less than 48 hours can be cardioverted without prior anticoagulation, but there are no randomized trial data to support this, and systematic embolic can occur in this situation. Anticoagulation therapy is so recommended for AF since the onset time of AF is often impossible to measure accurately [4]. There are certain types of atrial flutter all having rapid, regular atrial rates of generally 240–340 bpm. Typical atrial flutter is characterized by negative saw tooth waves, and reverse typical atrial flutter is characterized by positive flutter waves in ECG leads (also called counter-clockwise and clockwise flutter, respectively). After open heart surgery, commonly within a week, some patients show symptoms of atrial flutter. It is associated with chronic obstructive pulmonary disease (COPD), mitral valve or tricuspid valve disease and postsurgical repair of certain congenital cardiac lesions as well as enlargement of atria for any reason, especially the right atrium. Atrial flutter can be diagnosed from ECG. Most of the time, it may be difficult to identify atrial flutter since it is very low in amplitude in the ECG.

The acute atrial flutter treatment parallels the approach to acute AF. In order to slow down the ventricular response rate, drug therapy is used. Rapid and relatively regular rhythms refer to tachycardia that originates in the atria usually 130–250 bpm. Focus that characterizes atrial activation is a small area that starts rhythmically. Frequently in pulmonary veins, foci are found in the left atrium (LA) and in the right atrium (RA) foci can also occur at various sites in both atria. An abnormal P wave or a low amplitude P wave or a rapid atrial rate in the range from 160 to 240 bpm often characterizes ectopic. A high-grade block and ultimately heart failure are usually due to rates higher than 200 bpm. Intern presence of conduction block is demonstrated through AV node. A consistent termination of tachycardia is a useful sign of AV nodal dependence followed by a P wave without conduction to ventricles. With no reversible cause found, antiarrhythmic agents may provide effective treatment. Cardioversion is rarely helpful. Ranging from PVCs to VF are the ventricular arrhythmias [5,6] that result in sudden death. The presence or absence of structural heart diseases plays a major role in risk stratification. Management of potentially critical arrhythmias occurring in heart's structure appearing normal depends on the associated symptoms, hemodynamic consequences and long-term prognosis. It is important to have proper guidance while selecting management strategies that are appropriate and is provided by the ECG pattern of the ventricular arrhythmia. PVCs are frequently occurring in practice. Its significance depends on their frequency, the presence and severity of structural heart disease and presence of associated symptoms. In general, PVCs that occur in patients even without any structural heart disease are not so dangerous, and there is no risk of death. Such PVCs generally require no therapy, unless significant symptoms are exhibited. The presence of PVCs is associated with an increased risk of sudden death especially after an MI when their frequency of occurrence exceeds 10 per hour. Patients with MI and LVEF are at the greatest risk of sudden death. It is not recommended to treat PVCs with anti-arrhythmias unless hemodynamic compromise is associated. Mitral regurgitation (MR) is an abnormality when there is reverse flow of blood LV to LA. The enlargement of LA or LV due to chronic MR, consequently, results in increased amplitude of both the P waves and QRS complex. Also, the LA enlargement is associated with coarse fibrillatory waves if atrial fibrillation is present. The ECG may be entirely normal especially in acute MR when muscle ischemia or infarction is the reason for MR. Even the electrocardiogram (ECG) is also normal in case of patients with mitral valve prolapse (MVP) syndrome. Only if there is depression in ST-T-wave or inversion in T-wave, it indicates abnormality in MVP syndrome. MVP is also associated with false-positive exercise.

The MVP patients report higher incidences of arrhythmias. However, most of them do not exhibit danger to life and are not found to relate with symptoms of the patient.

Hemodynamic instability resulting due to a series of continuous ventricular impulses occurring at rate greater than 100 bpm and lasting for longer than 30 seconds is VT. In a duration of 24 hours, the ventricular storms occur with three sustained episodes of VT. Acute ischemia generally reflects VF. The likelihood of VT is more than 80% if there is any problem of heart disease. Using ECG differentiating VT from supraventricular tachycardia (SVT) [7,8] is difficult. For the prevention of recurrent VT and sudden death, in patients [9], long-term management is directed, which is usually a treatment involving therapy of anti-arrhythmias with implantation of internal cardioverter defibrillator [10,11]. Pacemaker leads are both unipolar and bipolar. In unipolar lead, anode is pacemaker generator and cathode is the catheter which has distal electrode. The unipolar lead completes the circuit using body tissue. Bipolar lead has two separate conductors as well as electrodes in the lead. Most of the new pacemaker systems nowadays use bipolar leads; unipolar leads are only occasionally used due to small diameter for LV pacing through the sinus. If pacemaker is inflected, it is essential to remove pacemaker leads and generator. Pacemaker has its own pros and cons. For quantitating cardiac arrhythmias and for diagnosing, ambulatory ECG recordings are helpful [12]. The only means of diagnosis is to record an arrhythmia when a patient experiences symptoms. Ambulatory ECG monitoring is now possible for long durations because of the technological advances in telemetric recording available in a wide variety of systems. An arrhythmia as the cause for the symptoms can be excluded if the normal rhythm is recorded during symptoms and has proven equally valuable. Asymptomatic arrhythmia detection using ambulatory ECG is useful in certain patients for detecting future cardiac events. Some of the significant applications include determining the changes in ST segment or T wave for detecting myocardial ischemia and HRV measurements. Depending upon individual patient's need, the appropriate long-term ECG recording system is chosen. Misinterpretation in diagnosis leads to inappropriate treatment. Every variety of cardiac arrhythmias is mimicked, and artifacts registered during prolonged ECG lead to misinterpretation. These artifacts occur at different levels of recording. Ablation is a reasonably first line therapy for most tachycardias, atrial flutter, AV node and VT [13–15].

One potential solution is recent development of wearable defibrillator. The patient is made to wear a vest. The vest is incorporated with electrodes and defibrillator which is fed by ECG, which is continuously analyzed. It initially delivers an audible and tactile alarm. The patient has to disable the device within 30 seconds if no VF is present. If the device is not disabled during the stipulated time, the defibrillator charges, and the patient gets a biphasic shock. Cardiovascular disorders cause syncope. A transient decrease in cerebral blood flow causes sudden loss of consciousness referred to as syncope [16]. Syncope occurs suddenly without warning or may precede with light headedness, dizziness, nausea, diaphoresis and blurred vision. This problem increases with age, and syncope is caused due to multiple reasons and hence is difficult to determine in more than half of the cases. It is associated with the highest risk of mortality, 30% within a year after diagnosis approaching 50% in over 5 years. Syncope has the lowest rate of mortality risk if it is not due to any heart-related issue. Hence, it is very important to distinguish whether syncope is heart-related or from other causes of loss of consciousness including seizures, hypoglycemia and trauma. One major task is to determine whether cause for syncope in patient is life threatening or not. Also, in addition, preciseness and accuracy in diagnosis are based on effective therapy. Patients need to minimize exposure to factors that provoke syncope, and measures should be taken to avoid it by lying down if the symptoms are experienced. It is preferable to lie down on the right side. Tight cloths should be avoided; especially losing around neck or waist is recommended.

Unnatural and unexpected death due to cardiac reason within a short duration of time from when symptoms are initiated is referred to as sudden cardiac death (SCD). Fatal arrhythmia causing cardiac arrest that occurs in the background of any disease related to heart may result in SCD. Worldwide, in most developed countries, overall cardiac mortality due to SCD is 50%. Observations say that from the onset of the symptoms, it takes hardly 2 hours for a patient to collapse, suppose 88% of the deaths are due to heart diseases, and 12% are due to sudden cardiac arrest. An approximate percentage of SCD that occurs outside the hospital environment is around 60%. The first event accounts for 85%–90% of SCDs, while the remaining is due to recurring events. Though SCD increases with age, still SCD accounts for sudden deaths in patients younger than 20 years of age by approximately 20%. Overall, SCD in infants, children, adolescents and young adults is rare. SCD rate in men is higher than in women; 70%–90% of SCDs occur in men. The risk of SCD increases in congenital conditions.

Circulatory abnormalities cause cardiac arrest due to abrupt termination of organized activity of the heart. Primary phenotypes due to cardiac rhythm and conduction abnormalities cause genetic disorders that affect ion regulators and their channels. This characteristic disease of the heart conduction system is an autosomal dominant called as familial block. The chance of occurrence of congenital heart disease (CHD) ranging from moderate to severe forms are six per 1000 live births. Most patients with complex CHD would not survive to adulthood without early medical or surgical treatment. Surgical and medical advances have dramatically improved prognosis; roughly, the CHD patients who actually reach adulthood is more than 85%. However, there are many cases wherein the adult patients with CHD may never require any intervention of surgery. Every year, on an average, around 50,000 patients are expected to have the problem of MI which is postoperative, and the cause of around 40,000 deaths is due to cardiac events. Either myocardial ischemia or arrhythmias are often related to most perioperative cardiac morbidity and mortality. A careful observation of history of the patient, physical examination and review of resting 12-lead ECG can be helpful in identifying the increased risk of adverse perioperative cardiac events in majority of patients. Recommendations of American College of Cardiology (ACC) and American Heart Association (AHA) designate classification of risk factors into three groups: major, intermediate and minor. The rise in the prevalence of obesity worldwide is becoming a threat which is nullifying the recent advances in cardiovascular disease prevention. Obesity is the mother of different complications associated with cardiovascular events and cause of the greatest morbidity and mortality. A step ahead is the situation becoming worst leading to further increase in mortality among patients where obesity precedes diabetes. However, the one out of several problems that relate with obesity is diabetes. Hypertension [17–19] and systemic inflammation are among other problems. Recently, metabolic syndrome is a new term trending in the cardiovascular field which groups all the above-mentioned factors together representing multiple risk factors. This syndrome does not include but is strongly associated with other complications of obesity like fatty liver, cholesterol gallstones, sleep apnea and polycystic ovarian syndrome. Cardiovascular specialist places more emphasis on metabolic syndrome and its early diagnosis and treatment.

As a result of the focus on metabolic syndrome, people are giving more priority to physical activities and promotion of weight control, thus encouraging the health efforts of public. This demands a need of change in the scenario where investments on preventive measures can reconfigure our health care systems. A prevalence of diabetes is higher nowadays. The developing world in near future will be highly impacted by diabetes epidemic. A substantial increase in diabetes in developing countries is a contribution of increased urbanization, westernization and economic growth. Prevalence rates of diabetes among young populations is rapidly increasing in developing countries; earlier, diabetes was more common in elderly populations. A very strong risk factor causes CFD as well as stroke is diabetes mellitus, whether type 1 or type 2. Around 80% of all deaths are among diabetic patients in comparison to 30% among nondiabetic. Diabetic education must be provided to every patient suffering with diabetes [20]. Recommendation for glucose testing varies from individual to individual and varies depending on the current degree of control. Hypoglycemia is caused potentially in patients who are on medication. Patients need to be well aware of the food intake, exercise regimes and circumstances that are going to affect blood glucose levels and also how they can modify the behavior for an optimal glycemic control. Actually, it is very challenging on the clinical front to prevent and manage cardiovascular complications. Glycemic control, however, is difficult to manage for patients with long-term diabetes.

Valvular diseases are more common. Mitral valve prolapse is frequent. Valvular diseases typically present with nodules and fibrosis of leaflet, annulus and apparatus. Patients with symptomatic or severe valvular diseases require surgical intervention. Although any of the four valves may be affected, commonly occurring valvular abnormalities are associated with mitral valve, resulting in mitral regurgitation. The next is aortic valve abnormalities. Valvular lesions are asymptomatic but not uncommon. 2D echocardiography is used for detection and diagnosis. Patients with clinically symptomatic and hemodynamically significant valve disease often require valve replacement surgery.

3.5 HEART ABNORMALITIES IN WOMEN

The importance of CVD and its prevention in women is day by day gaining significance in public and also among physicians. Recently, an updated guideline for CVD prevention in women is given by an expert panel, and sex differences are being increasingly explored. Women's lower work capacity and oxygen uptake than men are due to less physical activities [21,22]. This leads to increase in women's cardiac output significantly, thereby increasing the heart rate. It has been observed in various studies that women who have a habit of walking have less chances of CHD when compared to women who don't walk regularly (at least an hour). The benefits of cardiac rehabilitation programs after MI are equal for both men and women. Most of the time, women are either not referred cardiac rehabilitation, or they restrict themselves to participate in such activities. The risk factors for CVD in women include importance of menstrual cycle and menopause but are still not properly understood. The risk for CVD and osteoporosis is higher in women with early menopause after gynecologic surgery. But women smokers are at a greater risk of CVD with young age of menopause. Although it has been disclosed through surveys that after menopause hormonal therapy decreases the risk of CVD, women using hormones tended to be healthier, due to reportedly less tobacco exposure, greater levels of exercise and readier access to medical care. Women's Health Initiative (WHI) suggests the risk of CHD is reduced in women who after menopause begin hormonal therapy. Migraine headaches, especially those with aura, are an evolving risk factor for CVD. Further, stroke risk is very high for women than for men among adults of age in between 45 and 54 years. Also, as long as we speak of, receiving pacemakers or taking anticoagulants for AF is not very common in women than men. After suicide, the most common reason for maternal death is heart diseases (as second). Maternal death is a major determinant of fetal death. Pregnant women [23] with heart diseases are informed to take extra measures of diagnostics and therapies in view of fetal safety as an important consideration. Ultimately, maternal health is the highest priority. Sometimes when the mother is at risk, the doctors recommend termination or interruption of pregnancy. For those who continue face-specific issues for newborn such as potentially jeopardized nourishment of the infant due to maternal illness, chances are that milk feeding transmits cardiac medication to the infant and finally the fear that due to heart disease we may have potential loss of the mother. Thus, patients suffering from heart diseases when conceive require the expertise of most care providers and in fact exceed the capabilities of any single care provider. Best care is to be given by an experienced team that includes counsellors, primary care provider, obstetricians, cardiologists, anesthesiologists and pediatricians. Any women contemplating pregnancy with heart disease should be educated by experienced care providers before conception. Each method of birth control has its advantages and disadvantages, which are more crucially applicable to women who are heart patients. ECG is safe, but ST-T wave variations are difficult to interpret during pregnancy. Depression is common even in normal pregnancy. A true axis deviation represents heart disease; however, a left-ward shift arises during pregnancy. The valve lesion which is difficult to tolerate during pregnancy is mitral stenosis. In general, mitral regurgitation is well tolerated during pregnancy. If it is severe, LV dysfunction [24] valve repair is recommended before pregnancy. Congenital heart disease is also commonly encountered in child-bearing women, with greater than 10% overall maternal complications during pregnancy. Each abnormality is unique, but some issues apply to all. Due to abnormalities of heart, the maternal morbidity and mortality risk in pregnant women are very high. The potential targets for treatment and prevention are represented by risk factors like cardiac and vascular aging. Lack of exercise increases the risk factor with age in comparison to healthy persons.

Many researchers have investigated the automated classification of heart beats. The classification methods and their types are based on a variety of features. Generally included heartbeat features are ECG morphology, temporal features, correlation of beats and summits. The requirement of classification process is to obtain an intelligent model which can classify any heartbeat signal into a specific type of heartbeat. Deep learning is also a vastly employed technique in recent research studies for ECG beats' classification. To reduce high mortality rate due to heart diseases, some countries have built tele-ECG system for early detection and monitoring of patients with heart abnormalities. Neural networks and support vector machine (SVM) algorithms are also frequently used in classification because of higher accuracy in results. Much higher accuracies are achieved in classification using deep neural networks (DNN) according to latest research studies. Convolutional neural networks are also used for ECG beat type classification. Machine learning algorithms are also very popular for classification of heart beats. The basic requirement for this classification is huge database comprising records of ECGs of different patients with different pathological problems for accomplishing computational analysis. The algorithms basically work with extraction of features and using these features for classification. The acquired datasets are usually split into training and testing data normally 70%–80% and 20%–30%, respectively. The built model needs to be test validated on different datasets. Optimal values for required parameters are obtained with cross validation.

ECG analysis based on neural networks classification is a commonly used technique for different types of ECG signals. The method involves loading ECG signal and preprocessing it and then classifies them into classes. The output which is taken from classifiers carries a predictive feature. Automatic or computer-aided classification of ECG demands accuracy which is comparable to that of gold standards that refer to the opinion of a cardiology expert. Recently, in the field of biomedical signal and image processing, neural networks are probably preferred for this application which are coupled with high levels of performance. Neural networks [25–27] are structures consisting of a parallel interconnected network of processing elements called channels which distribute information using unidirectional signal channels. These channels further branch into more than one connection that are collateral. The processing elements or channels produce mathematical output. The entire processing carried out within these channels is completely local to the processing elements which means it only depends on current values of the input signals. The inputs to processing elements are from impinging connections, and the output also depends upon stored values in the local memory of the processing elements. Fuzzy logic, on the other hand, corresponds to heterogenous family of formalism that are capable of modelling uncertain and vague information successfully and processing them. Fuzzy logic is a complementary method to neural network-based methods. The fuzzy logic has an advantage of human readable representation of interpreting predictions symbolically. This does not necessarily mean that the analysis and interpretation of fuzzy logic is ultimate, accurate and efficient. Actually, the significance of fuzzy logic is because it gives transparent and more interpretable results. Analysis and prediction of time series are important and widely used in many practical applications. For final diagnosis of disorders of heart, the diagnostic code stored in the ECG monitors is considered relatively reliable in clinical practices.

3.6 SUMMARY

Educating people about early access to emergency services when a patient develops acute chest pain can help save life. Attention must be paid to the role of weight reduction, diet, exercise and medications. Hence, preventing heart diseases is no doubt a lifelong commitment to control blood pressure, high cholesterol and diabetes. Stress is a normal part of life but if left unmanaged can lead to emotional, psychological and physical problems including heart diseases, high blood pressure, chest pain or irregular heartbeats. Several studies have also linked stress to changes in the way blood clots, which increases the risk of heart attack. The way people handle stress is also equally important, like in ways that make bad situations worse by reacting with feelings of anger, guilt, fear, hostility and anxiety. It's always better to face life's challenges with ease, learn to relax, sleep well and have a positive attitude, which is a good defense against stress and heart abnormalities. Further, with a positive attitude, it is possible to view stress as a challenge rather than a problem. So, keep yourself away from all negativities. Particularly, in this pandemic situation of COVID 19, positive attitude can only keep all of us in control when there are inevitable changes in life. A positive attitude defines telling ourselves there are things we can do to improve certain situations and admitting that sometimes there's nothing we can do so stay calm, stop worrying and breathe deeply. Reflect on your choices, assume we can get through the situation and try to be objective, realistic and flexible, think about positive solutions and choose one that is most acceptable and feasible. Also think about outcomes and learn from every situation, how to manage time effectively but be realistic and flexible. Relaxing is a learned skill to cope with stress. It's something more than sitting back and being quiet; rather, it's an active process involving techniques that can calm the body and mind. True relaxation requires becoming sensitive to basic needs for peace, self-awareness and thoughtful reflection. Once you find a relaxation method that works for you, practice it every day at least an hour, maybe prayer, meditation, yoga or simple brisk walking. Lastly, if we wish to change the dangerous scenario of the world, it is possible only if we be a part of the change we want and change this world by rectifying our inward because it is always the inward that precedes the outward.

REFERENCES

1. Lipinski M.J., Froelicher V.F. ECG exercise testing. In: Fuster V., Walsh R.A., Harrington R.A., et al., eds. *Hurst's The Heart.* 13th ed. New York, NY: McGraw-Hill. 2011; 16:371–387.
2. Shaw L.J., Berman D.S., Maron D.J., et al. Prognostic value of gated myocardial perfusion SPECT. *J Nucl Cardiol* 2004; 11:171–185.
3. Hsu L.F., Jais P., Sanders P., et al. Catheter ablation for atrial fibrillation in congestive heart failure. *N Engl J Med* 2004; 351:2373–2383.
4. Oral H., Scharf C., Chugh A., et al. Catheter ablation for paroxysmal atrial fibrillation: segmental pulmonary vein ostial ablation versus left atrial ablation. *Circulation* 2003; 108:2355–2360.

5. Rho R.W., Page R.L. Ventricular arrhythmias. In: Fuster V., Walsh R., Harrington R.A., et al. *Hurst's The Heart.* 13th ed, New York, NY: McGraw-Hill; 2011, 42:1006-1024.
6. ACC/AHA/ESC 2006 Guidelines for Management of Patients with Ventricular Arrhythmias and the Prevention of Sudden Cardiac Death. 2006; 48:e247–e346. Available at www.content.onlinejacc.org/cgi/content.
7. Brugada P., Brugada J., Mont L., Smeets J., Andries E.W. A new approach to the differential diagnosis of a regular tachycardia with a wide QRS complex. *Circulation* 1991; 83:1649–1659.
8. Lee K.W., Badhwar N., Scheinman M.M. Supraventricular tachycardia.2008; 33:467–546 Part I Current Problems in Cardiology Curr Probl Cardiol . doi:10.1016/j.cpcardiol.2008.06.002.
9. Buxton A.E., Lee K.L., Fisher J.D., et al. A randomized study of the prevention of sudden death in patients with coronary artery disease. *N Engl J Med* 1999; 341:1882–1890.
10. Reddy V.Y., Reynolds M.R., Neuzil P., et al. Prophylactic catheter ablation for the prevention of defibrillator therapy. *N Engl J Med* 2007; 357:2657–2665.
11. Prystowsky E.N., Fogel R.I. Approach to the patient with cardiac arrhythmias. In: Fuster V., O'Rourke R.A., Walsh R.A., et al. eds. *Hurst's the Heart.* 13th ed. New York, NY: McGraw-Hill; 2011; 39:949–962.
12. Myerburg J.R., Chaitman B.R., Ewy G.A., et al. Training in electrocardiography, ambulatory electrocardiography, and exercise testing. *J Am Coll Cardiol* 2008; 51:384.
13. Stevenson W.G., Friedman P.L., Kocovic D., et al. Radiofrequency catheter ablation of ventricular tachycardia after myocardial infarction. *Circulation.* 1998; 98:308–314.
14. Moss A.J., Zareba W., Hall W.J. Prophylactic implantation of a defibrillator in patients with myocardial infarction and reduced ejection fraction (MADIT II). *N Engl J Med* 2002; 346:877–883.
15. Bardy G.H., Lee K.L., Mark D.B., et al. Amiodarone or an implantable cardioverter-defibrillator for congestive heart failure. *N Engl J Med* 2005; 352:225–237.
16. Krahn A., Klein G., Yee R., et al. Use of an extended monitoring strategy in patients with problematic syncope. *Circulation.* 1999; 99:406–410.
17. Atkins G.B., Rahman M., Wright Jr. J.T. Diagnosis, and treatment of hypertension. In: Fuster V., Walsh R.A., Harrington R.A., et al., eds. *Hurst's The Heart.* 13th ed. New York, NY: McGraw-Hill; 2011; 70:1585–1605.
18. European Society of Hypertension–European Society of Cardiology. 2003 European Society of Hypertension-European Society of Cardiology guidelines for the management of arterial hypertension. 2003; 21:1011–1053.
19. Bonow R.O., Carabello B., Chatterjee K., et al. ACC/AHA 2006 guidelines for the management of patients with valvular heart disease: Erratum appears. *Circulation* 2007; 115: e409.
20. Lichtenstein A.H., Appel L.J., Brands M., et al. Diet and lifestyle recommendations revision 2006: A scientific statement from the American Heart Association Nutrition Committee. *Circulation.* 2006; 114:82–96.
21. Gibbons R.J., Balady, G.J., Bricker J.T., et al. ACC/AHA 2002 guideline update for exercise testing—summary article. *Circulation* 2002; 106:1883–1892.
22. Redberg R.F., Taubert K., Thomas G., et al. American Heart Association, Cardiac Imaging Committee consensus statement: The role of cardiac imaging in the clinical evaluation of women with known or suspected coronary artery disease. *Circulation* 2005; 111:682–696. doi:10.1161/01.CIR.0000155233.67287.60.
23. Hung L., Rahimtoola S.H. Prosthetic heart valve and pregnancy. *Circulation* 2003; 107: 1240–1246.
24. Solomon S.D., Zelenkofske S., McMurray J.J., et al. Sudden death in patients with myocardial infarction and left ventricular dysfunction, heart failure, or both. *N Engl J Med* 2005; 352:2581–2588.

25. Bajaj V. and Sinha G.R. *Modelling and Analysis of Active Bio-potential Signals in Healthcare*, Volume 1, IOP Publishing August 2020. https://iopscience.iop.org/book/978-0-7503-3279-8.
26. Sinha G.R. and Suri J. *Cognitive Informatics, Computer Modelling and Cognitive Science, Volume 1: Theory, Case Studies and Applications*, Elsevier, 2020. https://www.elsevier.com/books/cognitive-informatics-computer-modelling-and-cognitive-science/sinha/978-0-12-819443-0.
27. Sinha G.R. and Suri J. *Cognitive Informatics, Computer Modelling and Cognitive Science, Volume 2: Applications to Neural Engineering, Robotics and STEM*, Elsevier, 2020. https://www.elsevier.com/books/cognitive-informatics-computer-modelling-and-cognitive-science/Sinha/978-0-12-819445-4.

4 Diagnosis of Parkinson's Disease Using Deep Learning Approaches
A Review

Priyanka Khanna, Mridu Sahu, and Bikesh Kumar Singh
National Institute of Technology, Raipur

CONTENTS

4.1 INTRODUCTION

Parkinson's disease (PD), narrated in 1817 by physician James Parkinson, is stated as long-standing, progressive and neurodegenerative illness that influences individuals worldwide [1]. Increase in PD patients worldwide is a worrying sign. As stated in ADPA (American Parkinson's Disease Association), presently, one million Americans and around ten million individuals globally suffer from PD [2]. Around four to six million people above the age of 50 years suffer from PD [3]. There are many neurodegenerative disorders like tumors, trauma, epilepsy, Alzheimer's and dementias, and among all, the second most common disability is PD [4]. Diagnosis of PD at an advanced stage is easier, but effectual medical treatment still remains challenging. Thus, it demands the early diagnosis of PD. It is generated due to deficiency of the chemical substance dopamine (regulates control of movement), which is generated in a tiny portion of the brain substantia nigra. Symptoms of PD can be categorized as motor and nonmotor symptoms. Motor symptoms are also known as "classic Parkinson's triad", and its disorders are akinesia/bradykinesia, muscles rigidity and resting tremor. Nonmotor symptoms are initially asymptomatic and can remain underestimated for a long time. Nonmotor symptoms include anxiety, apathy, sleep disorder, depression, cognitive deficit, visual and olfactory disturbance, weight loss and digestive disorder [5,6]. As stated by Movement Disorder Society – Unified Parkinson's Disease Rating Scale (MDS-UPDRS), level and characteristics of motor impairments are evaluated [7]. Noninvasive methods and clinical tests are required for early diagnosis of PD. Recently, several deep learning approaches are used for accessing motor symptoms of patients for timely diagnosis of PD and its treatment, and different modes of input like speech, handwriting, gait and EEG signals have been used.

In many cases, people suffering from PD remain undiagnosed. One of the usual signs found in PD is voice impairments; the two main vocal impairments due to PD are dysphonia in which a person is not able to generate normal vocal sounds and dysarthria when a person is hardly able to pronounce words. Speech processing is one of the methods in clinical settings to detect PD and is preferred as it is noninvasive. As the severity of PD increases, patients' voice shutters. Phonation, articulation, prosody and intelligibility are few dimensions of speech impairment among PD patients [8]. Deep learning and ubiquitous computing are the emerging technologies in computing and information system, and at the intersection of both lies the speech-based health analysis [9].

PD can be diagnosed by one more noninvasive method, that is the movement of handwriting dynamics. Trembling, little pressure and reduced continuity enlist some of the characteristics shown in handwriting of PD patients [10]. Peak acceleration and stroke size, i.e., micrographia, deficiency in learning new movements specially in handwriting, is exhibited by PD patients [11].

According to researchers, micrographia exhibits in 63% of PD patients [12]. Different parameters like visual attributes of handwriting, kinematics and pressure features and many different approaches are considered for PD detection through handwriting dynamics. The most common and distressing symptom of PD is gait which causes difficulty in body movements [13,14]. There are different stages of gait and level of severity according to UPDRS scores [15]. Gait transition appears with patient walking movements. Transitions are segmented because of the existence of the elementary frequency of the signal [16,17].

Electroencephalogram (EEG) signals are also considered for detection of PD as it is associated with brain disorder. Other brain disorders like Alzheimer's, epilepsy, schizophrenia and autism can also be diagnosed using the EEG signals [18,19]. Due to the presence of nonlinear properties of EEG signals, it can differentiate between PD patients and healthy controls [20–67].

Deep learning (DL) is defined as a subgroup of machine learning, constructively combining feature extraction and classification process [21]. DL contains multiple stacks of neurons, helping to deal with unstructured data like speech and audio signals. In this chapter, review has been conducted to compare the increasing impact of deep learning techniques for PD diagnosis.

4.2 OBJECTIVE OF THE REVIEW

The objective of writing this chapter is as follows:

a. To throw light on automatic and timely diagnosis of Parkinson's diseases using deep learning.
b. To present an outlook and comparison in data acquisition, preprocessing, feature selection and classifiers.
c. To compare the accuracy of classifiers based on deep learning approaches on different types of data corpus like speech, handwriting, gait and EEG signals.

4.3 LITERATURE REVIEW

To predict patients with PD, lot of research work has been done, and various machine learning techniques, neural networks and hybrid systems have been used. Speech data corpus "Parkinson telemonitoring voice dataset" was created by M.A Little et al., collected in collaboration with around ten medical centres in the US and Intel corporation. For recording speech signal, he introduced a telemonitoring device. Research work carried on this data corpus is discussed here; Nilashi et al. [22] proposed a system combination of support vector regression and adaptive neuro fuzzy inference system speculating the PD. Tsanas et al. [23] made use of signal processing algorithms to extract voice features from 6000 samples; among these, useful features were selected and mapped to UPDRS using classification and regression. In a survey paper by Das et al. [24], four classification methods regression, decision tree, neural networks and DMNeural were applied for analysis. Among all classifiers, the best result was obtained with neural networks. Polat [25] proposed a model to diagnose the PD patients using k-nearest neighbor (KNN) and fuzzy c-mean clustering. Hariharan et al. [26] proposed an intelligent system using Gaussian mixture model-based feature weighting for feature preprocessing: PCA, LDA, SFS and SBS for feature selection and LS-SVM, PNN and GRNN methods for classification, eventually diagnosing PD. Sarkar et al. collected a speech corpus "Parkinson speech dataset with multiple types of sound recording" in collaboration with Cerrahpasa Faculty of Medicine, Istanbul University, Neurology Department. Shugaiv et al. [27] used KNN and SVM classifiers using LOSO (leave one subject out) and S-LOO (summarized leave one out). Most of the studies use SVM for classification measured in terms of ROC curves, true positive and false positive. Sakar and Kursun [28] implied that a feature selection based on mutual information and selected features is fed to SVM applied along with LOSO as a cross-validation scheme to avoid bias.

Most of the PD patients also face difficulty in handwriting, that is, patients are not able to sign legibly. Most of the work of handwriting focuses on kinematics and pressure, but they require temporal information and for acquiring it which equipment like digitized tablets and electronic pens can be used. Drotar et al. [29] evaluated various online features like kinematics measurements. The Mann-Whitney *U* test filter and relief algorithm are applied for feature selection and support vector machine (SVM) for classification. Drotar et al. [30] include conventional kinematics, spatio-temporal handwriting, novel handwriting measures based on entropy, signal energy and empirical mode. Support vector machine classifier with radial Gaussian kernel was used for feature selection. Drotar et al. [31] introduced pressure features which put pressure on the writing surface other than conventional kinematics features. Ensemble Adaboost classifier, SVM and K-NN are used for features extraction and to discriminate healthy control from PD patients. In literature survey, discussions related to handwriting task different ways are used to select features. Graca et al. [32] introduced an android application that combines gait and handwriting data.

Apart from vocal impairment and handwriting issues, PD patients also suffer from muscular movement disorder, and various wearable sensors are used to detect such disorders. Pastorino et al. [33] used wireless and wearable accelerometers for detection of bradykinesia, and classification is done using SVM. Arash Salarian et al. [34] used a sensor to predict the frequency of tremor and bradykinesia in PD patients. Sensing unit is tied to the forearms, which include a miniature gyroscope. Daphne G.M. Zwartjes et al. [35] proposed a novel ambulatory monitoring system that analyzes current motor task of the patient and severity related to bradykinesia, tremor and hypokinesia. Decision tree classifier is used as an activity classifier. Shyamal Patel et al. [36] used a support vector machine for classification to estimate the extremity of bradykinesia, quiver and dyskinesia recorded using an accelerometer. Recent research has also promoted multimodal assessment of PD; information is considered from speech, handwriting and gait. Juan Camilo Vasquez Correa [16] proposed multimodal assessment from speech signal, handwriting images and gait signal. Convolutional neural network is used for classification of PD patients and healthy control. Evaluation metrics used for assessment are accuracy, sensitivity, specificity, precision and F-score [11,37].

4.4 DEEP LEARNING FRAMEWORK

Deep learning (DL) is a category of machine learning that lies in the intersection of neural networks, optimization, artificial intelligence, signal processing, etc. DL has emerged strongly in every field of research [38]. It has gained popularity as it can incorporate massive amounts of training data and improves system accuracy and robustness in many health-related domains. DL is also referred to as deep architecture and ranks features in a way that high-level features are described in respect of lower-level features [38,39]. DL combines feature extraction and classification processes effectively. This section introduces deep learning as a breakthrough in the detection of neurodegenerative disease in the latest avant-grade technique.

Deep belief networks (DBN) and stacked Encoder made an evolution in DL. DBN comes under deep generative models, composed of stack of restricted Boltzmann machines (RBMs). DBN is a greedy learning approach, which improves complexity straight to the dimensions and depth of the networks [40]. Some of the revolutions in DL like dropout, a regularization technique to alleviate overfitting, has also promoted researchers toward DL. In limited amounts of training data like speech domain, use

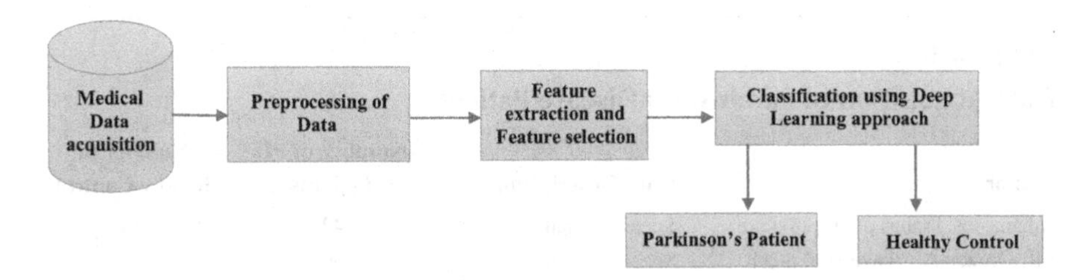

FIGURE 4.1 Deep learning framework.

of rectified linear units (ReLu) plays an important role. Other breakthroughs in the field of deep learning are end-to-end learning paradigms like convolution neural network (CNN) and recurrent neural network (RNN). CNN learns robust features directly from raw waveform, and RNN supports the temporal dynamics related with time series data (e.g. speech) [9]. Effective result can be obtained from CNN on large training datasets. Figure 4.1 shows the steps involved in medical image processing using deep learning approaches. The prognosis of Parkinson's disease through DL method is comprised of the following steps:

a. Data acquisition (speech data, handwriting data, gait and EEG signals).
b. Preprocessing of data (removal or reduction of artifacts).
c. Feature selection (reducing or removing of unwanted features).
d. Classification (validating the performance by using DL classifiers).

4.4.1 Data Acquisition

Data acquisition is an important and primary step for diagnosis. In this chapter review, data acquisition is in the form of speech signal, handwriting images, gait signal and EEG signals. Different types of smart devices and wearable technologies are available for data acquisition. For early diagnosis of different health conditions, smart technologies based on DL play a key role. For recording of speech (raw signals), various types of microphones are available and used for research purposes like Intel AHTD telemonitoring system [23], dynamic omnidirectional microphone shure, SM63L [41], Trust microphone MC-1500 [27], and Electromagnetic Articulograph [43]. For acquisition of handwriting data devices tablets are used like tablet Wacom cintiq 13-HD [16], Wacom cintiq 12wx graphics tablet [44] and Biometric pen [45]. Gait movements can be captured by eGait system [16], wearable sensors [46] and wrist-based sensors SNUMAP [47]. EEG signals can be captured by Emotiv EPOC neuroheadset [48] and 20 AG-AGCI electrodes set [68]. Table 4.1 describes the multimodal data acquisition for detection of Parkinson's disease.

In Parkinson telemonitoring voice dataset [23], a large database of 200 recordings from 42 PD patients is recorded using the Intel AHTD (telemonitoring system). AHTD is used to ease motor impairment symptoms, by enabling internet measurement of PD. Data are collected at the patient's home, using AHTD device, patient voice is recorded, and universal serial bus is used to store data. Corpus includes audio recording of sustained phonation's and running speech tests of each patient. New Spanish

TABLE 4.1
Data Acquisition of Parkinson's Disease Patients

Author	Data Description	Number of PD Patients	Number of Healthy Controls
Athanasios Tsanas et al. [23]	Speech signal	42	NR
J.R. Orozco Arroyave et al. [41]	Speech signal	50	50
Shugaiv et al. [27]	Speech signal	20	20
Soengjun Hahm and Jun Wang [43]	Speech signal	02	NR
Caliskan et al. [49]	Speech signal	23	8
Amina Naseer et al. [11]	Handwriting image	37	38
Pereira et al. [45]	Handwriting image	14	21
Pedram Khatamino et al. [44]	Handwriting image	57	15
Han Byul Kim et al. [47]	Gait signal	92	95
Marc Bachlin et al. [50]	Gait signal	8	2
Chun xiao Han et al. [68]	EEG signal	15	15
Shu Lih Oh et al. [48]	EEG signal	20	20
Rajamanickam Yuvaraj et al. [51]	EEG signal	20	20

speech corpus database [41] comprises a speech recording of 100 patients (50 PD and 50 healthy controls). This corpus is of Spanish native speakers which includes sustained phonations of the vowels, reading text, monologue, etc. Dynamic omnidirectional microphone (shure, SM 63L) is used for audio recording. Parkinson's speech dataset with multiple types of sound recording corpus used in [27] comprises 20 PD patients (6 male, 14 female) and 20 healthy controls (10 female, 10 male). PD patients were tested and asked to utter sustained vowels 'a' and 'o' (three times). Recording is done by a Trust MC-1500 microphone, having frequency range between 50 and 13 KHz. TIMIT corpus [43] comprises simultaneous recording of speech articulatory data of 1 male and 1 female British English speaker. Articulatory data were collected using an Electromagnetic Articulograph. In [49], "Oxford Parkinson's disease dataset" is composed of speech recording (23 PD patients and 8 healthy controls), along with 23 attributes and 195 instances. Another corpus included in this paper is of "Parkinson's speech dataset with multiple types of sound recordings"; it contains 20 PD patients and 20 healthy controls and includes specimen for training and testing dataset.

PaHaw (Parkinson's diseases handwriting) corpus [11] is collected using digitized tablets in which handwriting specimen of 37 PD patients and 38 healthy controls are recorded. Each participant performed eight handwriting tasks. Coordinates of the pen trajectory and status are used by digitized tablet. The handwritten dataset [44] contains time-series information of handwriting spiral tests of 57 PD patients and 15 healthy controls. Stability Test, Static Spiral Test (SST) and Dynamic Spiral Test (DST) are performed to evaluate motor activities of each individual. Dataset is captured using Wacom cintiq 12WX graphics tablet. Handwriting test [45] is performed with biometric pen (sensors are located at four points) on 14 PD patients and 21 healthy controls. No drawing test is performed; only the signals produced are captured through movements.

In corpus [47], a wrist sensor is used to record tremor signal using device SNUMAP which is equipped with an accelerometer and gyroscope. The test is performed among 92 PD patients and 95 healthy controls. In corpus [50], a wearable assistant is used to measure patient's movement having a symptom of freezing of gait (FOG). Totally, ten patients were tested and performed different walking postures. Eight patients were diagnosed with freezing of gait, during analysis in the laboratory, 237 FOG events were identified by a professional physiotherapist.

Diagnosis of neurodegenerative diseases is usually examined with electroencephalogram (EEG) signals. In [68], EEG signals are captured with 20 Ag-Agci electrodes set, by following international 10–20 systems on a Bio-logic Ceegraph-vision system. Corpus comprises 15 PD patients and 15 healthy controls. In [48], EEG signals of 20 PD patients and 20 healthy controls are recorded for diagnosis of PD. Recording was taken for 5 minutes in resting state using EMOTIV EPOC neuroheadset of 14 channels. In [51], EEG signals of 20 PD patients and 20 healthy controls were recorded in a resting state, and initially the participants were instructed to avoid body movements. Signals were recorded for 5 minutes using 14-channel EMOTIV EPOC neuroheadset.

4.4.2 Preprocessing

During acquisition of signals, some glitches affect the analysis of signals, and these glitches are known as artifacts. Preprocessing is a process of elimination or reduction of artifacts. It is a key step, and different preprocessing methods that can be applied on raw data are binarization, normalization, data augmentation, transformation, sampling, noise removal, etc. Binarization is a type of preprocessing technique; it is a process of conversion of numerical feature vector into a Boolean vector. With respect to digital image processing, gray scale image is converted into binary image in binarization. Normalization can be defined as scaling of range before further processing of data. There are many normalization techniques like Z-score, decimal scaling, Min-Max, etc. DL algorithms work on raw data so noisy patterns need to be corrected as preprocessing step. Data in healthcare are very confidential, sensitive and hard to collect, so size of dataset is usually small. To incorporate small size data in DL, preprocessing steps like data augmentation are used.

Srishti Grover et al. [52] performed min-max normalization column-wise on Parkinson UCI telemonitoring dataset; it has been normalized in the range from 0 to 1. Ali H. AL-Fatwani et al.'s [53] corpus has 195 samples recorded from 31 people (23 PD patients and 8 healthy controls) that have real values that are normalized to zero mean and unit variance. Pereira et al. [45] used biometric pen with four sensors for recording handwriting data; signals generated are transformed into images. Each image is resized to a squared matrix, rescaled and normalized to gray scale and time series images as a preprocessing step. PaHaw handwriting dataset [11] contains unwanted information and can affect the diagnosis. As a preprocessing step, noise is removed by applying a median filter, and the result is converted into gray scale. Large numbers of instances are required for training the networks in deep neural network and if dataset size is not enough, the data augmentation technique is used. Different types of data augmentation techniques which can increase the size of the dataset are rotations, flipping and contours. Unsharp masking is also performed to sharp the original image. Amina Naseer et al. [11] have taken handwriting dataset MNIST, and preprocessing methods like changing size of image, digit image channelization are used. Images of MNIST dataset are converted from 2D to 3D to make it fit for AlexNet architecture. Han Byul Kim et al. [47] used wrist-based sensor; acceleration and gyroscope data are used for analysis. The data are recorded by EEG signals [68] according to the international 10–20 system contain artifacts. Using a cut-off frequency of 0.5–55 Hz, filtering is done to take out artifacts caused due to noise. Table 4.2 describes the preprocessing techniques for detection of PD.

4.4.3 Feature Selection

After preprocessing, signals can be further processed for particular application. Feature selection is reducing the redundant features to improve the classification accuracy. In [52], after preprocessing using min-max normalization voice features are selected, 16 biomedical voice measures are selected as features for classification. Caliskan et al. [49] used automated features on speech dataset. In [43], features like Jitter, Shimmer, log HNR, Rfilt, Rasta, MFCC, Harmonicity and spectral Rolloff are not disabled. 2400 articulatory features are selected to test Parkinson's condition estimation. Zhang [54] used time frequency features on voice data to select features. Pereira et al. [45] used pen-based features, and signals generated by this pen are recorded for differentiating PD patients and healthy controls. Soltanzadeh and Rahmati [37] used visual features on handwriting image. In this study, effectiveness of visual attribute is assessed between graph motor impressions to distinguish between PD patients and healthy controls. Various representations are used to train the network to improve feature learning and later features are combined. Table 4.3 describes the feature selection techniques applied in the literature for diagnosis of PD using DL.

TABLE 4.2
Preprocessing Techniques for Detection of PD

Author	Data Description	Preprocessing Method
Srishti Grover et al. [52]	Speech signal (Parkinson telemonitoring voice dataset)	Min-Max normalization
Ali H. Al-Fatlawi et al. [53]	Speech signal (Parkinson telemonitoring voice dataset)	Normalization (zero mean and unit variance)
Amina Naseer et al. [11]	Handwriting image (PaHaw dataset)	Median filter, data augmentation, unsharp masking.
Amina Naseer et al. [11]	Handwriting image (MNIST dataset)	Resizing, channelization
Pereira et al. [45]	Handwriting image	Resizing, rescaling, normalization (conversion to gray scale image, time series image)
Han Byul Kim et al. [47]	Gait signal	Filtering (high pass filter)
Chun xiao Han et al. [68]	EEG signal	Filtering Elbert method

TABLE 4.3
Feature Selection Techniques for Detection of PD

Author	Data Description	Features
Zhang [54]	Speech signal	Time frequency features
Caliskan et al. [49]	Speech signal	Automated features
Srishti Grover et al. [52]	Speech signal	Voice features
Soengjun Hahm and Jun Wang [43]	Speech signal	Quasi articulatory features
Pereira et al. [45]	Handwriting image	Pen-based features
Pereira et al. [56]	Handwriting image	Pen-based features
Pereira et al. [57]	Handwriting image	Automated features
Soltanzadeh and Rahmati [37]	Handwriting image	Automated visual features
Amina Naseer et al. [11]	Handwriting image	Automated visual features
Bjoern M. Eskofier et al. [46]	Gait signal	Automated features
Shu Lih Oh et al. [48]	EEG signal	Automated features

4.4.4 Classification

After feature selection, the next phase is the classification. It comes under the category of supervised learning, a problem of identifying the category to which new considerations will belong. Different methods used for classification are convolutional neural network (CNN), recurrent neural network (RNN), deep neural network (DNN) and deep belief network (DBN).

4.4.4.1 Convolution Neural Network (CNN)

Convolutional neural network (CNN) concerning the primary cortex of cats comes under the class of DL neural network. It is formed on Hubel and Wiesel's architecture. CNN uses 2D convolutional layer and learns features from input data, basically used in images. It comprises input layer, output layer and multiple hidden layers with each layer increasing the complexity of the features. The hidden layer contains convolutional layers, ReLu layers, pooling layers and fully connected layers. In convolution layer, features apply a convolution operation to the input layer and passes information to the succeeding layer. The cluster of neurons is combined into a single neuron in pooling layer, and every neuron in one layer connects to the other in the succeeding layer in fully connected layers. Different types of CNN architecture are available, and among all, AlexNet has got success in various classification tasks in health domains. Figure 4.2 demonstrates the architecture of convolutional neural network.

CNN Algorithm

Step 1: CNN starts with an input image.
Step 2: Applying different filters on input image resulting in feature map.

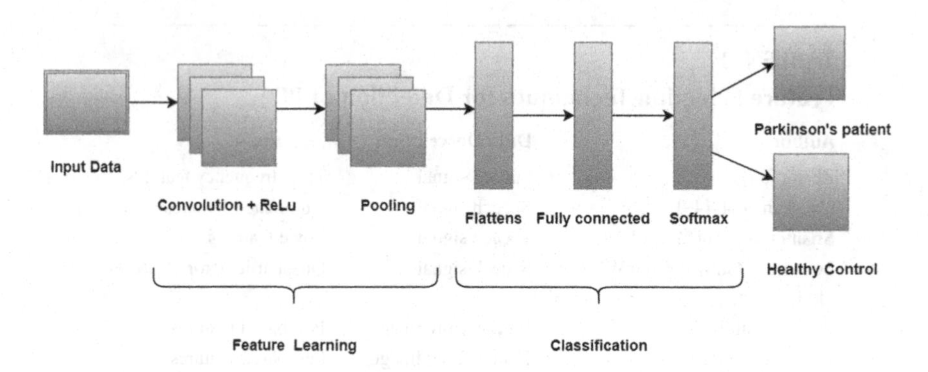

FIGURE 4.2 Convolutional neural network architecture.

Step 3: Applying ReLu activation function results in increase of nonlinearity.
Step 4: Feature map is used with pooling layer.
Step 5: Conversion of pooled images into one long vector.
Step 6: Input the vector into fully connected artificial neural network.
Step 7: Training forward propagation and back propagation for multiple epochs till neural network is trained and feature detector is acquired.

Pereira et al. [45] extracted pen-based features and applied convolutional neural network, which in this information is processed through a set of layers, learning an unlike and quality representation. In this work, smart pen is used for recording handwriting data, and signals generated by pen are converted into images. Meander and spiral images are further transformed into time series images. Classification of meander and spiral images are done using CNN, and both the dataset of meander and spiral are composed of 308 images; among them, 224 are PD patients, and 84 are healthy controls. Two image resolutions of 64×64 and 128×128 are considered. Different CNN architectures like ImageNet, CIFAR-10 and LeNet are used and compared with the baseline approach of the OPF classifier. Average accuracy of spiral dataset with 75% training and 25% testing data is 80.19% (ImageNet architecture), and accuracy of Meander dataset with 75% training and 25% testing data is 85% (ImageNet architecture). Soltanzadeh and Rahmati [37] used pretrained CNN for classification; it is used in cases where training data are limited known as transfer learning. In transfer learning, fully connected layers are removed. For enhancement of classification, two-light fusion technique is used. CNN is limited to linear data, so initial data are given to CNN, and the result is given through nonlinear transforms. Support vector machine (SVM) is fed combined with the feature vector of each task. According to the number of tasks, weight is adjusted, for diagnosis of Parkinson's patients and healthy controls.

Amina Naseer et al. [11] applied 25-layered deep convolutional neural networks on PaHaw handwriting corpus along with SVM classifier. Once the AlexNet is trained for classification, healthy controls and PD images are distinguished. Using AlexNet fine-tune-image net approach, transfer learning on spiral pattern accuracy recorded is 98.28%. It is observed that spiral images are more informative than letters, words or sentences for detection of PD. Pedram Khatamino et al. [44] applied CNN on handwriting dataset. Data are fed to CNN in the form of a square matrix and evaluated using 128×128 pixels image resolution. Proposed CNN architecture is composed of two convolutional, two max pooling, two fully connected layers and two binary classification are considered for PD patients and healthy controls. Dropout of 50% is used between two FC layers, and the model is tested using K-Fold cross validation and leave one out cross validation. Obtained accuracy is 88% for the proposed model.

Bjoern M. Eskofier et al. [46] used CNN on gait data, composed of an input layer, two convolutional neural network layers, ReLu as an activation function, max pooling, two fully connected layers and a soft max output layer [58]. Max pooling layers learn features in the convolution layer toward variation of the location and time scan in the input signal [59]. Fully connected layers contain 64 ReLus with bias to extract features that fit for classification. Dropout is applied to avoid overfitting. Softmax layer (output layer) contains neurons equivalent to the number of classes. Accuracy obtained on applying DNN on gait data is 90.9%. Han Byul Kim et al. [47] used CNN on a wrist module for data analysis, composed of three convolution layers, and ReLu as an activation function, after each convolution dropout is used to avoid overfitting. The optimal structure using a grid search is obtained, where the number of kernels and layers is varied.

4.4.4.2 Deep Belief Network (DBN)

Deep belief network is a type of deep neural network, containing multiple processing layers modelling high-level abstraction in data with complex network [60]. DBN is a class of generative graphical model with multiple hidden units composed of unsupervised networks like restricted Boltzmann machines (RBMs) or autoencoders. It is composed of a visible layer, hidden layer and an output layer. DBN key characteristics are its greedy learning approach that optimizes DBM weight with respect to time complexity, linear to the dimension and depth of the network [40].

Ali H. Al-Fatlawi et al. [53] used deep belief network (DBN) for classification on Parkinson telemonitoring voice dataset. Network considered in this work is a stack of two restricted Boltzmann machines; it consists of a visible layer to receive the input. It considered 16 features hence giving 16 neurons as an input and one unit as an output (two probabilities in output PD patient or healthy control). Between input and output layers are two hidden layers which play a key role in processing data providing high accuracy with no overfitting. Accuracy obtained using the DBN model is 94%. Figure 4.3 demonstrates the architecture of deep belief network.

4.4.4.3 Deep Neural Network (DNN)

Deep neural network (DNN) is a deep architecture model with multiple hidden layers which incorporate a huge number of neurons. Hidden layers can apprehend nonlinear relationship; thus, adding more hidden layers can deal with complex problems. In DNN, core unit is the artificial neuron unit, and weights are fully connected and are initialized using supervised or unsupervised techniques. DNN comprises two main parts: stacked autoencoder and SoftMax classifier. Assimilating hidden layers with immense neurons in a DNN improves the modelling capabilities resulting in closely optimal configurations [61].

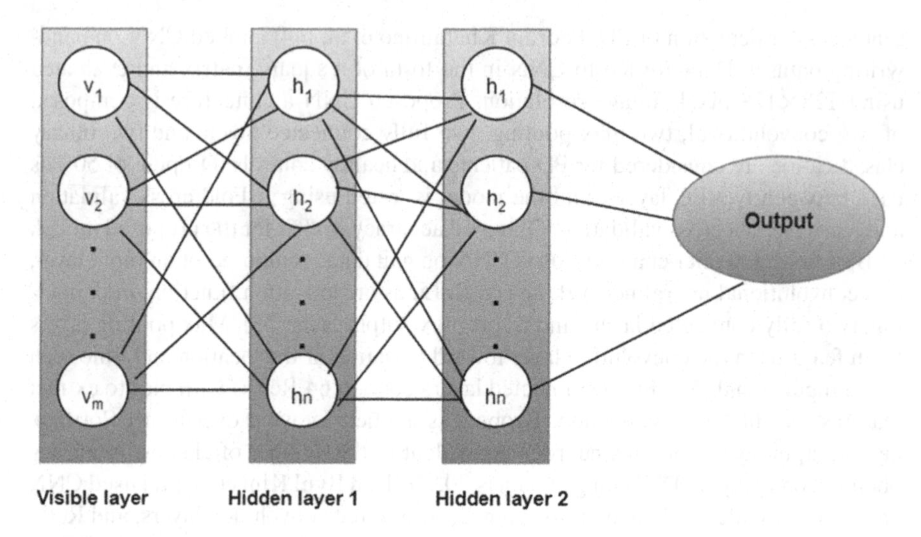

FIGURE 4.3 Deep belief network architecture.

Srishti Grover et al. [52] applied DNN on Parkinson telemonitoring voice dataset. DNN comprises input, hidden and output layer and according to the number of features, the number of neurons is given to the input layer, whereas the output neuron gives binary classification, severe and nonsevere. Accuracy obtained for total UPDRS score is 94.42% for training data and for motor UPDRS score is 83.367%. Caliskan et al. [49] used DNN on "Oxford Parkinson's disease dataset" and "Parkinson's speech dataset with multiple types of sound recording". DNN classifier combines SAE network and softmax classifier, and it is used to perform classification of the PD patients. It comprises a visible layer, hidden layer and output layer. Limited-memory BFGS is used as an optimization algorithm for training in this proposed work. Features of speech signal are taken as input and output is binary classification that is PD patient or healthy control. First, AE is trained with a speech dataset which is sent to both input and output of AE. The output of the hidden layer of trained AE trains the second AE, and its output is given as the input of softmax classifier. To construct DNN, SAE and trained softmax layer are combined. Ten-fold cross validation is performed, and accuracy obtained of proposed DNN for OPD dataset is 93.79% and for PSD dataset is 68.05%.

Table 4.4 describes the literature survey of performance classification of DL for detection of PD. Figure 4.4 demonstrates the comparison of accuracy of deep learning classifiers based of speech data. Figure 4.5 demonstrates the comparison of accuracy of DL classifiers of handwriting data.

4.5 CHALLENGES AND OPPORTUNITIES

In spite of promising results obtained using deep architectures in clinical setting, there remain several challenges and unsolved issues. Some of the crucial issues related to DL in healthcare for diagnosis of neurodegenerative disease are discussed below:

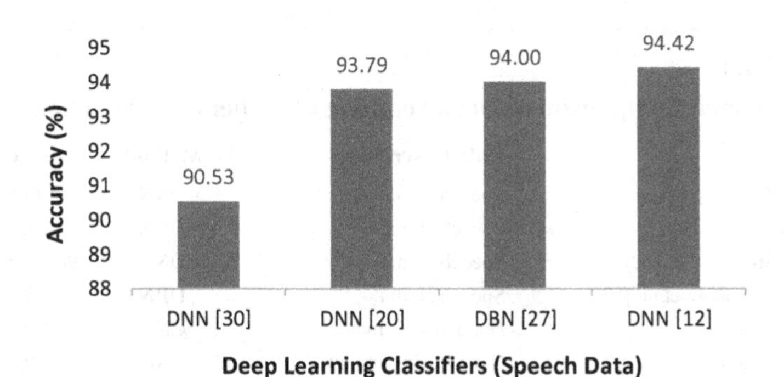

FIGURE 4.4 Comparison of accuracy using deep learning classifiers (speech signal).

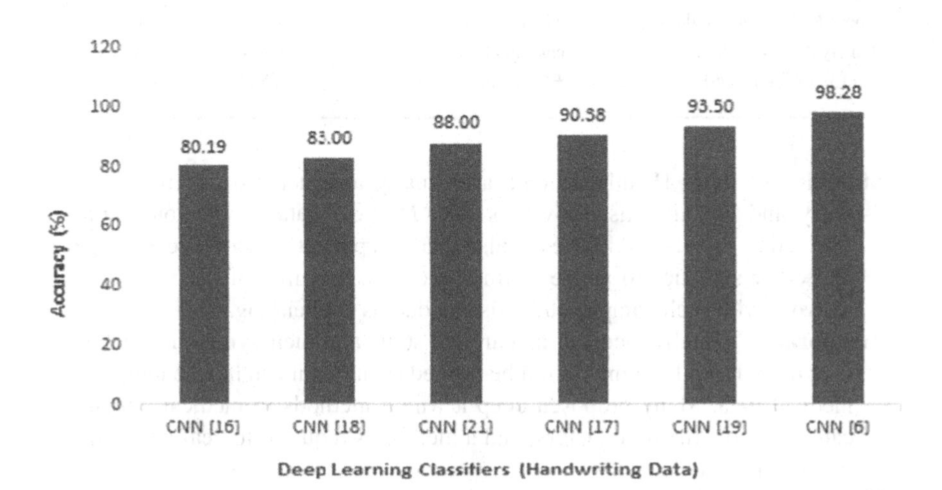

FIGURE 4.5 Comparison of accuracy using deep learning classifiers (handwriting image).

Imbalanced data: Small and imbalanced medical corpus usually leads to the problem of model overfitting. Techniques like data augmentation are used in recent literature to handle data imbalance [11]. In data augmentation, multiplicity of data can be increased without accumulating the new data. Data augmentation techniques like cropping, flipping and rotation are used to generate new data.

Acquisition and size of data: Extensive collaboration is required from hospital to acquire patient's data, for further applying of techniques for early diagnosis of disease and improving health care. Gathering of medical data is at times very challenging. Deep learning is a data hungry approach; it requires large datasets. Understanding medical data, its variability and lots of patient's data to train robust deep learning model is difficult. The database collected so far for neurodegenerative disease are usually small, which limits the effectiveness of classification algorithms.

TABLE 4.4
Performance Comparison of Deep Learning Classifiers for Detection of PD

Author	Data Description	Method	Accuracy (%)
Zhang [54]	Speech signal	DNN	90.53
Caliskan et al. [49]	Speech signal	DNN	93.79, 68.05
Srishti Grover et al. [52]	Speech signal	DNN	94.42, 83.36
Ali H. Al-Fatlawi et al. [53]	Speech signal	DBN	94
Pereira et al. [45]	Handwriting image	CNN	80.19
Pereira et al. [56]	Handwriting image	CNN	90.38
Pereira et al. [57]	Handwriting image	CNN	93.50
Soltanzadeh and Rahmati [37]	Handwriting image	CNN	83
Pedram Khatamino et al. [44]	Handwriting data	CNN	88
Amina Naseer et al. [11]	Handwriting data	CNN	98.28
Bjoern M. Eskofier et al. [46]	Gait signal	CNN	90.9
Han Byul Kim et al. [47]	Gait signal	CNN	85
Shu Lih Oh et al. [48]	EEG signal	CNN	88.25

Standard of data: Healthcare data are usually unstructured, heterogenous, noisy and contain missing values [62]. Medical data are not only constrained to signals and images; it also includes patient's history, gender, age and other statistics to arrive at finer decision. Training of deep learning network with such complex and missing data is challenging.

Temporality: Usually medical data are not static and their symptoms change over time. Deep learning should be trained such that it can handle temporal medical data. Many proposed deep learning methods in medical domain cannot handle the time factors, and a method is required to deal with temporal healthcare data.

Heterogeneous data: In medical imaging, classification is usually a binary task like normal versus healthy control, benign versus malignant. There may be case when both cases are heterogenous; this can lead to exclusion of most common normal subclasses. For this, deep learning system can be converted into multiclass system by providing details of all possible subclasses.

Technology constraint: In some cases, input of full image is required in deep learning to avoid patch classification. But at times, it is restricted due to memory constraint. It can be solved by advancement in GPU technology.

Blackbox: Deep learning methods are considered as 'black boxes' especially in medical data where wrong prediction can cause serious consequences. Several research studies have been done to predict wrong prognosis. Models used in deep learning are continuous; working process and why it provides better result are still not clear [63].

The challenges mentioned above promote future research opportunities to improve health care. The following points discussed below provide some potential research avenues based on deep learning.

Well-designed and feature enriched corpus: A well-designed and large corpus can be created for detection of PD which allows the fair assessment of different approaches. Corpus collected can be multimodal like acquisition of speech, handwriting, gait and others. While designing a database for ND, certain points should be considered like cardinality of the set and an acceptable dimension. Due to the limitation on the number of patients, the number of features extracted from each patient should be increased. The effective integration of multimodal data acquisition and processing data source separately with the appropriate deep learning approach can lead to a novel method.

Data augmentation: Data augmentation technique is used in deep learning [11] to handle small size data corpus (speech data). Unsupervised architecture like generative adversarial networks (GANS) can be used to increase multiplicity of data [64]. GANS consists of generative model which participate against a discriminative model. Continuous medical timeseries can be generated by using GANS in the healthcare domain [65].

Transfer learning: Different wearable sensors have been used in literature to capture gait movements. For enhancing the prediction accuracy of PD patients, deep learning models like long short-term memory (LSTMs) and recurrent neural networks (RNNs) can be used. RNNs can also be tested on speech health domain. Initially, RNNs were used for one-dimensional data, eventually applied to images also. 'Pixel RNNs' are used as autoregressive models in images [66]. DL works effectively with large datasets; due to unavailability of large medical dataset, techniques like transfer learning can be used.

4.6 CONCLUSION

This chapter provided an analysis of effect of deep learning in health domain and its overcomings on machine learning techniques in terms of accuracy in multimodal data (speech, handwriting, gait and EEG signals) for detection of PD. Analysis done in this chapter would help researchers to find novel topics and research gaps that have not been covered yet. Multimodal data can be used in diagnosis of neurodegenerative disease. It has been observed that not much work is done in speech domain using recurrent neural networks; exploration can be conducted using deep RNN model, mainly long short-time memory (LSTM). Feature extraction method like linear predictive coding (LPC) can be put to use to extract features from speech signals. It can be contemplated that the continuing progress and evolution in the ever-present computing devices has the capacity in providing large amounts of data, which in turn will lend support to the scholars and scientists working in the field of speech-health domain [42–55]. In our comparative study on speech corpus [52], DL neural network outperformed with accuracy of total UPDRS score of 94.42% for training data and for motor UPDRS score accuracy is 83.367. CNN applied on handwriting data [11], used Alexa-net architecture along with transfer learning and recorded accuracy of 98.28% on spiral pattern. Additional DL models like Google-net, res-net and VGG can be used as the future work on handwriting corpus. During analysis of gait data, different types of wearable sensors were used; DL proved as a potential approach in analysis of wearable sensor data. CNN classifier applied in [46] has achieved an accuracy of 90.9% on gait data using sensors. Innovation of wearable sensors has enabled monitoring of patients at home leading to easier data acquisition. It has been observed that CNN is widely used in ND disease and outperformed in many medical analysis challenges. Along with the exact CNN architecture, other aspects like preprocessing, augmentation techniques and expert knowledge is also important to get promising results.

REFERENCES

1. Parkinson, James. "An essay on the shaking palsy." *The Journal of neuropsychiatry and clinical neurosciences* 14, no. 2 (2002): 223–236.
2. Lücking, Christoph B., Alexandra Dürr, Vincenzo Bonifati, Jenny Vaughan, Giuseppe De Michele, Thomas Gasser, Biswadjiet S. Harhangi et al. "Association between early-onset Parkinson's disease and mutations in the parkin gene." *New England Journal of Medicine* 342, no. 21 (2000): 1560–1567.
3. Agarwal, Akshata S., and Kishori S. Degaonkar. "Detection of brain diseases using EEG and speech signal." *International Journal of Computer Applications* 149, no. 9 (2016): 1–5.
4. Sinha, G. R., and Jasjit S. Suri. "Introduction to cognitive science, informatics, and modeling." In: *Cognitive Informatics, Computer Modelling, and Cognitive Science*, pp. 1–12. Academic Press, Cambridge, MA, 2020.
5. Chaudhuri, K. Ray, Daniel G. Healy, and Anthony H.V. Schapira. "Non-motor symptoms of Parkinson's disease: diagnosis and management." *The Lancet Neurology* 5, no. 3 (2006): 235–245.
6. Weintraub, Daniel, Cynthia L. Comella, and Stacy Horn. "Parkinson's disease–Part 2: Treatment of motor symptoms." *The American Journal of Managed Care* 14, no. 2 Suppl (2008): S49–58.
7. Goetz, Christopher G., Barbara C. Tilley, Stephanie R. Shaftman, Glenn T. Stebbins, Stanley Fahn, Pablo Martinez-Martin, Werner Poewe et al. "Movement disorder society-sponsored revision of the Unified Parkinson's Disease Rating Scale (MDS-UPDRS): Scale presentation and clinimetric testing results." *Movement Disorders: Official Journal of the Movement Disorder Society* 23, no. 15 (2008): 2129–2170.
8. Hlavnička, Jan, Roman Čmejla, Tereza Tykalová, Karel Šonka, Evžen Růžička, and Jan Rusz. "Automated analysis of connected speech reveals early biomarkers of Parkinson's disease in patients with rapid eye movement sleep behaviour disorder." *Scientific Reports* 7, no. 1 (2017): 1–13.
9. Cummins, Nicholas, Alice Baird, and Bjoern W. Schuller. "Speech analysis for health: Current state-of-the-art and the increasing impact of deep learning." *Methods* 151(2018): 41–54.
10. De Stefano, Claudio, Francesco Fontanella, Donato Impedovo, Giuseppe Pirlo, and Alessandra Scotto di Freca. "Handwriting analysis to support neurodegenerative diseases diagnosis: A review." *Pattern Recognition Letters* 121(2019): 37–45.
11. Naseer, Amina, Monail Rani, Saeeda Naz, Muhammad Imran Razzak, Muhammad Imran, and Guandong Xu. "Refining Parkinson's neurological disorder identification through deep transfer learning." *Neural Computing and Applications* 32, no. 3 (2020): 839–854.
12. Letanneux, Alban, Jeremy Danna, Jean-Luc Velay, François Viallet, and Serge Pinto. "From micrographia to Parkinson's disease dysgraphia." *Movement Disorders* 29, no. 12 (2014): 1467–1475.

13. Bloem, Bastiaan R., Jeffrey M. Hausdorff, Jasper E. Visser, and Nir Giladi. "Falls and freezing of gait in Parkinson's disease: A review of two interconnected, episodic phenomena." *Movement Disorders: Official Journal of the Movement Disorder Society* 19, no. 8 (2004): 871–884.
14. Hannink, Julius, Thomas Kautz, Cristian F. Pasluosta, Karl-Günter Gaßmann, Jochen Klucken, and Bjoern M. Eskofier. "Sensor-based gait parameter extraction with deep convolutional neural networks." *IEEE Journal of Biomedical and Health Informatics* 21, no. 1 (2016): 85–93.
15. Camps, Julia, Albert Sama, Mario Martin, Daniel Rodriguez-Martin, Carlos Perez-Lopez, Joan M. Moreno Arostegui, Joan Cabestany et al. "Deep learning for freezing of gait detection in Parkinson's disease patients in their homes using a waist-worn inertial measurement unit." *Knowledge-Based Systems* 139(2018): 119–131.
16. Vásquez-Correa, Juan Camilo, Tomas Arias-Vergara, Juan Rafael Orozco-Arroyave, Björn Eskofier, Jochen Klucken, and Elmar Nöth. "Multimodal assessment of Parkinson's disease: a deep learning approach." *IEEE Journal of Biomedical and Health Informatics* 23, no. 4 (2018): 1618–1630.
17. Camps, Julià, Albert Samà, Mario Martín, Daniel Rodríguez-Martín, Carlos Pérez-López, Sheila Alcaine, Berta Mestre et al. "Deep learning for detecting freezing of gait episodes in Parkinson's disease based on accelerometers." In: Ignacio Rojas, Gonzalo Joya, Andreu Catala (eds.) *International Work-Conference on Artificial Neural Networks*, pp. 344–355. Springer, Cham, 2017.
18. Ullo, Silvia Liberata, Smith K. Khare, Varun Bajaj, and G. R. Sinha. "Hybrid computerized method for environmental sound classification." *IEEE Access* 8(2020): 124055–124065.
19. Mandal, Sunandan, Manvendra Thakur, Kavita Thakur, and Bikesh Kumar Singh. "Comparative investigation of different classification techniques for epilepsy detection using EEG signals." In: *Advances in Biomedical Engineering and Technology*, pp. 413–424. Springer, Singapore, 2020.
20. Mohdiwale, Samrudhi, Mridu Sahu, G. R. Sinha, and Vikrant Bhateja. "Statistical wavelets with harmony search based optimal feature selection of EEG signals for motor imagery classification." *IEEE Sensors Journal* (2020). doi:10.1109/JSEN.2020.3026172.
21. Saba, Luca, M. Agarwal, Siva Skandha Sanagala, Suneet K. Gupta, G. R. Sinha, A. M. Johri, N. N. Khanna et al. "Brain MRI-based Wilson disease tissue classification: An optimised deep transfer learning approach." *Electronics Letters* 56 (2020): 1395–1398.
22. Nilashi, Mehrbakhsh, Othman Ibrahim, and Ali Ahani. "Accuracy improvement for predicting Parkinson's disease progression." *Scientific Reports* 6, no. 1 (2016): 1–18.
23. Tsanas, Athanasios, Max A. Little, Patrick E. McSharry, and Lorraine O. Ramig. "Accurate telemonitoring of Parkinson's disease progression by noninvasive speech tests." *IEEE Transactions on Biomedical Engineering* 57, no. 4 (2009): 884–893.
24. Das, Resul. "A comparison of multiple classification methods for diagnosis of Parkinson disease." *Expert Systems with Applications* 37, no. 2 (2010): 1568–1572.
25. Polat, Kemal. "Classification of Parkinson's disease using feature weighting method on the basis of fuzzy C-means clustering." *International Journal of Systems Science* 43, no. 4 (2012): 597–609.
26. Hariharan, Muthusamy, Kemal Polat, and Ravindran Sindhu. "A new hybrid intelligent system for accurate detection of Parkinson's disease." *Computer Methods and Programs in Biomedicine* 113, no. 3 (2014): 904–913.
27. Shugaiv, Erkingul, Asli Kıyat-Atamer, Erdem Tüzün, Feza Deymeer, Piraye Oflazer, Yesim Parman, and Gulsen Akman-Demir. "Case report Coexistence of Guillain-Barré syndrome and Behçet's disease." *Clinical and Experimental Rheumatology* 31, no. 77 (2013): S88–S89.

28. Sakar, C. Okan, and Olcay Kursun. "Telediagnosis of Parkinson's disease using measurements of dysphonia." *Journal of Medical Systems* 34, no. 4 (2010): 591–599.
29. Drotár, Peter, Jiří Mekyska, Irena Rektorová, Lucia Masarová, Zdeněk Smékal, and Marcos Faundez-Zanuy. "A new modality for quantitative evaluation of Parkinson's disease: In-air movement." In *13th IEEE International Conference on Bioinformatics and Bioengineering*, pp. 1–4. IEEE, 2013. Chania, Greece.
30. Drotár, Peter, Jiří Mekyska, Irena Rektorová, Lucia Masarová, Zdeněk Smékal, and Marcos Faundez-Zanuy. "Decision support framework for Parkinson's disease based on novel handwriting markers." *IEEE Transactions on Neural Systems and Rehabilitation Engineering* 23, no. 3 (2014): 508–516.
31. Drotár, Peter, Jiří Mekyska, Irena Rektorová, Lucia Masarová, Zdeněk Smékal, and Marcos Faundez-Zanuy. "Evaluation of handwriting kinematics and pressure for differential diagnosis of Parkinson's disease." *Artificial Intelligence in Medicine* 67(2016): 39–46.
32. Graça, Ricardo, Rui Sarmento e Castro, and Joao Cevada. "Parkdetect: Early diagnosing parkinson's disease." In *2014 IEEE International Symposium on Medical Measurements and Applications (MeMeA)*, pp. 1–6. IEEE, 2014. Lisboa, Portugal.
33. Pastorino, Matteo, Jorge Cancela, María Teresa Arredondo, Mario Pansera, Laura Pastor-Sanz, Federico Villagra, María A. Pastor, and J. A. Martin. "Assessment of bradykinesia in Parkinson's disease patients through a multi-parametric system." In *2011 Annual International Conference of the IEEE Engineering in Medicine and Biology Society*, pp. 1810–1813. IEEE, 2011. Boston, MA, USA.
34. Salarian, Arash, Heike Russmann, Christian Wider, Pierre R. Burkhard, Franios J.G. Vingerhoets, and Kamiar Aminian. "Quantification of tremor and bradykinesia in Parkinson's disease using a novel ambulatory monitoring system." *IEEE Transactions on Biomedical Engineering* 54, no. 2 (2007): 313–322.
35. Zwartjes, Daphne G.M., Tjitske Heida, Jeroen P.P. Van Vugt, Jan A.G. Geelen, and Peter H. Veltink. "Ambulatory monitoring of activities and motor symptoms in Parkinson's disease." *IEEE Transactions on Biomedical Engineering* 57, no. 11 (2010): 2778–2786.
36. Patel, Shyamal, Konrad Lorincz, Richard Hughes, Nancy Huggins, John Growdon, David Standaert, Metin Akay, Jennifer Dy, Matt Welsh, and Paolo Bonato. "Monitoring motor fluctuations in patients with Parkinson's disease using wearable sensors." *IEEE Transactions on Information Technology in Biomedicine* 13, no. 6 (2009): 864–873.
37. Soltanzadeh, Hasan, and Mohammad Rahmati. "Recognition of Persian handwritten digits using image profiles of multiple orientations." *Pattern Recognition Letters* 25, no. 14 (2004): 1569–1576.
38. Nassif, Ali Bou, Ismail Shahin, Imtinan Attili, Mohammad Azzeh, and Khaled Shaalan. "Speech recognition using deep neural networks: A systematic review." *IEEE Access* 7(2019): 19143–19165.
39. Sinha, G. R. "Study of assessment of cognitive ability of human brain using deep learning." *International Journal of Information Technology* 9, no. 3 (2017): 321–326.
40. Hinton, Geoffrey, Li Deng, Dong Yu, George E. Dahl, Abdel-rahman Mohamed, Navdeep Jaitly, Andrew Senior et al. "Deep neural networks for acoustic modeling in speech recognition: The shared views of four research groups." *IEEE Signal Processing Magazine* 29, no. 6 (2012): 82–97.
41. Orozco-Arroyave, Juan Rafael, Julián David Arias-Londoño, Jesús Francisco Vargas-Bonilla, Maria Claudia Gonzalez-Rativa, and Elmar Nöth. "New Spanish speech corpus database for the analysis of people suffering from Parkinson's disease." In *LREC*, pp. 342–347. 2014.
42. Istepanian, Robert S.H., and Turki Al-Anzi. "m-Health 2.0: New perspectives on mobile health, machine learning and big data analytics." *Methods* 151(2018): 34–40.

43. Hahm, Seongjun, and Jun Wang. "Parkinson's condition estimation using speech acoustic and inversely mapped articulatory data." In *Sixteenth Annual Conference of the International Speech Communication Association*. 2015.
44. Khatamino, Pedram, İsmail Cantürk, and Lale Özyılmaz. "A deep learning-CNN based system for medical diagnosis: An application on parkinson's disease handwriting drawings." In *2018 6th International Conference on Control Engineering & Information Technology (CEIT)*, pp. 1–6. IEEE, 2018. Istanbul, Turkey.
45. Pereira, Clayton R., Silke A.T. Weber, Christian Hook, Gustavo H. Rosa, and Joao P. Papa. "Deep learning-aided Parkinson's disease diagnosis from handwritten dynamics." In *2016 29th SIBGRAPI Conference on Graphics, Patterns and Images (SIBGRAPI)*, pp. 340–346. IEEE, 2016. Sao Paulo, Brazil.
46. Eskofier, Bjoern M., Sunghoon I. Lee, Jean-Francois Daneault, Fatemeh N. Golabchi, Gabriela Ferreira-Carvalho, Gloria Vergara-Diaz, Stefano Sapienza et al. "Recent machine learning advancements in sensor-based mobility analysis: Deep learning for Parkinson's disease assessment." In *2016 38th Annual International Conference of the IEEE Engineering in Medicine and Biology Society (EMBC)*, pp. 655–658. IEEE, 2016.
47. Kim, Han Byul, Woong Woo Lee, Aryun Kim, Hong Ji Lee, Hye Young Park, Hyo Seon Jeon, Sang Kyong Kim, Beomseok Jeon, and Kwang S. Park. "Wrist sensor-based tremor severity quantification in Parkinson's disease using convolutional neural network." *Computers in Biology and Medicine* 95(2018): 140–146.
48. Oh, Shu Lih, Yuki Hagiwara, U. Raghavendra, Rajamanickam Yuvaraj, N. Arunkumar, M. Murugappan, and U. Rajendra Acharya. "A deep learning approach for Parkinson's disease diagnosis from EEG signals." *Neural Computing and Applications* 32 (2018): 1–7.
49. Caliskan, Abdullah, Hasan Badem, Alper Basturk, and Mehmet Emin Yuksel. "Diagnosis of the Parkinson disease by using deep neural network classifier." *Istanbul University-Journal of Electrical & Electronics Engineering* 17, no. 2 (2017): 3311–3318.
50. Bächlin, Marc, Meir Plotnik, Daniel Roggen, Inbal Maidan, Jeffrey M. Hausdorff, Nir Giladi, and Gerhard Troster. "Wearable assistant for Parkinson's disease patients with the freezing of gait symptom." IEEE Transactions on Information Technology in Biomedicine 2009, 14, no. 2, 436–446.
51. Yuvaraj, Rajamanickam, U. Rajendra Acharya, and Yuki Hagiwara. "A novel Parkinson's disease diagnosis index using higher-order spectra features in EEG signals." *Neural Computing and Applications* 30, no. 4 (2018): 1225–1235.
52. Grover, Srishti, Saloni Bhartia, Abhilasha Yadav, and K. R. Seeja. "Predicting severity of Parkinson's disease using deep learning." *Procedia Computer Science* 132(2018): 1788–1794.
53. Al-Fatlawi, Ali H., Mohammed H. Jabardi, and Sai Ho Ling. "Efficient diagnosis system for Parkinson's disease using deep belief network." In *2016 IEEE Congress on Evolutionary Computation (CEC)*, pp. 1324–1330. IEEE, 2016.
54. Zhang, Y. N. "Can a smartphone diagnose parkinson disease? A deep neural network method and telediagnosis system implementation." *Parkinson's Disease* 2017 (2017): 6209703.
55. Sewall, Gregory K., Jack Jiang, and Charles N. Ford. "Clinical evaluation of Parkinson's-related dysphonia." *The laryngoscope* 116, no. 10 (2006): 1740–1744.
56. Pereira, Clayton R., Danillo R. Pereira, Joao P. Papa, Gustavo H. Rosa, and Xin-She Yang. "Convolutional neural networks applied for parkinson's disease identification." In: A. Holzinger (eds.) *Machine Learning for Health Informatics*, pp. 377–390. Springer, Cham, 2016.
57. Pereira, Clayton R., Danilo R. Pereira, Gustavo H. Rosa, Victor H.C. Albuquerque, Silke A.T. Weber, Christian Hook, and João P. Papa. "Handwritten dynamics assessment through convolutional neural networks: An application to Parkinson's disease identification." *Artificial Intelligence in Medicine* 87 (2018): 67–77.

58. Dong, Chao, Chen Change Loy, Kaiming He, and Xiaoou Tang. "Image super-resolution using deep convolutional networks." *IEEE Transactions on Pattern Analysis and Machine Intelligence* 38, no. 2 (2015): 295–307.
59. Boureau, Y.-Lan, Jean Ponce, and Yann LeCun. "A theoretical analysis of feature pooling in visual recognition." In *Proceedings of the 27th International Conference on Machine Learning (ICML-10)*, pp. 111–118. 2010.
60. Deng, Li, and Dong Yu. "Deep learning: Methods and applications." *Foundations and Trends in Signal Processing* 7, no. 3–4 (2014): 197–387.
61. Collaboration, Skin Imaging. "Machine Learning and Health Care Disparities in Dermatology." (2018).
62. Miotto, Riccardo, Fei Wang, Shuang Wang, Xiaoqian Jiang, and Joel T. Dudley. "Deep learning for healthcare: Review, opportunities and challenges." *Briefings in Bioinformatics* 19, no. 6 (2018): 1236–1246.
63. Dey, Nilanjan, Amira S. Ashour, and Surekha Borra, eds. *Classification in BioApps: Automation of Decision Making*. Vol. 26. Springer, Berlin, 2017.
64. Goodfellow, Ian, Jean Pouget-Abadie, Mehdi Mirza, Bing Xu, David Warde-Farley, Sherjil Ozair, Aaron Courville, and Yoshua Bengio. "Generative adversarial nets." In: Thomas G. Dietterich, Suzanna Becker and Zoubin Ghahramani (eds.) *Advances in Neural Information Processing Systems*, pp. 2672–2680. MIT Press, Cambridge, MA, 2014.
65. Xiao, Cao, Edward Choi, and Jimeng Sun. "Opportunities and challenges in developing deep learning models using electronic health records data: A systematic review." *Journal of the American Medical Informatics Association* 25, no. 10 (2018): 1419–1428.
66. Litjens, Geert, Thijs Kooi, Babak Ehteshami Bejnordi, Arnaud Arindra Adiyoso Setio, Francesco Ciompi, Mohsen Ghafoorian, Jeroen Awm Van Der Laak, Bram Van Ginneken, and Clara I. Sánchez. "A survey on deep learning in medical image analysis." *Medical Image Analysis* 42 (2017): 60–88.
67. Mohdiwale, Samrudhi, Mridu Sahu, G. R. Sinha, and Silvia Liberata Ullo. "Cognitive and biosensors: An overview." In: G. R. Sinha (ed.) Advances in Modern Sensors Physics, Design, Simulation and Applications, pp. 9–1, 9–22. IOP Publishing Ltd., Bristol, 2020.
69. Han, Chun-Xiao, Jiang Wang, Guo-Sheng Yi, and Yan-Qiu Che. "Investigation of EEG abnormalities in the early stage of Parkinson's disease." *Cognitive Neurodynamics* 7, no. 4 (2013): 351–359.

5 Classifying Phonological Categories and Imagined Words from EEG Signal

Ashwin Kamble and Pradnya H Ghare
Visvesvaraya National Institute of Technology

Vinay Kumar
Motilal Nehru National Institute of Technology

CONTENTS

5.1 INTRODUCTION

The most basic and growing way of communication is via word transfer. Vocal speech alongside physical gestures is people's means of communication for their everyday lives. Individuals with complete paralysis lose their ability to speak and struggle to engage with the external world. Human interaction with the external world is a research field that supports people suffering from neurological disorders and paralysis. In the same way, people with speech impairments inspire researchers to focus on imagined word recognition. Decoding imaginary thoughts or sentences is a great boon to the neurologically impaired individuals.

Brain computer interface (BCI) is a technology that gives individuals with neurological disorders a medium of contact to communicate their feelings and thoughts to a great extent, improving the quality of rehabilitation [1]. BCI analyzes the brain's electrophysiological signals and produces commands that represent the mental activity of the user. BCI system has applications in assisting the people with motor disabilities, identifying the emotional states of the individuals, and observing the mental state of an individual while in pain. For these applications, various techniques have been used for the recording the activities of the brain and design a BCI system to assist the individuals. Functional magnetic resonance imaging (fMRI), functional near-infrared imaging (fNIR), electrocorticography (ECoG), electromyography (EMG), magnetoencephalography (MEG), and electroencephalography (EEG) are the neuroimaging techniques that have been used by the researchers to record brain activities.

MEG is a nonacoustic method for capturing the speech imagery data. Despite having moderate spatial resolution and high temporal resolution (as compared to EEG), no positive results have been published for this method [2]. ECoG is an invasive method, which involves electrodes implanted in the scalp. fMRI studies have greatly contributed to the research on language comprehension and language production [3–6]. But the poor temporal resolution of fMRI and fNIR makes them poor choices for imagined speech classification. The limitations like low temporal resolution, high cost for data acquisition, low portability, and a large amount of time for a subject to sit in the lab for data acquisition limit the use of these neuroimaging techniques for use in laboratory and clinics only.

Among these neuroimaging techniques, EEG has been commonly used for the design of BCI system for various applications. The motivations of using EEG over the other neuroimaging techniques and EEG signals being the most popular preference for researchers are [7–9] as follows: (i) EEG signal has a noninvasive nature, (ii) portability of the EEG devices is high as compared to the other, (iii) EEG acquisition devices are relatively cheaper, and (iv) EEG signals recorded have a good temporal resolution and can be used as a communication tool when used with BCI. EEG is a technique that uses electrodes in various positions on the scalp to measure electric impulses generated throughout the brain cortex.

By considering the advantages of EEG signals, researchers have started using EEG signals for designing the BCI system for various applications such as classification of alertness and drowsiness [10], emotion recognition [11], and classification of schizophrenia [12]. Raw EEG signals captured from the scalp need to be processed before it is given to the BCI system. Also, EEG signal has nonstationary nature which makes it difficult to analyze in either time domain or frequency domain separately. Raw EEG signals are decomposed to extract the meaningful information content in the signal.

Clinical studies have been conducted to identify EEG signals generated by motor movements. The motor movements such as the hand movement, foot movement, and tongue movement can be classified and separated easily from each other. Hence, these actions are considered to design a BCI system. In contrast to this, the EEG signals generated by the mental imagination task can be used to design a BCI system that can help treat the mental disorders [2] and provide people with a means of communication with the disabilities [13–15]. Motor imagination task means the process of the imagination of movement of body parts such as hand, foot and tongue, without actually moving them. Most of the existing work focused on classification of movement produced by hand and foot such as right hand, right leg, left hand, and left leg. Data collected from these movements are used to design a BCI system. As these movements are limited in number, a limited number of control signals are generated by a BCI system. This limited number reduces the capability of a BCI system that can be used to control a large number of control signals to support real-world applications.

To increase the number of control signals of a BCI system, it was proposed that instead of classifying only motor imagery task, other mental imagination tasks such as visual imagination and speech imagination can also be employed to design a BCI system. Visual imagination refers to generating the image of an object in the brain without actually seeing it. The visual imagination task was highly investigated by the researchers.

The concept of reading one's thoughts, which is commonly referred to as imagined speech or covert speech, is not a unique concept. Much of the research is being done in the field of BCI for word recognition. Being an invasive technology, ECoG has shown the most success for word recognition, but showing no clear indication of the mechanism for language processing [16]. Equally, ECoG is favored by its better spatial resolution and time resolution over EEG, but the EEG is favored because its implementation is non-invasive, portable, and relatively cheaper. The most important aspect is to provide a non-invasive design because the final product should be portable and ready to be used by others. While ECoG is typically more effective in capturing imagined speech than EEG, EEG work has had its own success.

EEG has been widely used by the researchers to recognize and classify the imagined speech. In 2009, M. D'Zmura et al. [17] experimented with four participants for syllabic speech imaging without the involvement of muscle movement, using two syllables */ba/* and */ku/*. The study shows that EEG signal generated from brain cortex is highly contaminated with the EMG signals. The source of these EMG signals is eye and head muscle movement. The Hilbert transform was used to extract the features from the wavelet envelopes of theta, beta, and alpha bands. The imagined syllables were then classified using matched filters. Results show that the beta band is found to be the most informative frequency band as compared to the delta and alpha band and showed discriminatory features with the highest accuracy of 62%–87%. The same syllables, */ba/* and */Ku/*, collected from seven subjects have been classified by [18]. K Brigham et al. developed an autoregressive (AR) coefficient and k-nearest neighbors (k-NN)-based algorithm to achieve the binary classification accuracy of 61%. As noted, relatively higher accuracy reported in [17] may have been reached due to the additional presence of motor imagery. By considering the suitability of the Huang Hilbert transform (HHT) [19] to the nonstationary and nonlinear signals over Fourier transform, Deng et al. [20] performed the classification of the same two syllables */ba/*, */ku/* using HHT. The experiment was performed on seven subjects to collect data for the imagined class for syllables */ba/* and */ku/*. Raw data were decomposed in mutually orthogonal components using a second-order blind identification algorithm. A Bayesian classifier was used for the classification task. The highest classification accuracy reported is 72.6%. Empirical mode decomposition (EMD) has been selected, as the time and frequency resolution is adaptive and does not reliably project data. The results show that the temporal domain produces information, which is much significant as compared to that of other domains. It also shows that temporal domain activity during imagined speech has a similarity to that of speech itself.

DaSalla et al. [21] used a support vector machine (SVM) to classify three tasks, the imagination of */a/*, */u/* and no action or rest state. Data were collected from three English-speaking subjects. Binary classification was performed between */a/* and *rest*, */a/* and */u/*, and */u/* and *rest*. Features were extracted using Common Spatial Pattern (CSP) method and classification performed with nonlinear SVM. The overall accuracies were reported in the range of 56%–82%. The data were made open access which were then used by Anaum Riaz et al. [22], along with the other two datasets. The other two datasets are data collected from two subjects for mouthing the vowels with 20 electrodes and dataset collected by considering electrodes carrying significant information. CSP method was used for dimensionality reduction. Mel Frequency Cepstral Coefficient (MFCC) and log variance Auto-Regressive (AR) coefficient techniques were used for feature extraction. SVM, kNN, and Hidden Markov Model (HMM) were used for classification. A pairwise classification is then performed by the use of these features and obtained significant results in terms of classification accuracy. It was found that out of total electrodes, the electrodes that are placed on the motor cortex, Broca's area, and Wernicke's area are giving significant information for the classification task. Idrees and Farooq [23] used four level wavelet decomposition methods to extract the features to investigate the dominance of information from delta, beta, and theta bands over the other information present in the raw signal. The feature set was reduced and the features with maximum information used for the classification. The classification was performed as a 'combination of tasks' and 'pairwise classification' using a linear classifier. The proposed method shows that delta, beta, and theta bands can be used for speech classification with an accuracy of 65%–82.5% for 'pairwise classification', which is higher than that in [21], and 82.25% for 'combination of tasks'.

N. Rehman [24] proposed Multivariate Empirical Mode Decomposition (MEMD) for analyzing multivariate results by considering the finding in [25] suggesting that EMD has problem in mode mixing and mode misalignment. MEMD was used in [26] to extract brain signals relating to imagined speech. Intrinsic mode functions (IMF) which showed dominant information in alpha band were selected, and analysis was performed on */a/*, */i/*, */u/* from seven subjects. Results show that MEMD can extract more useful information from EEG. Taking into account the findings of [24], Jongin Kim et al. signals than other algorithms and IMF2 have significant information for imagined speech in the alpha band.

In a study in 2011, Xuemin Chi et al [27] experimented on five subjects to record EEG data with 52 electrodes to discriminate five phonemes. Data were recorded for different vocal articulations in overt speech production (*jaw tongue, nasal, lip, fricative*). A binary classification accuracy of 80% was achieved on single-day data, and two-way classification has achieved an accuracy of 70% on overall trials.

C. H. Nguyen, [28] has come up with a Riemannian manifold features-based approach for the classification of four separate sets of prompts: vowels (*/a/*, */i/* and */u/*), short words ("*in*" and "*out*"), long words ("*cooperate*" and "*independent*"), and short-long words ("*in*" and "*cooperate*"). Data were recorded from 15 subjects. As the data were recorded from 62 electrodes, it was necessary to reduce the dimensionality of the data. Hence, the CSP method was applied using the toolbox provided in [29]. CSP pattern infers that brain function was focused on the left frontal, middle, and parietal sections of the brain that were centered on Broca's area, the motor cortex, and wernicke's area during the imagined speech task. These results suggest that Broca's area, the motor cortex, and Wernicke's area are considered to be most responsible for the production of speech, as suggested in [22]. The reported accuracies for the vowel class, short words class, long words class, and short-long words are 49.2%, 50.1%, 66.2%, and 80.1%, respectively.

In a study in 2018, M. N. I. Qureshi et al. [30] experimented on eight subjects and recorded a dataset for the imagination of five different words which a person can use in a daily routine. Different feature extraction methods were used for the classification of five words. Covariance-based connectivity measures and maximum linear cross-correlation-based connectivity measures were used for the feature extraction. The experiment was performed separately on all electrode data and data from the electrode which monitor the language processing area, i.e., Broca's area and Wernicke's area. It was found that data from Broca's area and Wernicke's area give better classification accuracy. This again supports the findings provided in [22,29]. The resulted classification accuracies are 40.30% for multiclass classification and 87.90% for binary classification.

Mohanchandra et al. [31] used a multiclass support vector for classifying five different words namely, "*water*", "*help*", "*thanks*", "*food*", and "*stop*". The dimensionality of the EEG data was reduced by using the Subset Selection Method (SSM) that is based on a set of principal representative features (PRF). A new set of variables called PRF is generated by the subset process. The initial variables are a linear combination of every PRF. All PRF are orthogonal, and no redundant information is available.

Cooney et al. [32] used a feature set obtained from Mel Frequency Cepstral Coefficients (MFCC), and classification was performed using SVM classifier to classify the 11 prompts in the KARAONE dataset [33]. Zhao et al. [33] generated a database of 11 prompts, i.e., seven phonemic prompts *(/iy/, /uw/, /piy/, /tiy/, /diy/, /m/, /n/)* and four words (i.e., *pat*, *pot*, knew, and gnaw). In combination with speech audio data and facial features, Zhao used sequentially designed features from ICA decomposed EEG data to achieve the classification accuracy for phonological categories based on the articulatory stages. Pengfei Sun [34] used the dataset provided in [33] to classify the phonological categories and 11 words using a neural network (NN)-based EEG-speech (NES) framework. However, the results obtained for classifying the imagined speech from the EEG data alone, as stated in [34], are not satisfying on precision and reliability. Pramit Saha et al. [35,36] used deep learning architecture to work on the dataset provided in [33] and improved the results for all the categories suggested in [33]. Jerrin et al. [37], stated that the lower accuracy could have resulted from a greater number of choices and used Daubechies-4 (db4) wavelet for the feature extraction along with Deep Belief Network (DBN) as a classifier to obtain the average accuracy of 57.1%.

Cooney et al. [38] used dataset presented in [39] to perform binary classification on words (pairs of words) and achieved the highest classification accuracy of 65.67%

using Convolutional Neural Network (CNN). Cooney et al. [40] performed multi-class classification on imagined vowels presented in [22] using the Transfer Learning approach. Two different TL methods were used. TL1 required training the CNN on all source data to fine-tune CNN input layers before target data were applied. TL2 used the same technique; later layers of the CNN were fine-tuned. Such TL approaches have been contrasted with a non-TL teaching methodology with the same CNN architecture.

Different methods are proposed to classify the imagined words in the literature. Some methods have directly used the raw signal and extracted features from it. Some used FFT which suffers from time-frequency localization. The model proposed by the abovementioned techniques in the literature has been constrained by its efficiency in terms of classification accuracy. That's why there is an urgent need of an efficient model for the classification of phonological categories and recognition of imagined words to help the people suffering from the neurological disorder and complete paralysis. Hence, in this chapter, we propose EMD and wavelet transform-based system to recognize the imagined words. The motivation for using EMD is that it is adaptive, decomposes the one-dimensional signal into number of sub-bands, and has been widely used by the researchers for various applications such as detection of schizophrenia patients using EEG signals [14], classifying the seizure and non-seizure signals [41], classifying the motor imagery EEG signals for BCI applications [13], and classifying the EEG signals of alcoholic and nonalcoholic individuals [42]. Wavelet transform, on the other hand, is another effective technique which has been used by the researchers for various applications such as motor imagery signal classification [14], drowsiness detection [43], emotion detection [44], classification of schizophrenia patients [45], and classification of sleep stages [46]. The literature survey on imagined speech classification is provided in Table 5.1.

5.2 METHODOLOGY

This study performs the classification of phonological categories and imagined words using EEG data. We worked on the database presented in [33] to obtain better accuracy results using wavelet decomposition and EMD decomposition.

We conducted preprocessing for removing the artefacts from the source signals. After preprocessing, the reconstructed data were further decomposed separately using wavelet decomposition and EMD to get the meaningful information present in the data and extract the statistical features. Extraction and selection of features are the most crucial and inherent part of every automated framework to assist the decision-making. After decomposing the data, statistical features were extracted from wavelet decomposed and EMD decomposed data separately. A Kruskal Wallis test was performed to separate the highly discriminative features from the available feature set. Out of the total features, some features were discarded having a high probability value.

This comparative classification study was carried out by dividing the data into two categories. Category 1 has the EEG data collected from the entire brain, and category 2 has the EEG data obtained only from the electrodes observing the brain's language processing area, i.e., Broca's area, Wernicke's area, and motor cortex [30].

TABLE 5.1
Literature Survey on Imagined Speech Classification

Publication	Words Considered	Decomposition Method	Results(%)	Classifier
[17]	*/ba/, /ku/*	Hilbert transform	62–87	Matched filters
[18]	*/ba/, /ku/*	AR coefficients	61	k-NN
[20]	*/ba/, /ku/*	Hilbert transform	72	Bayesian classifier
[21]	*/a/, /u/* and no action	CSP	56–82	SVM
[23]	*/a/, /u/* and no action	Wavelet	65–82.5	Linear classifier
[26]	*/a/, /i/, /u/*	MEMD	68–74	LDA
[27]	*jaw, tongue, nasal, lip, fricative*	-	70	Naive Bayes and LDA
[28]	Vowels, long words, short words, and short-long words	CSP	49.2, 50.1, 66.2, and 80.1, respectively	Riemannian manifold
[30]	"*Go*", "*back*", "*left*", "*right*", "*stop*"	Independent component analysis (ICA), covariance-based features, maximum linear cross-correlation, phase only time-series of ICA components,	40.30 for multiclass and 87.90 for binary classification	ELM
[31]	"*water*", "*help*", "*thanks*", "*food*", and "*stop*	-	77.6 (average of all five words)	SVM
[32]	*(/iy/, /uw/, /piy/, /tiy/, /diy/, /m/, /n/)* and words (i.e., *pat*, *pot*, knew, and gnaw)	MFCC	44.79	SVM
[34]	*(/iy/, /uw/, /piy/, /tiy/, /diy/, /m/, /n/)* and words (i.e., *pat*, *pot*, knew, and gnaw)	-	69.8 (average)	NN-based NES framework
[36]	*(/iy/, /uw/, /piy/, /tiy/, /diy/, /m/, /n/)* and words (i.e., *pat*, *pot*, knew, and gnaw)	-	87.96	DBN
[37]	*(/iy/, /uw/, /piy/, /tiy/, /diy/, /m/, /n/)* and words (i.e., *pat*, *pot*, knew, and gnaw)	Wavelet	57.1	DBN
[38]	*/a/,/e/,/i/,/o/,/u/*	Wavelet	65.67	CNN

The results of the analysis demonstrate the potential of the proposed method to correctly decipher the imagined words and phonological categories in the EEG dataset for each of the five categories. In comparison, in terms of accuracy for classifying the phonological categories and imagined words, the findings of the proposed method surpass those of most state-of-the-art methods.

The rest of the chapter is structured accordingly: the Materials and Methods section explains the methods for the acquisition of EEG data, processing the EEG data, extraction of features, and classification methods. The Result section presents the classification accuracies obtained and compares results obtained from different classifiers for different decomposition methods. The chapter concludes with the Result and Discussion section discussing the better decomposition method.

5.2.1 Dataset

The database used for the proposed framework has been taken from the Toronto Rehabilitation Institute database which is publically available [33]. Eleven subjects participated in the experiment to perform the overt and imagined. This study used EEG data associated only with the imagination task. Seven phonemic prompts (*/iy/, /uw/, /piy/, /tiy/, /diy/, /m/, /n/*) and four words (i.e., *pat*, *pot*, *knew*, and *gnaw*) were imagined by the participants, and the EEG data were recorded. EEG recording used

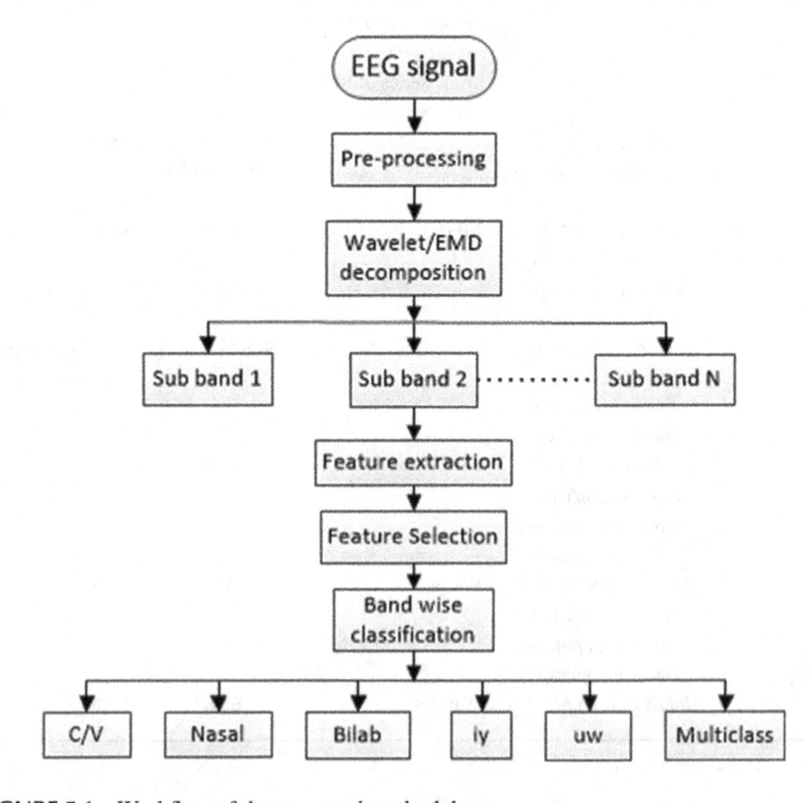

FIGURE 5.1 Workflow of the proposed methodology

a 64-channel Neuroscan Quick-Cap, and the electrode placement has followed the 10–20 system. Data were sampled at 1024 Hz. Out of the total data recorded, only 4.5 seconds of data are considered for further processing.

The EEG data were preprocessed using Python 3.7.2. Raw EEG data are band-pass filtered (fourth-order Butterworth filter, 1–50 Hz) as this band includes all the frequency components used in research associated with EGG.

5.2.2 Wavelet Decomposition

The reconstructed time series data were then decomposed using a discrete wavelet transform. Instead of concatenating the data obtained from different channels, every channel is considered as a separate input [47]. This is considered because the signals from every channel have a high correlation. Wavelet decomposition was applied to every channel separately. The data were decomposed using the Daubechies-4 (db4) wavelet with eight levels. Coefficients from only five bands, i.e., one approximation and four details are taken into consideration as these coefficients refer to delta, theta, alpha, beta, and gamma bands of EEG signal, and the rest are neglected. Figure 5.2 shows the decomposed data of word */diy/* for single trial of subject 1 for channel 1.

5.2.3 Empirical Mode Decomposition

EMD is an adaptive method and can be used for time-frequency analysis of nonstationary and nonlinear univariate signals [48]. The reconstructed time series data were then decomposed using EMD decomposition. First proposed by Huang et al [48] in 1998, EMD views the signal as a superposition of fast oscillations on slow oscillations [49], which can precisely be decomposed into a series of basic and intrinsic oscillations on a dynamic feature time scale without the requirement of a priori knowledge about the device. This decomposition is adaptive and became suitable for the nonstationary and nonlinear processes, producing a set of intrinsic mode functions [50].

Every channel is considered as a separate input. EMD decomposition was applied to every channel separately. Data were decomposed into a number of IMFs. Every channel produces a different number of IMFs, and then the data for the least number of IMFs are considered for further processing (Figure 5.3).

5.2.4 Channel Selection

The key objective of the channel selection procedure is to lessen the computational difficulty of any processing activity conducted on EEG signal. The appropriate channels are chosen to extract the essential features. This reduces the level of overfitting that could arise from the usage of unwanted channels. This leads to boost the performance and to decrease the setup time required in particular applications [51].

This study investigates the dominance of information collected from the electrodes placed on the area responsible for language processing. This entire data collection was divided into two parts: one containing data from all the electrodes and second containing data collected from the electrodes placed on the left inferior

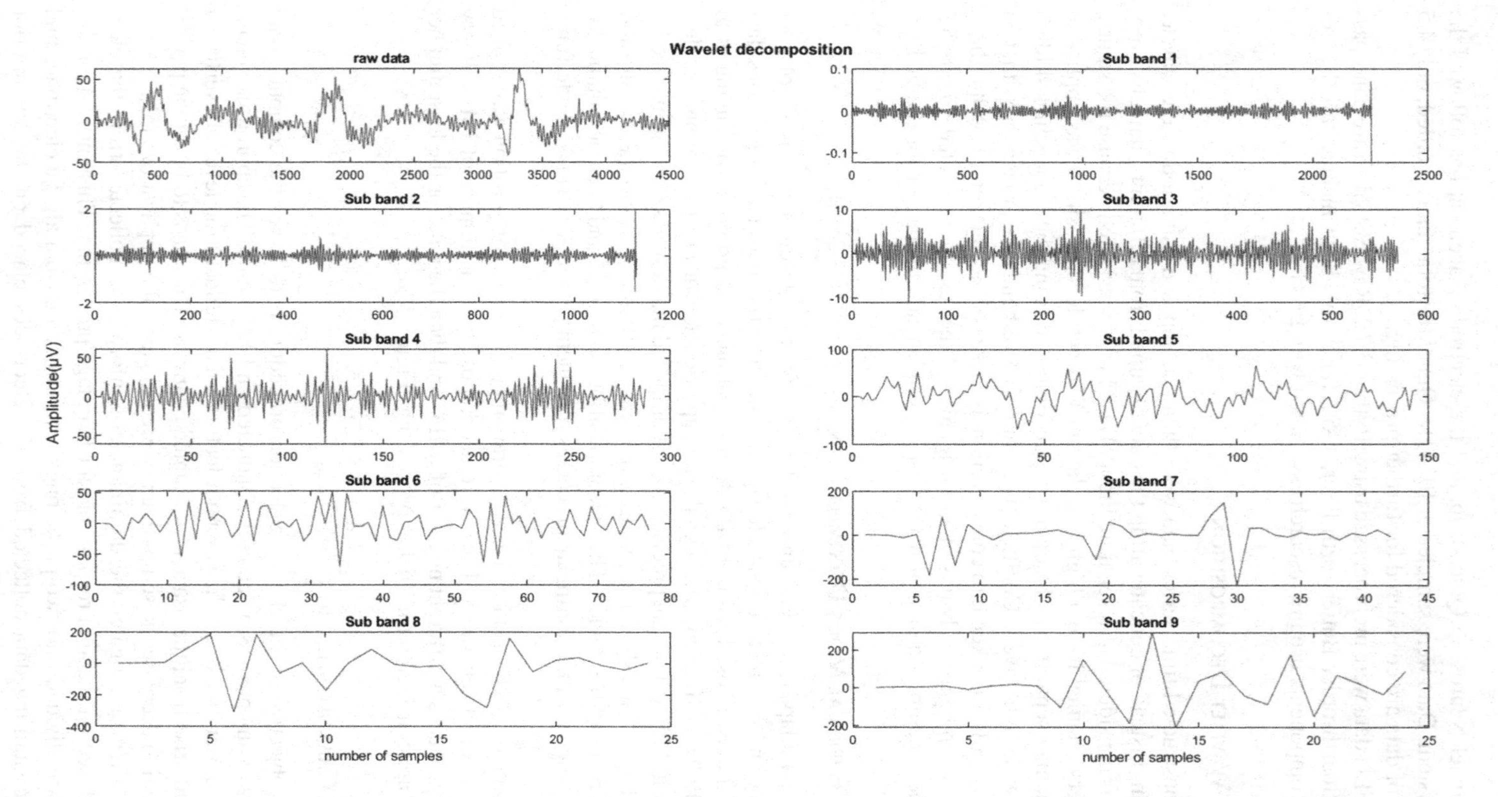

FIGURE 5.2 Wavelet decomposition of raw data of word */diy/* for single trial of subject 1 for channel 1. (The figure represents raw data and the wavelet coefficients)

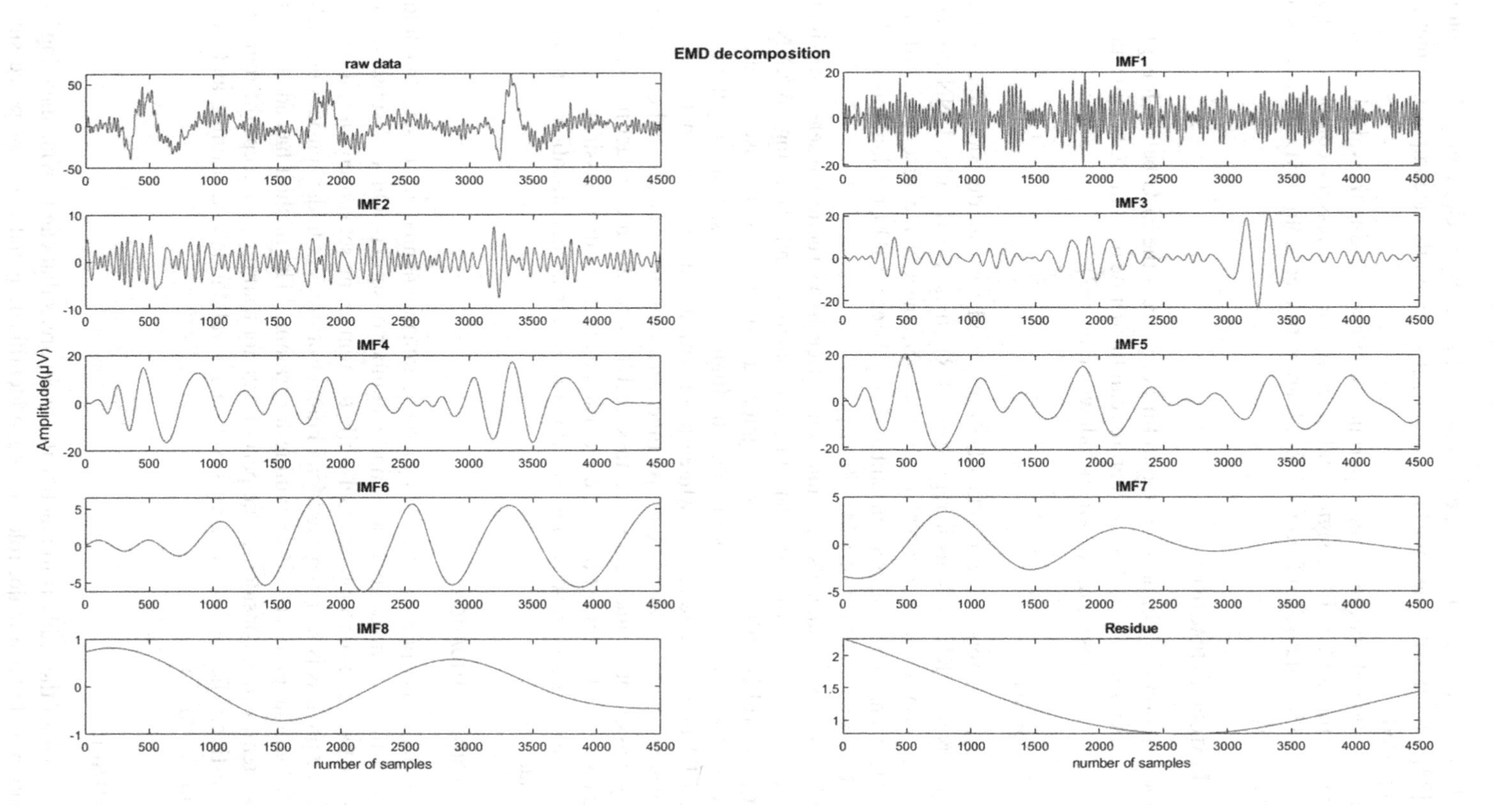

FIGURE 5.3 EMD decomposition of raw data of word */diy/* for single trial of subject 1 for channel 1. (The figure represents raw data and the IMFs.)

frontal lobe (Broca's area), left superior temporal lobe (Wernicke's area), and motor cortex [38]. The classification for both parts by using both the decomposition methods is reported.

The extraction of features is an important step for separating the valuable details contained in the surface EEG signal and deleting the unnecessary component and interferences [52]. Statistical features [52–57] are extracted from each band and each IMF separately.

5.2.5 Feature Extraction

Feature extraction is an important step to further process the EEG before it is given for the classification task. Extracted features can further be used in BCI applications. The statistical features extracted are as follows (Table 5.2).

5.2.6 Classifiers

In this study, different types of classifiers are used such as decision tree (DT), weighted k-NN (WKNN), logistic regression (LR), linear SVM, cubic k-NN, cosine k-NN, course k-NN, medium k-NN, medium k-NN, fine k-NN, course tree, medium tree, fine tree, ensemble bag tree, ensemble boosted trees (EBT), random forest (RF), and fine Gaussian SVM (FG-SVM) [58–61].

The DT classifier makes its decision using a tree-like structure to select the right one from a group of two based on human behavioral understanding. WKNN is another powerful classifier that uses weighted sum of associated classes, where the variable is assigned to the class that has the highest weight sum among the target classes. EBT doesn't quite require whitening or normalization of the input elements. Since they are powered by custom loss functions, they are versatile and can target arbitrary classification and regression tasks. EBT generates a compact model with fewer parameters for almost the same precision as that of other classifiers. Logistic regression uses a sigmoid activation function for the binary classification using non-linear relationship.

5.2.7 Cross Validation

Cross-validation is a process of dividing a set of data into number of subsets. In *k*-fold cross-validation, the data are divided into *k* number of subsets. Out of *k* subsets, *k*-1 subsets are used as training the model while the remaining set is used for testing the model. The process is then repeated for *k* number of times (*k* folds) considering each subset for validation once and remaining for training. The method has advantages over a system, which considers some part of data for training and keeps the remaining for testing. The method uses each subset for validation and training and as a validation set for once.

5.3 RESULT

The objective of the study is to identify the brain areas that can provide meaningful information and play a major role in speech identification and language processing.

TABLE 5.2
List of Features Extracted from the Wavelet and EMD Decomposed Data

Sr no	Feature	Mathematical Description
1	Enhanced Mean Absolute Value (EMAV) (F1) [57]	$\text{EMAV} = \frac{1}{N}\sum_{i=1}^{N}\left\|x(i)^{p}\right\|$ $p = 0.75$ if $i \geq 0.2N$ & $i \leq 0.8N$ $= 0.50$ otherwise
2	Enhanced wavelength (EWL) (F2) [57]	$\text{EMAV} = \frac{1}{N}\sum_{i=2}^{N}\left\|\left(x(i) - x(i-1)\right)^{p}\right\|$ $p = 0.75$ if $i \geq 0.2N$ & $i \leq 0.8N$ $= 0.50$ otherwise
3	Mean absolute value (MAV) (F3)	$\text{MAV} = \frac{1}{N}\sum_{i=1}^{N}\left\|x(i)\right\|$
4	Slope sign change (SSC) (F4)	$\text{SSC} = \sum_{i=2}^{N-1}\left[f\left[\left(x(i) - x(i-1)\right) * \left(\left(x(i) - x(i+1)\right)\right)\right]\right]$ $f(x) = 1$ if $x(i) \geq$ threshold $= 0$ otherwise
5	Zero crossing (ZC) (F5)	$\text{ZC} = \sum_{i=1}^{N-1} sgn\left(x(i) * x(i+1)\right) \cap \left\|x(i) - x(i+1)\right\|$ $sgn(x) = 1$ if $x(i) \geq$ threshold $= 0$ otherwise
6	Waveform length (WL) (F6)	$\text{WL} = \sum_{i=1}^{N-1}\left\|x(i+1) - x(i)\right\|$
7	Root mean square value (RMS) (F7)	$\text{RMS} = \frac{1}{N}\sum_{i=1}^{N}x(i)^{2}$
8	Average amplitude change (AAC) (F8)	$\text{AAC} = \frac{1}{N}\sum_{i=1}^{N-1}\left\|x(i+1) - x(i)\right\|$
9	Difference absolute standard deviation value (DASDV) (F9)	$\text{DASDV} = \sqrt{\frac{1}{N-1}\sum_{i=1}^{N-1}\left(x(i) - x(i-1)\right)^{2}}$
10	Log detector (F10)	$\text{LG} = \exp\left(\frac{1}{N}\sum_{i=1}^{N}\log\left(\left\|x(i)\right\|\right)\right)$

(Continued)

TABLE 5.2 (*Continued*)
List of Features Extracted from the Wavelet and EMD Decomposed Data

Sr no	Feature	Mathematical Description
11	Modified mean absolute value type 1 (MAV1) (F11)	$MMAV1 = \frac{1}{N}\sum_{i=1}^{N} w(n)\lvert x(i)\rvert$ $w(n) = 1$ if $0.25N \le n \le 0.75N$ $= 0.5$ otherwise
12	Modified mean absolute value type 2 (MAV2) (F12)	$\text{MMAV2} = \frac{1}{N}\sum_{i=1}^{N} w(n)\lvert x(i)\rvert$ $w(n) = 1$ if $0.25N \le n \le 0.75N$ $= 4n/N$ else if $0.25N > n$ $= 4(n - N)/N$ otherwise
13	Myopulse percentage rate (MYOP) (F13)	$\text{MYOP} = \frac{1}{N}\sum_{i=1}^{N} [x(i)]$ $f(x) = 1$ if $x(i) \ge$ threshold $= 0$ otherwise
14	Simple square integral (SSI) (F14)	$\text{SSI} = \sum_{i=1}^{N} x(i)^2$
15	Variance of EEG (F15)	$\text{VAR} = \frac{1}{N-1}\sum_{i=1}^{N} x(i)^2$
16	Willison amplitude (WA) (F16)	$\text{WAMP} = \frac{1}{N}\sum_{i=1}^{N-1} [f\lvert x(i) - x(i+1)\rvert]$ $f(x) = 1$ if $x(i) \ge$ threshold $= 0$ otherwise
17	Maximum fractal length (MFL) (F17)	$\text{MFL} = \log_{10}\left(\sqrt{\sum_{i=1}^{N-1} (x(i+1) - x(i-1))^2}\right)$
18	Integrated EEG(IEEG) (F18)	$\text{IEEG} = \sum_{i=1}^{N} \lvert x(i)\rvert$
19	Absolute value of the 3rd temporal moment (TM3) (F19)	$\text{TM3} = \left\lvert \frac{1}{N}\sum_{i=1}^{N} x(i)^3 \right\rvert$
20	Absolute value of the 4th temporal moment (TM4) (F20)	$\text{TM4} = \left\lvert \frac{1}{N}\sum_{i=1}^{N} x(i)^4 \right\rvert$

(*Continued*)

TABLE 5.2 (*Continued*)
List of Features Extracted from the Wavelet and EMD Decomposed Data

Sr no	Feature	Mathematical Description
21	Absolute value of the 5th temporal moment (TM5) (F21)	$\text{TM5} = \left\lvert \frac{1}{N}\sum_{i=1}^{N} x(i)^5 \right\rvert$
22	Mean (F22)	$\mu = \frac{1}{N}\sum_{i=1}^{N} x(i)$
23	Median (F23)	$\text{median} = x\left(\frac{N+1}{2}\right)$ if N is odd; $= \frac{x\left(\frac{N}{2}\right) + x\left(\frac{N}{2}+1\right)}{2}$ if N is even
24	Skewness (F24)	$s = \frac{\sqrt{\left[E\left(x(i)-\mu\right)^3\right]}}{\sigma^3}$
25	Kurtosis (F25)	$k = \frac{\sqrt{\left[E\left(x(i)-\mu\right)^4\right]}}{\sigma^4}$
26	Standard deviation (F26)	$\sigma = \sqrt{\frac{\sum_{i=1}^{N}\left[\left(x(i)-\mu\right)\right]^2}{N}}$
27	Minimum value (F27)	$\text{Minimum} = \min_{i=1}^{N} (x(i))$
28	Maximum value (F28)	$\text{Maximum} = \max_{i=1}^{N} (x(i))$

Dataset considered for the study was collected from 12 subjects for imagining of seven prompts (/iy/, /uw/, /piy/, /tiy/, /diy/, /m/, /n/) and four words (i.e., pat, pot, knew, and gnaw). Data were classified between various phonemic and phonological classes. Specifically, we considered five binary classification tasks: vowel-only vs. consonant (C/V), presence of nasal (± Nasal), presence of bilabial (± Bilab), presence of high-front vowel (±/iy/), and presence of high-back vowel (±/uw/) and lastly a multiclass classification considering 11 words.

Raw data were preprocessed using band pass filter to remove the eye blink and muscle movement artefacts present in the signal. Then wavelet decomposition with dB4 wavelet and eight levels is applied that decomposes the signal in detail and approximate coefficients with nine bands out of which only five bands (delta, theta, alpha, beta, gamma) are considered for the further process. Signal obtained from these five bands is then used for extracting features. Similarly, preprocessed data were decomposed using EMD decomposition. EMD decomposes data in the number of IMFs. These IMFs are considered for feature extraction and classification. A total of 28 features were extracted from the wavelet decomposed bands and EMD decomposed IMFs separately.

For successful classification of EEG signal, selecting feature vector with high variance is an important task. A Kruskal-Wallis (KW) test was performed for the binary classification, and post-hoc analysis was performed for the multiclass classification to get the probabilistic value (p) of each feature for each band of wavelet decomposed data and each IMF of EMD decomposed data. The feature matrix is formed for each class using the abovementioned features having $p < 0.05$. The feature matrix generated from the abovementioned features having $p < 0.05$ is then applied to the classifiers to classify the data.

The classification was performed in two categories: (i) for signals generated from all the electrodes, and (ii) for signals generated from electrodes placed at left hemisphere as this area belongs to speech processing, especially the Broca's area which is considered to be in relation with speech production and Wernicke's area which is functional in language processing. The data are classified into seven classes: C/V, bilabial, nasal, /iy/, /uw/, multiclass classification by considering all words for classification, and binary classification by considering one versus all. Performance parameters such as accuracy, sensitivity, specificity, and precision are calculated for the classifier showing the best results in terms of classification accuracy for all the classes.

5.3.1 Binary Classification Results

Results obtained for binary classification accuracy from different classifiers for five bands of wavelet decomposed signal are shown in Table 5.3 and compared with the results obtained for binary classification accuracy from the same classifiers for four IMFs of EMD decomposed signals for each category. Out of the total classifiers, for both wavelet and EMD decomposed signals, the ensemble bagged tree gives the highest classification accuracy as compared to the other classifiers. Also, it can be seen from the classification results of wavelet decomposed signals that theta band is giving the highest classification accuracy followed by the alpha band. Hence, it can be noted that the delta and alpha band are responsible for the imagination of speech. Also, it can be seen from the classification results of EMD decomposed signals, that IMF1 is giving the highest classification accuracy followed by the IMF2.

5.3.2 Multiclass Classification Results

Different classifiers are used to classify the wavelet and EMD decomposed data into 11 classes. The results obtained from different classifiers for wavelet and EMD decomposed data for each category are then compared. The ensemble bagged tree has shown better results than the other classifiers for both the wavelet decomposed signals and EMD decomposed signals. As mentioned above, theta band is showing the highest classification accuracy for multiclass classification. In the same way, IMF1 is proving to have dominant information for speech recognition (Figure 5.4 and Tables 5.4–5.6).

TABLE 5.3
Classification Accuracy (%) for Wavelet Decomposition of Data from All Electrodes and from the Electrodes Placed at Language Processing Area

Phonological Category	C/V									
	Category 1 (All Electrodes)					Category 2 (Electrodes from Language Processing Area)				
Classifiers	**Delta**	**Theta**	**Alpha**	**Beta**	**Gamma**	**Delta**	**Theta**	**Alpha**	**Beta**	**Gamma**
Weighted k-NN	85.23	88.78	88.08	87.20	85.37	83.91	87.71	87.15	86.61	85.57
Cubic k-NN	83.99	87.62	87.20	86.29	83.75	82.42	85.78	84.88	84.69	83.60
Cosine k-NN	84.42	87.92	87.37	86.66	84.47	82.68	86.15	85.51	85.32	84.39
Course k-NN	82.09	84.15	83.46	83.43	82.60	81.91	81.71	81.97	82.05	81.86
Medium k-NN	84.12	87.85	87.51	86.72	84.53	82.50	85.97	85.22	85.27	84.32
Fine k-NN	82.01	85.68	84.51	82.82	80.34	80.59	84.72	83.95	81.94	80.70
Logistic regression	81.86	81.85	81.86	81.86	81.86	81.84	81.81	81.84	75.30	81.43
Course tree	81.86	82.01	81.94	82.06	81.85	81.88	81.94	81.94	82.18	81.85
Medium tree	82.06	82.15	82.25	82.24	81.98	81.97	82.11	82.42	82.42	81.89
Fine tree	82.48	82.78	83.01	82.89	82.59	82.24	82.32	83.03	82.54	82.52
Ensemble bagged tree	87.46	89.69	89.52	88.80	88.37	85.14	87.75	87.75	87.42	86.78
Ensemble boost tree	81.93	82.09	82.12	82.13	81.97	81.91	82.06	81.96	82.23	81.90
Linear SVM	81.86	81.86	81.86	81.86	81.86	81.86	81.86	81.86	81.86	81.86
Phonological Category					**NASAL**					
Weighted k-NN	71.10	75.73	73.75	70.62	67.42	68.45	73.82	72.84	70.63	68.69
Cubic k-NN	67.82	73.29	70.89	67.05	63.93	64.46	69.56	68.10	66.62	64.97
Cosine k-NN	68.49	73.79	71.31	67.71	65.02	64.86	70.16	68.98	67.25	65.91
Course k-NN	65.27	68.36	66.99	66.02	65.08	63.69	64.65	64.55	64.74	64.51
Medium k-NN	68.11	73.55	71.33	67.78	64.96	64.64	69.75	68.81	67.04	66.00

(Continued)

TABLE 5.3 (*Continued*)
Classification Accuracy (%) for Wavelet Decomposition of Data from All Electrodes and from the Electrodes Placed at Language Processing Area

Phonological Category	C/V									
	Category 1 (All Electrodes)					Category 2 (Electrodes from Language Processing Area)				
Classifiers	**Delta**	**Theta**	**Alpha**	**Beta**	**Gamma**	**Delta**	**Theta**	**Alpha**	**Beta**	**Gamma**
Fine k-NN	70.08	74.76	72.61	69.05	65.24	67.69	73.11	71.54	68.63	66.65
Logistic regression	63.61	63.61	63.62	56.28	63.61	63.59	63.60	63.62	63.60	63.37
Course tree	63.62	63.92	63.68	63.61	63.68	63.71	63.85	63.80	63.68	63.70
Medium tree	64.38	64.53	64.10	63.86	64.38	64.14	64.06	63.98	63.68	64.31
Fine tree	65.33	65.86	66.07	64.78	65.29	64.91	65.16	65.75	65.24	65.20
Ensemble bagged tree	75.03	79.34	78.79	76.26	75.82	70.57	74.96	75.42	73.50	72.86
Ensemble boost tree	64.33	64.11	64.42	64.05	64.56	64.20	64.29	64.36	63.90	64.47
Linear SVM	63.15	63.15	63.15	63.15	63.15	63.63	63.61	63.63	63.64	63.61
Phonological Category	**BILABIAL**									
Weighted k-NN	72.07	76.13	74.00	70.89	68.15	70.31	74.17	73.35	70.98	68.68
Cubic k-NN	68.80	73.58	71.35	67.66	64.95	65.22	70.13	68.86	66.81	64.57
Cosine k-NN	69.28	74.12	71.99	68.31	66.04	65.79	70.61	69.76	67.77	65.70
Course k-NN	65.42	68.48	67.84	66.78	65.69	63.84	65.57	65.20	65.40	64.80
Medium k-NN	68.89	74.02	71.90	68.31	66.21	65.28	70.56	69.73	67.64	66.20
Fine k-NN	70.96	75.07	72.88	69.22	65.90	69.17	73.80	72.69	69.22	66.79
Logistic regression	63.61	63.61	63.61	36.48	63.61	63.63	63.60	63.59	63.62	63.14
Course tree	63.78	63.88	63.81	63.74	63.61	63.83	63.71	63.82	63.65	63.90
Medium tree	64.13	64.60	64.35	64.47	64.00	63.97	64.72	64.73	63.81	64.18
Fine tree	64.83	66.27	66.26	66.39	65.73	64.84	66.38	66.44	65.26	65.55

(*Continued*)

TABLE 5.3 (*Continued*)
Classification Accuracy (%) for Wavelet Decomposition of Data from All Electrodes and from the Electrodes Placed at Language Processing Area

Phonological Category	C/V									
	Category 1 (All Electrodes)					Category 2 (Electrodes from Language Processing Area)				
Classifiers	**Delta**	**Theta**	**Alpha**	**Beta**	**Gamma**	**Delta**	**Theta**	**Alpha**	**Beta**	**Gamma**
Ensemble bagged tree	76.04	79.53	79.22	77.07	76.67	71.40	75.65	76.19	74.22	73.24
Ensemble boost tree	63.95	65.49	64.41	64.03	64.27	64.05	65.23	64.47	63.92	64.12
Linear SVM	62.25	64.12	63.14	62.39	64.27	63.61	63.61	63.61	63.61	63.61
Phonological Category	IY									
Weighted k-NN	92.43	93.70	93.34	92.85	92.21	92.00	93.31	93.32	92.96	92.54
Cubic k-NN	91.87	93.34	93.11	92.19	91.54	91.04	92.18	92.26	91.87	91.66
Cosine k-NN	92.08	93.47	93.28	92.49	91.83	91.16	92.49	92.44	92.09	91.87
Course k-NN	91.00	91.48	91.41	91.14	91.09	90.95	90.96	90.95	90.95	90.95
Medium k-NN	91.93	93.44	93.23	92.43	91.82	91.07	92.35	92.49	92.11	91.94
Fine k-NN	89.83	91.20	90.49	89.27	88.19	89.11	90.93	90.22	89.21	88.65
Logistic regression	90.95	90.95	90.95	90.95	90.95	90.95	90.95	90.95	90.94	90.64
Course tree	90.95	91.02	90.96	91.11	90.95	90.95	91.05	91.01	91.08	90.95
Medium tree	91.04	91.06	91.15	91.23	91.06	90.98	91.06	91.08	91.27	91.03
Fine tree	91.35	91.35	91.69	91.68	91.56	91.06	91.22	91.61	91.45	91.27
Ensemble bagged tree	93.36	94.43	94.46	94.09	93.94	92.27	93.45	93.58	93.28	92.95
Ensemble boost tree	90.98	91.08	90.99	90.97	90.97	90.97	91.03	91.09	91.13	90.96
Linear SVM	90.95	90.95	90.95	90.95	90.95	90.95	90.96	90.95	90.95	90.95

(*Continued*)

TABLE 5.3 (*Continued*)
Classification Accuracy (%) for Wavelet Decomposition of Data from All Electrodes and from the Electrodes Placed at Language Processing Area

Phonological Category	C/V									
	Category 1 (All Electrodes)					Category 2 (Electrodes from Language Processing Area)				
Classifiers	**Delta**	**Theta**	**Alpha**	**Beta**	**Gamma**	**Delta**	**Theta**	**Alpha**	**Beta**	**Gamma**
Phonological Category					**UW**					
Weighted k-NN	92.89	94.55	94.16	93.49	92.82	92.04	94.09	93.97	93.25	92.68
Cubic k-NN	92.03	93.74	93.42	92.40	91.83	91.04	92.70	92.50	92.05	91.59
Cosine k-NN	92.21	93.84	93.58	92.70	92.31	91.13	92.78	92.78	92.31	91.83
Course k-NN	90.95	91.67	91.48	91.35	90.99	90.90	90.90	90.89	90.90	90.90
Medium k-NN	92.08	93.87	93.65	92.81	92.26	91.05	92.88	92.79	92.43	91.94
Fine k-NN	90.54	92.28	91.37	89.99	89.11	89.56	91.67	91.08	89.98	88.98
Logistic regression	90.90	90.90	90.90	90.90	90.90	90.88	90.83	90.80	82.76	90.43
Course tree	90.95	91.00	90.98	90.96	90.94	90.95	90.99	91.01	91.02	90.89
Medium tree	91.11	91.07	91.28	91.10	91.07	91.01	91.00	91.22	91.21	91.07
Fine tree	91.32	91.56	92.12	91.87	91.60	91.05	92.15	91.25	90.14	90.65
Ensemble bagged tree	93.48	94.72	94.61	94.33	94.16	92.37	93.73	93.72	93.51	93.33
Ensemble boost tree	90.97	90.99	91.06	91.00	90.92	91.00	91.02	90.94	90.96	90.91
Linear SVM	90.90	90.90	90.90	90.90	90.90	90.90	90.90	90.90	90.90	90.90
Category					**MULTICLASS**					
Weighted k-NN	46.01	46.08	46.13	46.15	46.05	39.89	40.09	40.09	40.33	40.25
Cubic k-NN	37.52	37.46	37.6	37.56	37.63	27.48	27.47	27.62	27.47	27.51

(*Continued*)

TABLE 5.3 (*Continued*)
Classification Accuracy (%) for Wavelet Decomposition of Data from All Electrodes and from the Electrodes Placed at Language Processing Area

Phonological Category	C/V									
	Category 1 (All Electrodes)					Category 2 (Electrodes from Language Processing Area)				
Classifiers	Delta	Theta	Alpha	Beta	Gamma	Delta	Theta	Alpha	Beta	Gamma
Cosine k-NN	38.77	38.75	38.76	38.69	38.79	28.8	28.6	28.49	28.83	28.68
Course k-NN	23.35	23.44	23.49	23.43	23.42	16.39	16.59	16.59	16.73	16.85
Medium k-NN	37.97	37.97	38.06	38.01	38	27.93	27.92	28.08	27.92	28.01
Fine k-NN	46.68	46.57	46.6	46.53	46.63	41.9	41.57	41.76	41.9	41.58
Course tree	10.06	10.02	10.08	10.06	10.03	10.06	10.02	10.1	9.97	10.04
Medium tree	11.71	11.73	11.71	11.72	11.63	11.39	11.26	11.18	11.27	11.23
Fine tree	12.95	13.08	13.07	13.17	13.05	13.57	13.37	13.7	13.32	13.64
Ensemble bagged tree	52.95	52.8	52.96	53.07	53.02	43.32	43.76	43.74	44.11	43.52
Ensemble boost tree	11.71	11.68	11.77	11.77	11.78	11.3	11.52	11.22	11.38	11.33

TABLE 5.4
Classification Accuracy (%) for EMD Decomposed of Data from All Electrodes and from the Electrodes Placed at Language Processing Area

Phonological Category	C/V							
	Category 1 (All Electrodes)				Category 2 (Electrodes from Language Processing Area)			
Classifier	**IMF 1**	**IMF 2**	**IMF 3**	**IMF 4**	**IMF 1**	**IMF 2**	**IMF 3**	**IMF 4**
Weighted k-NN	80.45	80.81	80.77	80.45	80.67	80.74	80.38	80.30
Cubic k-NN	81.03	81.03	81.22	81.22	81.40	81.36	81.25	81.33
Cosine k-NN	81.14	81.12	81.18	81.18	81.25	81.41	81.23	81.40
Course k-NN	81.85	81.86	81.87	81.90	81.86	81.86	81.86	81.84
Medium k-NN	81.20	81.14	81.27	81.25	81.33	81.31	81.29	81.26
Fine k-NN	72.83	72.51	72.49	72.40	72.32	72.13	72.04	71.93
Logistic regression	81.86	81.86	81.86	81.85	81.81	81.83	75.53	81.82
Course tree	81.86	81.86	81.86	81.85	81.84	81.85	81.86	81.83
Medium tree	81.84	81.84	81.84	81.83	81.73	81.81	81.80	81.79
Fine tree	81.74	81.77	81.78	81.84	81.39	81.36	81.45	81.45
Ensemble bagged tree	82.82	81.95	81.95	81.87	81.58	81.17	81.25	81.17
Ensemble boost tree	81.86	81.86	81.85	81.86	81.86	81.85	81.85	81.87
Linear SVM	81.18	81.86	81.86	81.86	81.18	81.86	81.86	81.86
Phonological Category	**NASAL**							
Weighted k-NN	61.33	60.94	60.60	60.03	61.24	61.30	60.31	60.00
Cubic k-NN	60.95	60.55	60.07	60.14	60.51	60.15	59.57	59.83
Cosine k-NN	61.13	60.61	60.30	60.27	60.22	60.26	59.86	59.70
Course k-NN	64.32	64.00	63.86	63.86	63.78	63.75	63.57	63.69
Medium k-NN	61.04	60.74	60.34	60.16	60.49	60.63	60.23	59.89
Fine k-NN	57.62	57.17	56.97	56.38	57.12	57.21	56.61	56.30
Logistic regression	63.61	63.61	63.61	63.61	63.60	63.62	63.58	63.58
Course tree	63.64	63.61	63.61	63.64	63.58	63.66	63.69	63.63
Medium tree	63.88	63.63	63.65	63.73	63.82	63.59	63.59	63.54
Fine tree	64.26	63.65	63.73	63.86	63.84	63.19	63.17	63.38
Ensemble bagged tree	65.78	63.58	63.10	62.51	62.49	61.79	61.11	60.73
Ensemble boost tree	64.00	63.61	63.63	63.74	63.86	63.65	63.70	63.63
Linear SVM	63.61	63.61	63.61	63.61	63.62	63.63	63.64	63.64
Phonological Category	**BILABIAL**							
Weighted k-NN	61.51	61.23	61.36	60.63	60.95	60.97	60.79	60.29
Cubic k-NN	60.95	60.56	60.78	60.34	60.18	60.43	60.36	60.50
Cosine k-NN	61.34	60.84	61.01	60.57	60.60	60.67	60.55	60.29
Course k-NN	64.57	64.18	64.34	63.99	63.92	63.97	63.95	63.91
Medium k-NN	61.13	60.78	60.93	60.40	60.49	60.45	60.38	60.34
Fine k-NN	57.29	57.44	57.52	56.80	56.77	56.99	56.35	56.11
Logistic regression	63.61	63.61	63.62	63.61	63.60	63.56	63.52	63.58
Course tree	63.61	63.61	63.61	63.61	63.64	63.61	63.66	63.68
Medium tree	64.12	63.69	63.81	63.70	64.20	63.60	63.75	63.70
Fine tree	64.41	63.61	64.06	63.95	64.02	63.22	63.57	63.51
Ensemble bagged tree	66.45	64.13	63.46	62.84	63.14	62.08	61.66	61.39
Ensemble boost tree	64.28	63.67	63.76	63.78	64.15	63.70	63.69	63.64
Linear SVM	63.61	63.61	63.61	63.61	63.61	63.61	63.61	63.61

(Continued)

TABLE 5.4 (*Continued*)
Classification Accuracy (%) for EMD Decomposed of Data from All Electrodes and from the Electrodes Placed at Language Processing Area

Phonological Category	C/V							
	Category 1 (All Electrodes)				Category 2 (Electrodes from Language Processing Area)			
Classifier	IMF 1	IMF 2	IMF 3	IMF 4	IMF 1	IMF 2	IMF 3	IMF 4
Phonological Category				IY				
Weighted k-NN	90.65	90.84	90.70	90.66	90.82	90.85	90.62	90.71
Cubic k-NN	90.81	90.83	90.84	90.87	90.84	90.81	90.80	90.77
Cosine k-NN	90.85	90.84	90.84	90.86	90.79	90.79	90.77	90.81
Course k-NN	90.95	90.95	90.95	90.95	90.95	90.95	90.95	90.95
Medium k-NN	90.84	90.84	90.85	90.86	90.84	90.82	90.80	90.83
Fine k-NN	84.51	84.63	84.53	84.54	84.62	84.23	84.48	84.17
Logistic regression	90.95	90.95	90.95	90.95	90.95	90.58	90.92	90.89
Course tree	90.95	90.95	90.95	90.95	90.95	90.90	90.98	90.95
Medium tree	90.92	90.94	90.92	90.94	90.87	90.86	90.83	90.87
Fine tree	90.88	90.85	90.83	90.86	90.49	90.56	90.47	90.59
Ensemble bagged tree	91.31	91.07	91.01	91.04	90.87	90.87	90.80	90.92
Ensemble boost tree	90.96	90.96	90.98	90.96	90.95	90.95	90.95	90.95
Linear SVM	90.95	90.95	90.95	90.95	90.95	90.95	90.95	90.95
Phonological Category				UW				
Weighted k-NN	90.61	90.76	90.82	90.63	90.84	90.74	90.68	90.62
Cubic k-NN	90.76	90.76	90.71	90.80	90.84	90.80	90.78	90.83
Cosine k-NN	90.79	90.76	90.81	90.85	90.79	90.79	90.79	90.87
Course k-NN	90.90	90.90	90.89	90.91	90.90	90.90	90.90	90.90
Medium k-NN	90.78	90.76	90.81	90.85	90.88	90.79	90.79	90.84
Fine k-NN	84.50	84.81	84.79	84.47	84.78	84.70	84.52	84.55
Logistic regression	90.90	90.90	90.90	90.90	90.90	90.80	82.16	82.73
Course tree	90.90	90.89	90.90	90.90	90.90	90.89	90.90	90.90
Medium tree	90.91	90.88	90.87	90.89	90.86	90.78	90.78	90.86
Fine tree	90.89	90.84	90.87	90.87	90.54	90.47	90.54	90.58
Ensemble bagged tree	91.39	91.09	91.10	91.12	90.95	90.81	90.80	90.80
Ensemble boost tree	90.90	90.90	90.90	90.90	90.90	90.90	90.90	90.92
Linear SVM	90.90	90.90	90.90	90.90	90.90	90.90	90.90	90.90
Phonological Category				MULTICLASS				
Weighted k-NN	19.49	18.53	17.42	16.38	16.94	17.02	16.96	16.96
Cubic k-NN	17.8	37.46	37.6	37.56	27.48	27.47	27.62	27.47
Cosine k-NN	17.39	16.44	16.07	15.83	15.31	15.4	15.46	15.04
Course k-NN	16.96	16.93	16.84	16.99	14.38	14.2	14.27	14.41
Medium k-NN	18.11	17.16	16.48	16	15.39	15.16	15.49	15.39
Fine k-NN	18.61	17.35	16.5	15.41	16.53	16.5	16.54	16.37
Course tree	10.41	10.48	10.37	10.46	10.32	10.45	10.53	10.44
Medium tree	12.45	11.91	11.38	11.82	11.59	11.91	11.95	12.59
Fine tree	14.29	14.26	14.27	14.26	13.9	13.7	13.83	13.9
Ensemble bagged tree	25.19	19.94	18.68	18.03	20.18	20.29	20.24	19.91
Ensemble boost tree	12.96	12.57	12.53	12.58	11.82	11.7	12.1	11.88

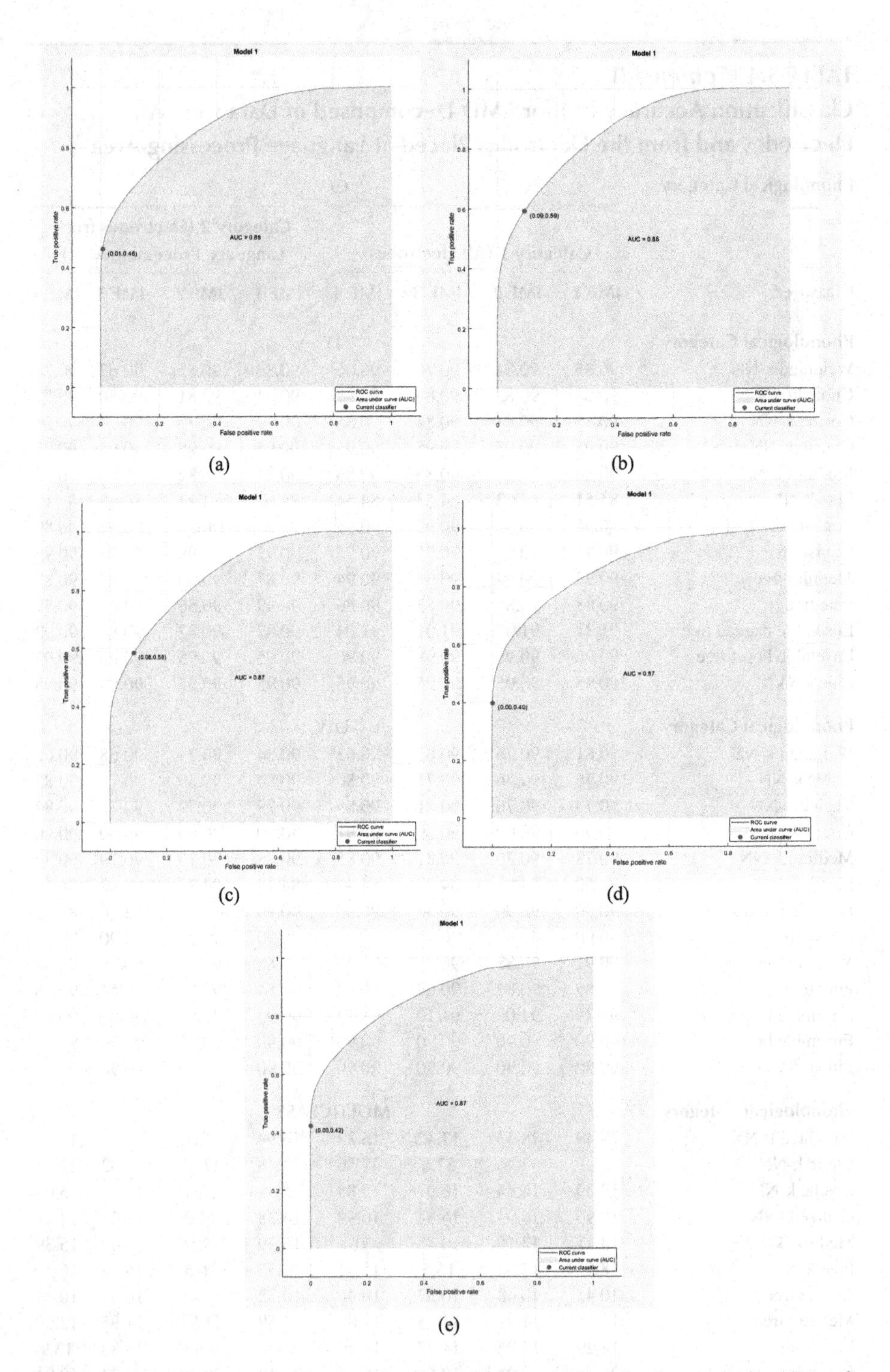

FIGURE 5.4 ROC curve for the classifier Ensemble Bagged Tree for the categories (a) vovel vs. consonant, (b) nasal, (c) bilab, (d) iy, and (e) uw

TABLE 5.5
Previous Results in Classification Accuracy (%)

Sr	Author	Method	c/v	Nasal	Bilab	Iy	Uw	Multi
1	Pengfei Sun [34]	DBN	87		–	–	82	–
		SVM	18	64	57	59	79	25
		NESG	41	74	71	76	87	58
2	[40]	SVM						50
		Dec tree						50
3	[45]	DBN						57
4	[43]		85.23	73.45	75.55	73.3	81.99	
5	[44]		89.16	78.33	81.67	87.20	85.00	
6	proposed		89.69	79.34	79.53	94.43	94.72	53.07

TABLE 5.6
Performance Parameters of the Best Classifier

	Performance Parameters			
Category	Accuracy (%)	Sensitivity (%)	Specificity (%)	Precision (%)
C/V	89.69	99.30	80.86	90.67
Nasal	79.34	90.88	59.25	72.64
Bilab	79.53	91.74	58.41	73.30
IY	94.43	99.86	39.81	96.18
UW	94.72	99.90	42.25	95.93

5.4 DISCUSSION AND CONCLUSION

Recognition of imagination word is a field of research for many researchers to assist the people suffering from neurological disorders and paralysis, i.e., complete locked-in state to communicate with their external environment. Keeping this thing in mind, we tried to recognize a task of the imagination of phonological categories and different words. This research work uses wavelet transform and EMD decomposition-based features for the binary and multiclass classification. The results from the different classifiers are analyzed, and it can be concluded that the ensemble bagged tree classifier is giving the best results for all the six categories, i.e., *C/V*, *nasal*, *bilab*, *iy*, *uw*, and multiclass. Bagging reduces the variance of a prediction by mixing various predictions from different models. This leads to improvement in the model efficiency and much stronger and accurate forecast. The highest classification accuracy for C/V, nasal, bilab, iy, uw, and multiclass is observed to be 89.69%, 79.34%, 79.53%, 94.43%, 94.72%, and 82.72%, respectively.

REFERENCES

1. S. K. Khare and V. Bajaj 2020 An evolutionary optimized Variational mode decomposition for emotion recognition, *IEEE Sensors Journal*, vol. 21, pp. 2035–2042.
2. J. Pearson, T. Naselaris, E. A. Holmes, and S. M. Kosslyn 2015 Mental imagery: Functional mechanisms and clinical applications, *Trends in Cognitive Sciences*, vol. 19, no. 10, pp. 590–602.
3. P. Indefrey and W.J.M. Levelt 2004 The spatial and temporal signatures of word production components, *Cognition*, vol. 92, pp. 101–144.
4. G. Hickok and D. Poeppel 2004 Dorsal and ventral streams: A framework for understanding aspects of the functional anatomy of language, *Cognition*, vol. 92, pp. 67–99.
5. G. Hickok and D. Poeppel 2007 The cortical organization of speech processing, *Nature Reviews Neuroscience*, vol. 8, pp. 393–402.
6. D. Poeppel, W.M.Idsardi and V. Wassenhove 2007 Speech perception at the interface of neurobiology and linguistics, *Philosophical Transactions of the Royal Society* B, vol. 363, pp. 1071–1086.
7. N. Kosmyna, J. T. Lindgren, and A. Lécuyer 2018 Attending to visual stimuli versus performing visual imagery as a control strategy for EEG-based brain-computer interfaces, *Scientific Reports*, vol. 8, no. 1, pp. 1–14.
8. L. F. Nicolas-Alonso and J. Gomez-Gil 2018 Brain computer interfaces, a review, *Sensors* vol. 12, no. 2, pp. 1211–1279.
9. E. T. Esfahani and V. Sundararajan 2012 Classification of primitive shapes using brain_ computer interfaces, *Computer-Aided Design*, vol. 44, no. 10, pp. 1011–1019.
10. V. Bajaj, S. Taran, S. K. Khare, and A. Sengur 2020 Feature extraction method for classification of alertness and drowsiness states EEG signals, *Applied Acoustics*, vol. 163, p. 107224.
11. S. K. Khare and V. Bajaj 2020 Time-frequency representation and convolutional neural network based emotion recognition, *IEEE Transactions on Neural Networks and Learning Systems*, pp. 1–9. In-press, DOI: 10.1109/TNNLS.2020.3008938.
12. S. Siuly, S. K. Khare, V. Bajaj, H. Wang and Y. Zhang 2020 A computerized method for automatic detection of schizophrenia using EEG signals, *IEEE Transactions on Neural Systems and Rehabilitation Engineering.* doi:10.1109/TNSRE.2020.3022715.
13. S. Taran, V. Bajaj, D. Sharma, S. Siuly, A. Sengur 2017 Features based on analytic IMF for classifying motor imagery EEG signals in BCI applications, *Measurement.* doi:10.1016/j.measurement.2017.10.067.
14. S. Taran and V. Bajaj 2018 Motor imagery tasks-based EEG signals classification using tunable Q wavelet transform, *Neural Computing and Applications.* doi:10.1007/s00521-018-3531.
15. S. K. Khare and V. Bajaj 2020 A facile and flexible motor imagery classification using electroencephalogram signals, *Computer Methods and Programs in Biomedicine*, vol. 197, p. 105722.
16. L. Sellami and T. Neubig 2019 Analysis of speech related EEG signals using emotivepoc+ headset, fast fourier transform, principal component analysis, and K-nearest neighbor methods, *International Journal of BiosenBioelectron*,vol. 5, no. 3, pp. 94–98. doi:10.15406/ijbsbe.2019.05.00160.
17. M. D 'Zmura, S. Deng, T. Lappas, S. Thorpe, and R. Srinivasan 2009 Toward EEG sensing of imagined speech. *International Conference on Human-Computer Interaction*, pp. 40–48.
18. K. Brigham and B. V. Kumar, 2010 Imagined speech classification with EEG signals for silent communication: A preliminary investigation into synthetic telepathy. *Proceedings of the 4th International Conference on Biomedical and Bioinformatics Engineering*, 2010, pp. 1–4.

19. N. E. Huang 2005 *Hilbert–Huang Transform and Its Applications*, Singapore: World Scientific.
20. S. Deng, R. Srinivasan, T. Lappas, and M. D'Zmura 2010 EEG classification of imagined syllable rhythm using Hilbert spectrum methods, *Journal of Neural Engineering*, vol. 7, no. 4, p. 046006.
21. C. S. DaSalla, H. Kambara, M. Sato, and Y. Koike 2009 Single-trial classification of vowel speech imagery using common spatial patterns, *Neural Networks*, vol. 22, no. 9, pp. 1334–1339.
22. A. Riaz, S. Akhtar, S. Iftikhar, A. A. Khan, and A. Salman, 2014 Inter comparison of classification techniques for vowel speech imagery using EEG sensors. *2nd International Conference on Systems and Informatics, ICSAI 2014*, pp. 712–717.
23. B. M. Idrees and O. Farooq, 2016 Vowel classification using wavelet decomposition during speech imagery. In *2016 3rd International Conference on Signal Processing and Integrated Networks (SPIN)*, Feb 2016, pp. 636–640.
24. N. Rehman and D. P. Mandic 2010 Multivariate empirical mode decomposition, *Proceedings of the Royal Society of London A*, vol. 466, pp. 1291–302.
25. H. Meng and L. Hualou 2012 Adaptive multiscale entropy analysis of multivariate neural data, *IEEE Transactions on Biomedical Engineering*, vol. 59, pp. 1–15.
26. J. Kim, S. K. Lee, and B. Lee 2014 EEG classification in a single-trial basis for vowel speech perception using multivariate empirical mode decomposition, *Journal of Neural Engineering*, vol. 11, no. 3, p. 036010.
27. X. Chi, J. B. Hagedorn, D. Schoonover, and M. D. Zmura 2011 EEG Based Discrimination of Imagined Speech Phonemes, *International Journal of Bioelectromagnetism*, vol. 13, no. 4, pp. 201–206.
28. C. H. Nguyen, G. K. Karavas, and P. Artemiadis 2017 Inferring imagined speech using EEG signals: A new approach using Riemannian manifold features, *Journal of Neural Engineering*, vol. 15, no. 1, p. 016002.
29. F. Lotte and C. Guan 2010 Regularizing common spatial patterns to improve BCI designs: Theory and algorithms, *IEEE Transactions on Biomedical Engineering*, vol. 58, no. 2, pp. 355–362.
30. M. N. I. Qureshi, B. Min, H. J. Park, D. Cho, W. Choi, and B. Lee 2018 Multiclass classification of word imagination speech with hybrid connectivity features, *IEEE Transactions on Biomedical Engineering*, vol. 65, no. 10, pp. 2168–2177, Oct. 2018.
31. K. Mohanchandra and S. Saha 2016 A communication paradigm using subvocalized speech: translating brain signals into speech, *Augmented Human Research*, vol. 1, no. 1, p. 3.
32. C. Cooney, R. Folli, and D. Coyle 2018 Mel frequency cepstral coefficients enhance imagined speech decoding accuracy from EEG, in *2018 29th Irish Signals and Systems Conference (ISSC)*. IEEE, pp. 1–7.
33. S. Zhao and F. Rudzicz 2015 Classifying phonological categories in imagined and articulated speech, in *ICASSP*, 2015. IEEE, pp. 992–996.
34. P. Sun and J. Qin 2017 Neural networks based EEG speech models, arXiv:1612.05369.
35. P. Saha, S. Fels, and M. Abdul-Mageed 2019 Deep learning the EEG manifold for phonological categorization from active thoughts, *ICASSP 2019-2019 IEEE International Conference on Acoustics, Speech and Signal Processing (ICASSP)*. IEEE, pp. 2762–2766.
36. P. Saha, M. Abdul-mageed and S. Fels 2019 SPEAK YOUR MIND! Towards Imagined Speech Recognition with Hierarchical Deep Learning, arXivPrepr. arXiv1801.05746V1, pp. 1–5.
37. J. T. Panachakel and T.V. Ananthapadmanabha 2019 Decoding imagined speech using wavelet features and deep neural networks, *IEEE 16th India Council International Conference (INDICON)*, 2019.

38. C. Cooney, A. Korik, R. Folli, D. Coyle 2019 Classification of imagined spoken word-pairs using convolutional neural networks, *Proceedings of the 8th Graz Brain-Computer Interface Conference 2019*. doi:10.3217/978-3-85125-682-6-62.
39. G. A. PresselCoretto, I. E. Gareis, and H. L. Rufiner 2017 Open access database of EEG signals recorded during imagined speech, *12th International Symposium on Medical Information Processing and Analysis*, p. 1016002.
40. C. Cooney, R. Folli, and D. Coyle 2019 Optimizing layers improves CNN generalization and transfer learning for imagined speech decoding from EEG, *2019 IEEE International Conference on Systems, Man and Cybernetics (SMC)*, Bari, Italy. October 6–9, 2019.
41. V. Bajaj and R. B. Pachori 2012 Classification of seizure and nonseizure EEG signals using empirical mode decomposition, *IEEE Transactions on Information Technology in Biomedicine*, vol. 16, no. 6, pp. 1135–1142.
42. A. Priya, P. Yadav, S. Jain, and V. Bajaj 2018 Efficient method for classification of alcoholic and normal EEG signals using EMD, *Journal of Engineering*, vol. 2018, no. 3, pp. 166–172. doi:10.1049/joe.2017.0878.
43. S. K. Khare and V. Bajaj 2020 Optimized tunable Q wavelet transform based drowsiness detection from electroencephalogram signals, *IRBM (2020)*. doi:10.1016/j.irbm.2020.07.005.
44. S. K. Khare, V. Bajaj and G. R. Sinha 2020 Adaptive tunable Q wavelet transform based emotion identification, *IEEE Transactions on Instrumentation and Measurement*. doi:10.1109/TIM.2020.3006611.
45. S. K. Khare, V. Bajaj, S. Siuly, and G. R. Sinha 2020 Classification of schizophrenia patients through empirical wavelet transformation using electroencephalogram signals. In V. Bajaj and G. R. Sinha (eds.) *Modelling and Analysis of Active Biopotential Signals in Healthcare*, vol. 1, ser. 2053–2563. Bristol: IOP Publishing, pp. 1–26.
46. S. K. Khare and V. Bajaj 2020 Constrained based tunable Q wavelet transform for efficient decomposition of EEG signals, *Applied Acoustics*, vol. 163, p. 107234.
47. T. Gandhi, B. K. Panigrahi and S. Anand 2011 A comparative study of wavelet families for EEG signal classification", *Neurocomputing*, vol. 74 (17), pp. 3051–3057.
48. N. E. Huang, Z. Shen, S. R. Long, M. C. Wu, H. H. Shih, Q. Zheng, N. C. Yen, C. C. Tung and Liu H H 1998 The empirical mode decomposition and the Hilbert spectrum for nonlinear and non-stationary time series analysis, *Proceedings of the. Royal Society A London*. doi:10.1098/rspa.1998.0193.
49. G. Rilling, P. Flandrin, and P. Goncalves 2003 On empirical mode decomposition and its algorithms. *Proceedings of the IEEE-EURASIP Workshop on Nonlinear Signal and Image Processing NSIP-03*, Grado, Italy, 8–11 June 2003.
50. Y. S. Lee, S. Tsakirtzis, A.F. Vakakis, L. A. Bergman, and D. M. McFarlan 2009 Physics-based foundation for empirical mode decomposition, *AIAA Journals*, vol. 47, pp. 2938–2963.
51. T. Alotaiby, F. E. Abd El-Samie, S. A. Alshebeili, and I. Ahmad 2015 A review of channel selection algorithm for EEG signal processing, *EURASIP Journal on Advances in Signal Processing*, vol. 2015, p. 66. doi: 10.1186/s13634-015-0251-9.
52. A. Phinyomark, P. Phukpattaranont, and C. Limsakul 2012 Feature reduction and selection for EMG signal classification, *Expert Systems with Applications*, vol. 39, pp. 7420–7431.
53. B. Hudgins, P. Parker, and R. N. Scott 1993 A new strategy for multifunction myoelectric control. *IEEE Transaction on Biomedical. Engineering*, vol. 40, no. 1, pp. 82–94.
54. W. T. Shi, Z. J. Lyu, S. T. Tang, T. L. Chia, and C. Y. Yang 2018 A bionic hand controlled by hand gesture recognition based on surface EMG signals: A preliminary study, *Biocybernetics and Biomedical Engineering*, vol. 38, no. 1, pp. 126–135.

55. D. Tkach, H. Huang, and T. A. Kuiken 2010 Study of stability of time domain features for electromyographic pattern recognition, *Journal of NeuroEngineering and Rehabilitation*, vol. 7, p. 21.
56. K. S. Kim, H. H. Choi, C. S. Moon, and C. W. Mun 2011 Comparison of k-nearest neighbor, quadratic discriminant and linear discriminant analysis in classification of electromyogram signals based on the wrist-motion directions, *Current Applied Physics*, vol. 11, no. 3, pp. 740–745.
57. T. Jingwei, R. A. Abdul, and M. S. Norhashimah 2019 Classification of hand movements based on discrete wavelet transform and enhanced feature extraction, *International Journal of Advanced Computer Science and Applications (IJACSA)*, vol. 10, no 6, 83–89.
58. S. L. Ullo, S. K. Khare, V. Bajaj, and G. R. Sinha 2020 Hybrid computerized method for environmental sound classification, *IEEE Access*, vol. 8, pp. 124055–124065.
59. S. K. Khare, V. Bajaj, and G. R. Sinha 2020 Automatic drowsiness detection based on variational nonlinear chirp mode decomposition using electroencephalogram signals, *Modelling and Analysis of Active Biopotential Signals in Healthcare*, vol. 1, pp. 5.1–5.25.
60. S. Taran, S. K. Khare, V. Bajaj, and G. R. Sinha, 2020 Classification of motor-imagery tasks from EEG signals using rational dilation wavelet transform. In: V. Bajaj and G. R. Sinha (eds.) *Modelling and Analysis of Active Biopotential Signals in Healthcare*, vol. 2, ser. 2053–2563. Bristol: IOP Publishing, pp. 1–14.
61. L. Breiman. 2001 Random forests, *Machine Learning*, vol. 45, no. 1, pp. 5–32.

6 Blood Pressure Monitoring Using Photoplethysmogram and Electrocardiogram Signals

Jamal Esmaelpoor
Islamic Azad University

Zahra Momayez Sanat
Tehran University of Medical Sciences

Mohammad Hassan Moradi
Amirkabir University of Technology

CONTENTS

6.1 INTRODUCTION

Cardiovascular disorders are condemned as the death cause of almost 50% of all people who die due to noncommunicable diseases [1]. Since blood pressure (BP) is one of the most important physiological parameters that reflect cardiovascular status, its continuous monitoring provides crucial information on an individual's health situation. It can be a true indicator of such problems as hypertension, asthma, heart attack, and chronic kidney diseases [2].

Several methods are available for BP monitoring. The main approaches are intra-arterial catheter insertion, auscultation, oscillometry, tonometry, and volume clamping [3].

Catheter insertion, which is known as the gold standard, was practiced for the first time in 1901 by Cushing in surgery rooms. This method provides an accurate reading of the beat-to-beat blood pressure, and it is suitable for patients who need constant monitoring of BP because of sudden changes, for instance, during vascular surgery or for those who receive medication to stabilize their BPs. Despite the accurate and continuous reading of BP that this method provides, due to its invasive nature, its application is limited to healthcare centers and for those patients who require very close monitoring [4]. Moreover, besides the pain and practical difficulties of this technique, the insertion of the cannula can cause infection and bleeding.

Auscultation and oscillometry are noninvasive methods that employ an inflatable cuff. Nicolai Korotkoff – a Russian army surgeon – invented Auscultation in 1905. In this approach, a cuff is closed around the brachial artery on the upper arm, and then, a mercury sphygmomanometer is used to measure pressure in the cuff. With the help of a stethoscope, a series of sounds are audible over the squeezed artery during the deflation, and the systolic and diastolic blood pressures are measured accordingly [5].

Marey introduced oscillometry in 1876 for the first time. In this method, the BP measurement is based on the detection of oscillations of the inflatable cuff during deflation. A pressure sensor inside the cuff detects these oscillations. As the pressure declines, the amplitude of the oscillations increases to a maximum that indicates mean arterial pressure. Then, the computer uses an algorithm designated by the manufacturing company to estimate diastolic and systolic blood pressures [6]. Although these noninvasive methods provide us with acceptable readings, since they are restricted to some minutes of intervals between two successive readings, they cause discomfort and fail to provide continuous monitoring.

To overcome these problems, many studies have concentrated on the topic in recent past years, and many commercial devices are introduced to the market to make blood pressure measurement continuously and noninvasively possible. Most of them are based on two techniques of applanation tonometry and volume clamping of the radial artery [7,8].

Applanation tonometry provides a reproducible and precise waveform of the aortic pressure noninvasively. Tonometry means measuring the pressure, while applanation refers to flatten. Radial artery applanation tonometry utilizes a portable tonometer (strain gouge pressure sensor, for instance) over the radial artery to flatten its surface by applying mild pressure. Then, the sensor measures the radial artery pressure. To calculate the central pressure from peripheral brachial blood pressure, some mathematical calculations should be applied to the measured pressure [9].

Volume clamping measures instant BP by employing a cuff and photoplethysmography sensor to maintain blood volume throughout the cardiac cycle. Multiple digital feedback loops control the pressure system to keep the blood flow constant. In this situation, the applied cuff pressure reveals BP [3].

Although tonometry and volume clamping techniques are noninvasive and provide a continuous reading of BP, they are most of the time too expensive and too complex to use. Therefore, their applications are restricted mostly to research environments.

Consequently, all these methods are invasive, noncontinuous, or manual. Therefore, many studies try to use some easy-access signals like photoplethysmogram (PPG) and electrocardiogram (ECG) to provide an ultra-convenient, cheap, and unintrusive method for continuous blood pressure monitoring. Here, we revise the theoretical background and proposed methods to achieve this goal.

6.2 PHYSIOLOGICAL MODELS

Photoplethysmography is an optical method to identify blood volume changes caused by the pressure pulse in the peripheral circulation system. This volume change is measured by illuminating the skin by the light from a light-emitting diode, and then, the transmitted or reflected light is detected by a photodetector [10]. Moreover, electrocardiography is the method of detecting electrical activities of the heart using electrodes placed on the skin. These electrical signals reveal the electrical excitations of the heart muscles during their depolarization and repolarization in each cardiac cycle [11]. Therefore, both ECG and PPG signals contain crucial information related to the cardiovascular system that is our system of interest for BP monitoring. This section provides a physiological model for blood pressure estimation.

6.2.1 BP Estimation Based on Pulse Transit Time

Pulse transit time (PTT) indicates the time for the pressure pulse to travel through vessels. In Figure 6.1a, the pressure pulse propagation is shown as the acute expansion of the arterial wall. Figure 6.1b also indicates that PTT is inversely correlated to BP and can be determined easily from the delay between proximal and distal arterial pulse waveforms. Therefore, PTT could make automatic, noninvasive, and cuff-less BP monitoring possible [3].

To find out the relationship between blood pressure and PTT, we employ a basic model for arterial wave propagation. Figure 6.2 shows the arterial vessel as a flexible and cylindrical tube. We neglect the viscous effects. Therefore, both wall viscosity and resistance against blood current are negligible. These assumptions are more realistic for central and peripheral arteries. The elasticity of the vessel is determined using compliance C, which is defined as the ratio between cross-section area changes and pressure changes (i.e., $C = {}^{dA}\!/_{dP}$). Compliance is defined by the tube geometry and the elastic modulus of the tube E. For a cylindrical tube, and by assuming

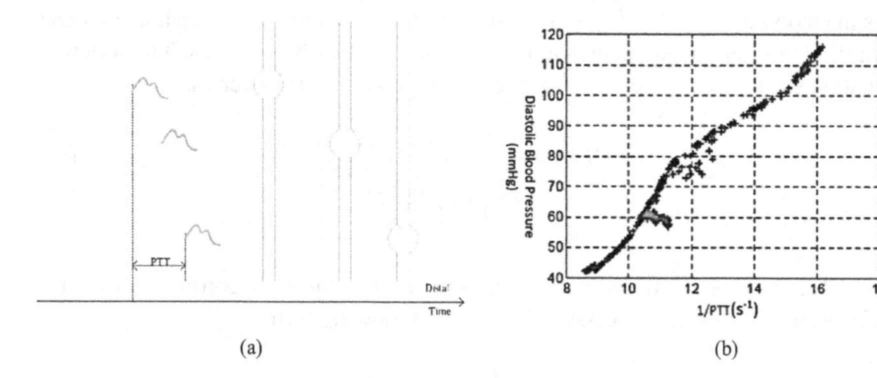

(a) (b)

FIGURE 6.1 (a) Pulse transit time (PTT) as the time delay for the pressure wave to travel a distance can be estimated from the timing between proximal and distal arterial waveforms; (b) the relationship between PTT and blood pressure. (Reproduced from [3] with permission.)

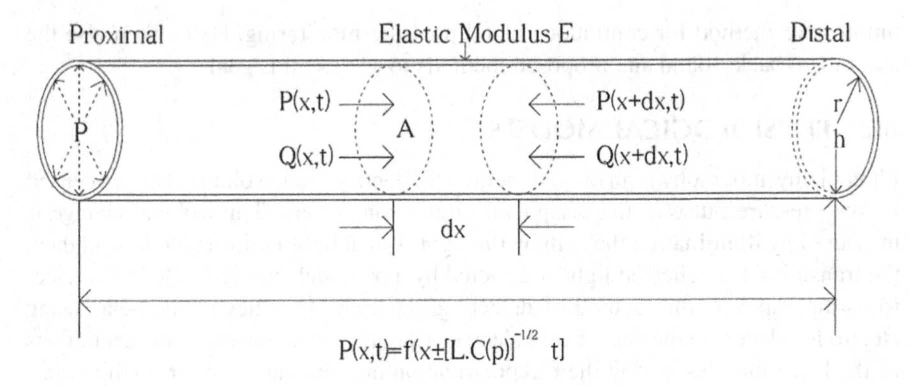

FIGURE 6.2 Wave propagation model in a central artery. (Reproduced from [3] with permission.)

constant E, Laplace's law defines $C = {2\pi r^3}/{(E.h)}$, where r is radial, and h is the wall thickness. Of course, elasticity (E) is not unique and is related to P as follows:

$$E(P) = E_0 \cdot e^{\alpha P} \tag{6.1}$$

where E_0 and α are positive and subject-specific parameters.

If the variations in A are negligible, the following equations result from applying the mass and momentum conservation rule:

$$\frac{d(Adx)}{dt} + Q(x) - Q(x+dx) = 0 \rightarrow \frac{\partial Q}{\partial x} + C(P) \cdot \frac{\partial P}{\partial t} = 0 \tag{6.2a}$$

$$A \cdot \left[P(x) - P(x+dx)\right] = \rho \cdot dx \frac{dQ}{dt} \rightarrow \frac{\partial P}{\partial x} + L \cdot \frac{\partial Q}{\partial t} = 0 \tag{6.2b}$$

In these equations, t and x refer to time and space, Q indicates volume flow rate, ρ is the blood density, $L = {\rho}/{A}$ is a constant that equals the arterial inertance for each unit of length, and C is dependent on P. C increases as P decreases. The following equation shows the relationship between C and P for central arteries.

$$C(P) = \frac{A_m}{\pi P_1 \left[1 + \left(\frac{P - P_0}{P_1}\right)^2\right]} \tag{6.3}$$

Here, A_m, P_0, and P_1 should be specified for each subject. According to Equation (6.2), pressure pulse in the vessel takes on the following form:

$$P(x,t) = f\left(x \pm {t}/{\sqrt{LC(P)}}\right) \tag{6.4}$$

Therefore, the velocity of the propagation known as *pulse wave velocity* (PWV) equals $\left[L \cdot C(P)\right]^{-1/2}$. Since C and P are inversely related (Equation 6.3), the pressure wave peak moves faster which could cause pressure discontinuity. The time for the wave to pass a length of l (PTT) is

$$\text{PTT} = l\sqrt{LC(P)} \tag{6.5}$$

As a result, considering the above hypotheses, PTT and BP are related to each other in an inverse relationship.

If we consider C as a constant, then PWV equation reduces to

$$\text{PWV} = \frac{1}{\sqrt{L \cdot C}} = \sqrt{\frac{AdP}{\rho dA}} = \sqrt{\frac{Eh}{2r\rho}} \tag{6.6}$$

These equations are known as Bramwell-Hill and Moens-Korteweg equations [3].

The real arterial system is not a mere tube. It has tapers, branches, and terminates with microvessels. The wave reflects in all sites of impedance mismatch, but it is most prominent at the arterial terminations. Figure 6.3a shows a vessel with a terminal

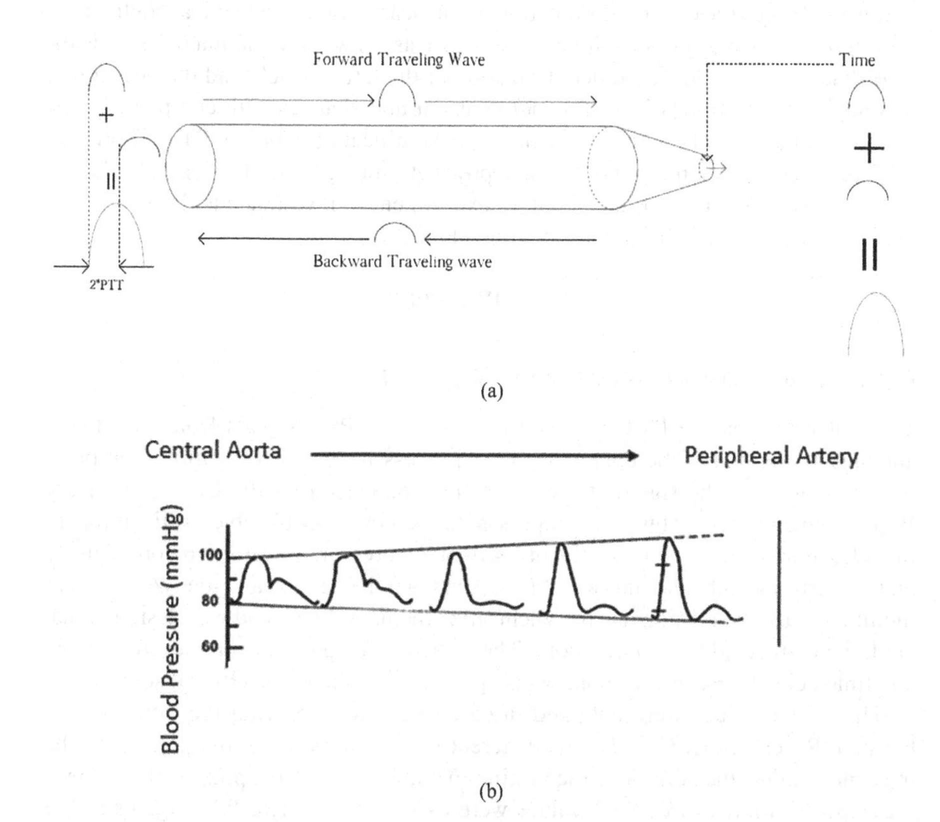

FIGURE 6.3 (a) A tube model with a terminal reflection site predicts that the BP waveform will be amplified when its distance increases from the heart. (b) Experimental BP waveforms that confirm these predictions. (Reproduced from [3] with permission.)

load of a microvessel. As the heart beats, a pressure wave starts traveling inside the tube. When it arrives at the tube end, part of the wave is reflected. Therefore, the BP waveform at a given site amplifies as the sum of these two components which enhances the amplitude of the waveform. This amplification has much less effect on the central pressure pulse. As a result, the pressure pulse should become more amplified when the distance from the heart increases. Figure 6.3b shows some experimental data indicating the higher amplification for waves when they become further away from the heart [3].

6.3 PULSE ARRIVAL TIME INSTEAD OF PULSE TRANSIT TIME

As it is described in the previous section, PTT can make continuous, noninvasive, and cuff-less BP monitoring possible. Some studies, however, propose to make the process even simpler by considering the time delay between the R-wave in ECG and the distal arterial pressure waveform instead of PTT. This time interval that is known as pulse arrival time (PAT) has attracted a lot of attention recently [12–14]. Since R-wave indicates the electrical excitation of the heart, not its mechanical contraction, PAT equals PTT plus pre-ejection period (PEP), as shown in Equation 6.7. PEP is the time delay between electrical depolarization of the left ventricle and the occurrence of ventricular ejection [15]. PEP is not constant and changes with contractility and afterload, and most of the time, constituting a significant fraction of PTT. Therefore, PAT, on the contrary, might not be an appropriate surrogate for PTT as an indicator of BP. Afterwards, we will carry out an experiment to investigate and compare the performance of these two important parameters.

$$\mathrm{PAT} = \mathrm{PTT} + \mathrm{PEP} \tag{6.7}$$

6.3.1 Performance Comparison: PAT vs. PTT

To be able to measure PTT, we need to record two PPG signals from two different sites of the body. The data acquisition process for our investigation took place in ICU units, and the signals were taken from patients after the Coronary Artery Bypass Surgery. The dataset encompasses 32 records from 14 subjects. Each record includes four signals: one ECG, the invasive blood pressure waveform recorded using an intra-arterial catheter, and two PPGs taken from the earlobe and toe. We used two monitors to record all signals. To synchronize them, an ECG lead was designed that could be connected to two monitors. Then, the ECG signal was employed to avoid any time delay between two monitors [16]. Figure 6.4 shows the clinical set-up.

Three PAT values were obtained in each cycle by measuring the time interval between R-peak in ECG and three different points on the PPG: the point with the maximum value, the point with the minimum amplitude, and the point with the highest slope. Similarly, three PTT values were extracted from two PPG signals of toe and earlobe based on three points with the highest amplitude, lowest amplitude, and the biggest slope on the waveforms. Figure 6.5 shows the definition of each of these parameters.

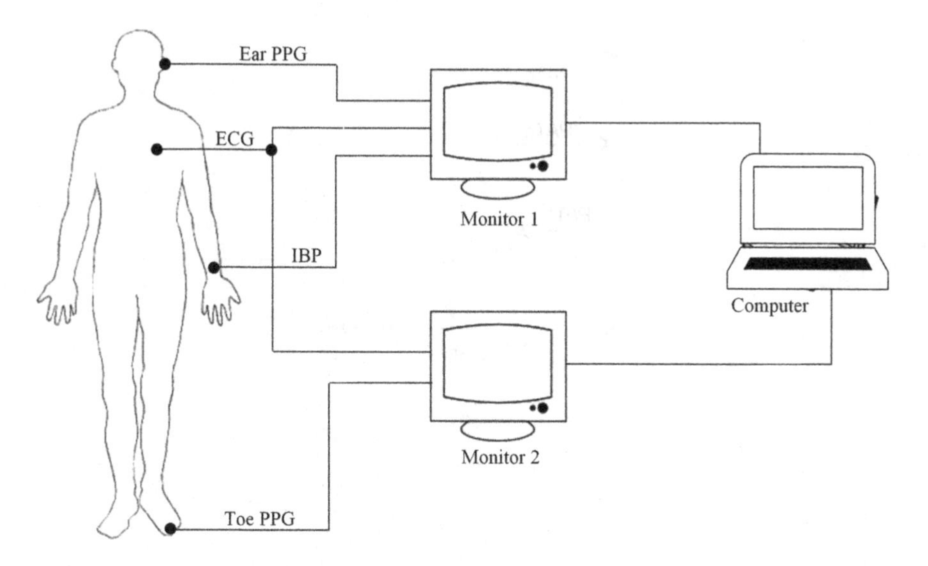

FIGURE 6.4 The clinical set-up to acquire data to compare PAT and PTT performance in BP estimation.

To estimate blood pressure based on PAT and PTT, the following models were considered:

$$BP = a_1 + \frac{a_2}{PAT^2} + a_3 \times BP_0 + a_4 \times HR \quad (6.8)$$

$$BP = a_1 + \frac{a_2}{PTT^2} + a_3 \times BP_0 + a_4 \times HR \quad (6.9)$$

where BP_0 is the primary blood pressure for each record, and HR is the heart rate measured per minute from R-R interval in ECG signal (Figure 6.5a).

After processing the raw data, 70% of cycles in each record were used for training, and 30% for testing. The Levenberg-Marquardt algorithm is utilized to find the parameters in each model and estimate BP from extracted features. The Levenberg–Marquardt algorithm (LMA) is a method to find the optimum solution of nonlinear least-square problems. Even though LMA, similar to the Gauss–Newton approach, is designed to solve an optimization problem without calculating the Hessian matrix, it is more robust. It means that in many cases, it can find the optimum point even if it starts far from the final desired destination [17].

Numerical results for all three possible PATs reveal a better performance for PAT measured as the time difference between R wave in ECG and the peak of the toe-PPG signal. Similarly, the BP estimation with the highest accuracy among the three possible choices of PTT was achieved by using the time difference between the peaks of two PPG signals. Table 6.1 presents the best results for both PAT and PTT based on the standard deviation (STD) and the root-mean-square of errors (RMSE) for the estimations of systolic and diastolic blood pressures in each cycle.

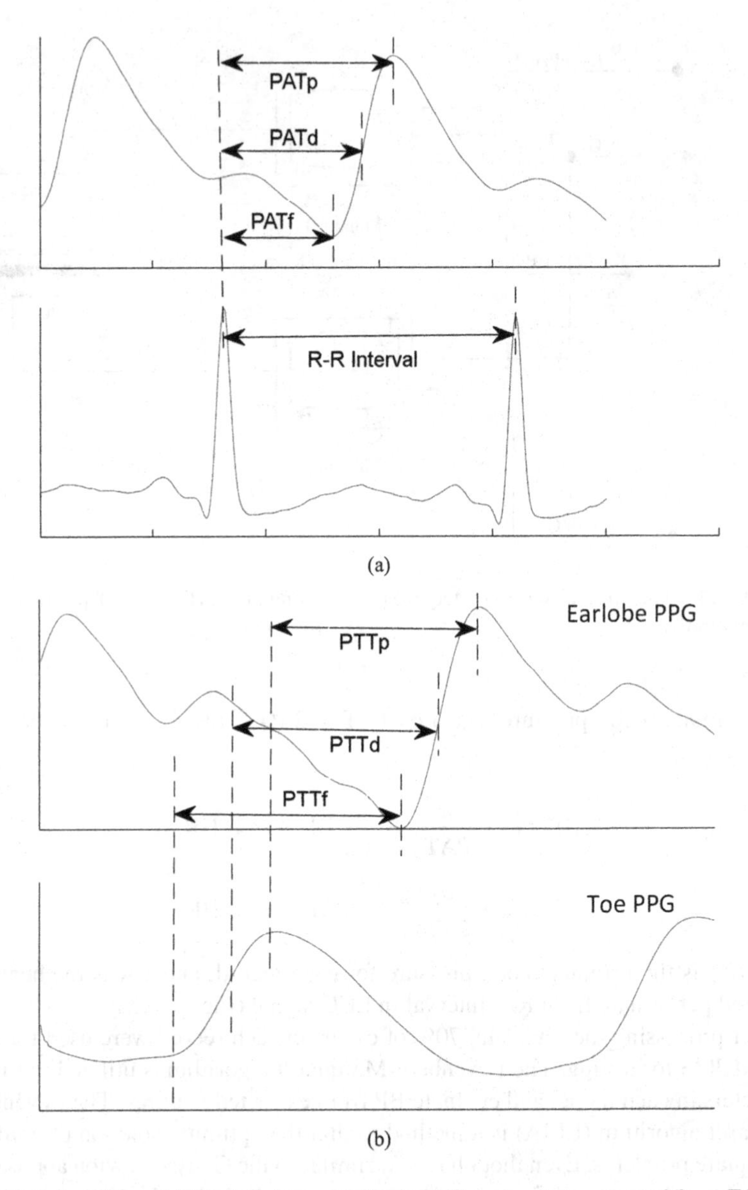

FIGURE 6.5 PAT and PTT definition. (a) Three PAT parameters extracted from ECG and PPG and (b) three PTT parameters extracted from two PPGs recorded from toe and earlobe.

These results show that PTT and its inverse are significantly superior to PAT and its reciprocal in BP prediction. The RMSE values for PTT are 3.75 and 1.59 mmHg for systolic and diastolic BPs, whereas the corresponding values for PAT are 4.43 and 1.96 mmHg. This experiment indicates that the contribution of PEP to PAT is considerable. Therefore, the use of the PAT instead of PTT as a marker of the vascular function for BP monitoring should be avoided [18].

TABLE 6.1
Best Results for BP Estimation Based on PTT and PAT Parameters

BP	Parameter	RMSE	STD
Systolic	PTT	3.75	2.33
	PAT	4.43	2.78
Diastolic	PTT	1.59	0.81
	PAT	1.96	0.93

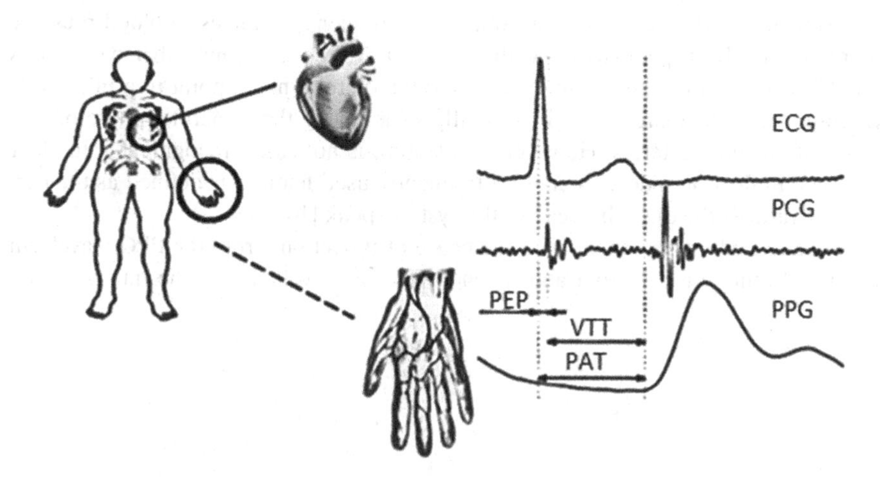

FIGURE 6.6 The vascular transit time (VTT) is the time difference between the first heart sound in PCG and the peak amplitude of the PPG signal at a finger. Like PTT, PEP is removed from all time-related measurements based on VTT.

Besides using two PPGs to measure PTT accurately, another approach is to use phonocardiography (PCG) instead of ECG. PCG can be considered as the graphical representation of the heart sounds. Due to the method used to record PCG, it is shown that the time-related parameters extracted from PCG are not distorted by PEP. Therefore, some studies utilize the transmission time delay between the first heart sound (S1) in PCG and the upstroke of PPG that is known as vascular transit time (VTT) for BP estimation [19]. Figure 6.6 shows measured VTT based on the PCG signal and a PPG waveform recorded from a finger.

6.4 BP ESTIMATION APPROACHES BASED ON PPG AND ECG

Cuffless blood pressure estimations based on ECG and PPG signals can be categorized into two different groups. One group includes those algorithms that rely on the manually extracted features such as PTT and PAT, while some are based on machine-learning algorithms for both automatic feature extraction and BP estimation from the signals.

Feature extraction refers to the reduction of the number of required resources to describe a set of data. During carrying out complex data analysis, one of the critical problems that might arise is the high number of variables involved. Besides computational difficulties and the necessity of a large amount of memory, too many variables may cause an algorithm to overfit training samples, and therefore, generalize poorly to new data. Feature engineering is a common term for constructing variables to tackle these problems while still describing the original data with sufficient accuracy [20].

PTT, HR, and PAT are among the most common features used in the literature [21,22]. Besides, many studies have defined other features to improve the accuracy of the estimation procedures. For example, as shown in Figure 6.7, pulse intensity ratio is defined as the peak intensity divided by the valley intensity $\left(\mathrm{PIR} = {}^{I_H}\!/_{I_L}\right)$. It is shown that this indicator can follow low-frequency changes in blood pressure more effectively in comparison with PTT [23]. Moreover, many other parameters are defined based on the diastolic peak and the dicrotic notch point in a PPG cycle (Figure 6.8a). The dicrotic notch is usually seen during the catacrotic phase of persons with healthy arteries. However, this feature is not easily recognizable in older subjects. Reflection index, as another frequently used feature, is defined as the percentage ratio of the diastolic peak to the systolic peak [10].

Since to find out the changes in the phase of inflections from the PPG waveform is difficult, many use its first and second derivatives to facilitate the interpretation

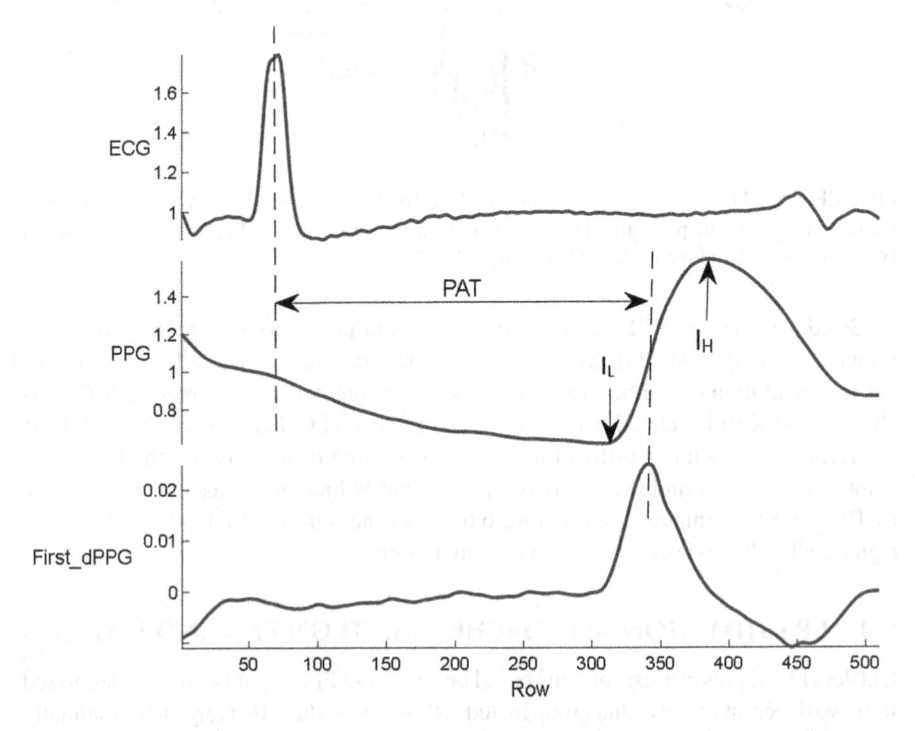

FIGURE 6.7 Pulse intensity ratio that is defined as the peak intensity divided by the valley intensity is shown to be more effective than PTT in tracking long-term variations in BP.

of the main PPG waveform [7,24]. Figure 6.8 shows the original PPG waveform and its first and second derivatives. The second derivative of PPG that is also known as acceleration plethysmogram is used more frequently in the literature to estimate some physiological parameters like arterial stiffness, aging, screening of arterio-sclerotic disease, and vascular performance. Figure 6.9 shows the most important

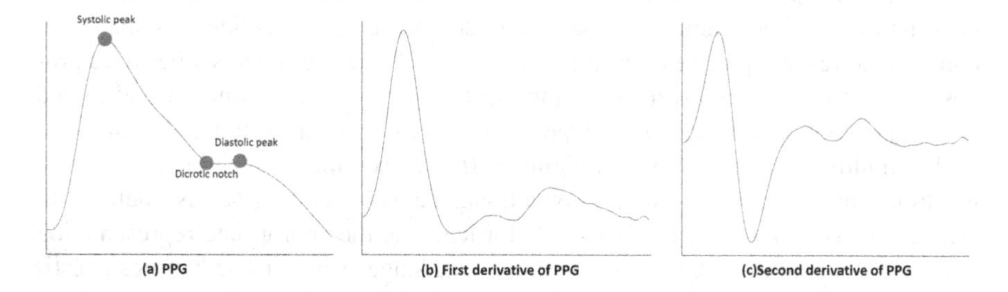

FIGURE 6.8 Besides PPG, its first and second derivatives are also used to extract many features for BP monitoring. (a) PPG waveform and some important points to define several features, (b) its first derivative, and (c) its second derivative.

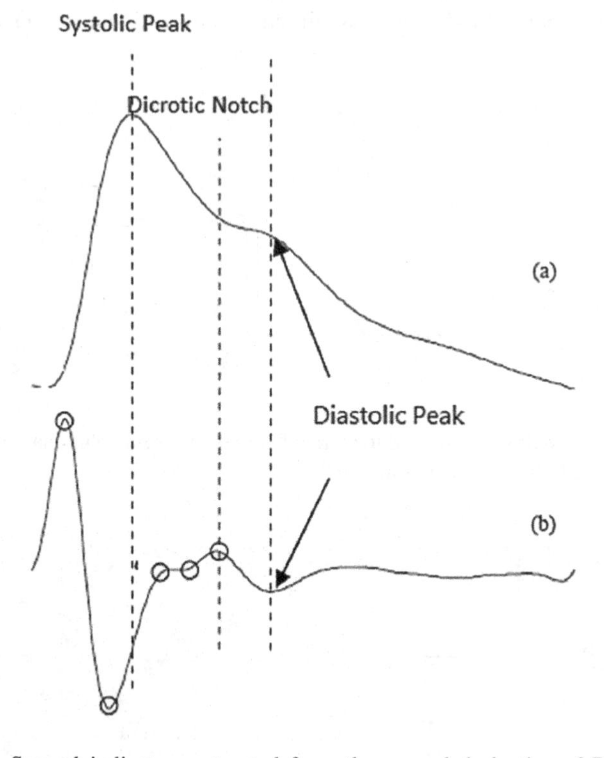

FIGURE 6.9 Several indicators extracted from the second derivative of PPG waveform (acceleration plethysmogram) are used to estimate some physiological parameters. (a) PPG waveform and (b) important points on the acceleration plethysmogram.

points in the waveform. In Section 6.4.1, we will discuss several of these handcrafted (manually extracted) features in more detail.

Although handcrafted features take advantage of human's prior knowledge in the issue and their ingenuity, it is highly recommended to make the learning approach less dependent on feature engineering to facilitate the application of machine learning and ease the way toward artificial intelligence [25]. Moreover, the reality that the shape of PPG might change considerably due to aging and some diseases highlights a restriction of using handcrafted features. These factors can make the extraction of some handcrafted features less precise or even impossible [2]. Therefore, some studies have proposed automatic feature extraction using machine learning techniques or end-to-end learning to represent the complete target system to carry out the estimation [26].

The multistage model shown in Figure 6.10 is an example of a model that extracts machine-learned features using convolutional neural networks (CNN) before BP estimation. The first stage is responsible for learning the appropriate representation of the input signal using CNNs, while the second stage utilizes these features to estimate both systolic and diastolic blood pressures using two long short-term memory (LSTM) networks [2]. CNNs have been successfully used in learning hierarchical representations of various datasets. LSTM networks are also very effective in capturing temporal dependencies.

Figure 6.11 also shows an end-to-end approach based on deep artificial neural networks to estimate blood pressures directly using PPG and ECG signals as its

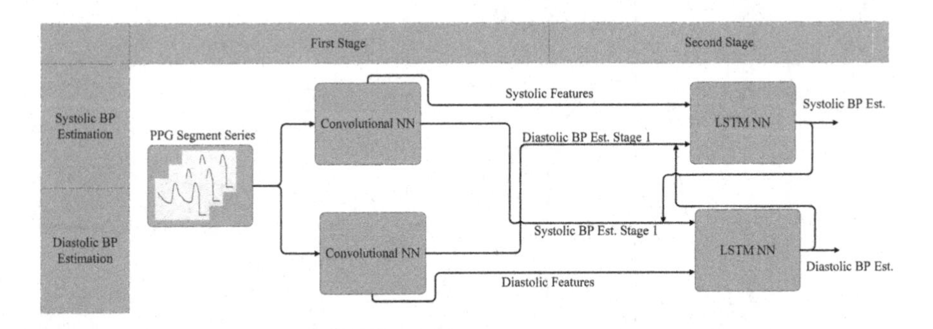

FIGURE 6.10 A multistage method to extract features using convolutional feature extractor and then estimate BPs using LSTM network.

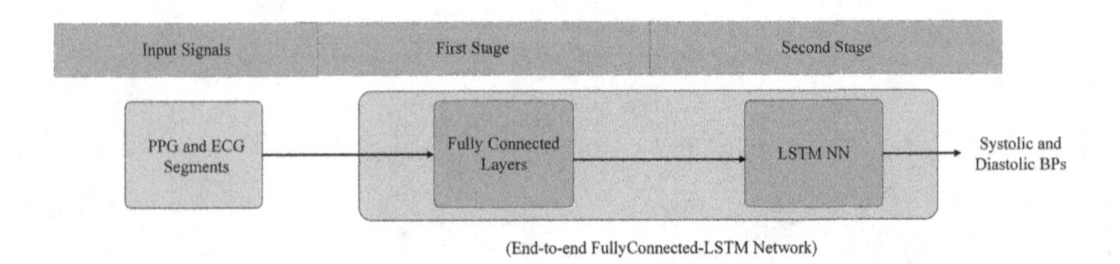

FIGURE 6.11 An end-to-end approach based on deep neural networks to monitor BP directly using PPG and ECG signals as its inputs.

inputs. The proposed architecture encompasses some fully connected layers in its lower hierarchy and LSTM layers in the upper hierarchy [27].

In the following two subsections, we propose and implement two sample methods for blood pressure estimation based on ECG and PPG signals. The first method is based on several handcrafted features that are frequently used in the literature. The second model, though, is an end-to-end approach based on LSTM deep neural networks. It takes raw signals after applying some preprocessing steps and provides BP estimations directly.

6.4.1 Estimation Based on Manual Features

Here, we extract several handcrafted features from some records and then use ensemble regression to estimate diastolic and systolic BP. The model steps are described as follows:

- **Data source:** We have selected 50 records from the Multiparameter Intelligent Monitoring in Intensive Care II (MIMIC-II) that is publicly available. Each record includes one PPG, one ECG, and invasive BP. Their sampling frequency is 125 Hz. Selected records include 14,508 cycles.
- **Preprocessing steps:** We up-sampled signals to 250 Hz to enhance time-domain accuracy. To alleviate different artifacts, for example, baseline wandering and respiratory components in low frequencies and electromyogram distortions and power-line harmonics in higher frequencies, a band-pass filter is applied to PPG and ECG signals to choose 0.48–40 Hz bandwidth. Moreover, since the quasi-DC component of PPG contains vital information about the average blood volume, we have also applied a narrow-band low-pass filter to retain this information [2,10]. We also carried out data normalization before extracting handcrafted features to let them have the same range. Since QRS complex occurrences are referred to as time references in the manual feature extraction procedure, we also detected them using a method introduced in [28]. The approach does not employ threshold or derivative operations like many other similar methods. However, the approach is inspired by the wide similarities between the ECG waveform and the integrated linear prediction residual (ILPR) in vocal signals [28]. Figure 6.12 summarizes all steps to preprocess ECG and PPG signals.
- **Feature extraction:** Twelve frequently used features are extracted from processed ECG, PPG, and PPG derivatives [7,23,29]. Three of them are HR, PIR, and PATp (PAT defined based on the peak amplitude) that were defined before. The rest are defined based on the points shown on the waveforms in Figure 6.13 as follows. We extracted each of them from both PPG and its first and second derivatives.

$$\text{AA} = \sum_{i=T(\text{Valley1})}^{T(\text{peak})} \left(I(i) - I(\text{Valley1})\right) \tag{6.10}$$

$$\text{DA} = \sum_{i=T(\text{Peak})}^{T(\text{Valley2})} \left(I(i) - I(\text{Valley2})\right) \tag{6.11}$$

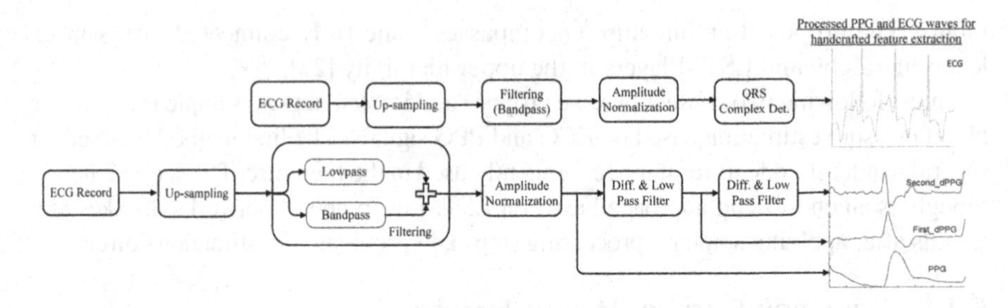

FIGURE 6.12 Preprocessing steps before manual feature extraction.

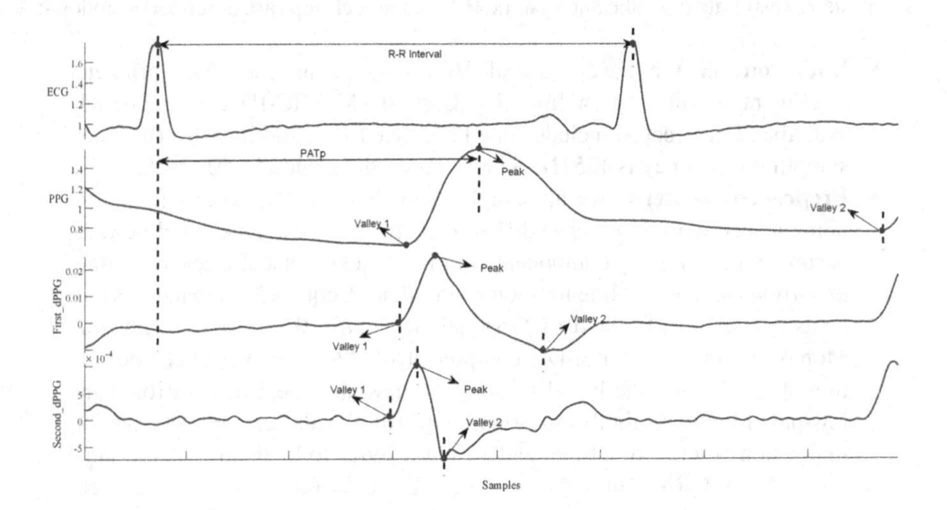

FIGURE 6.13 Critical points for manual feature extraction from ECG and PPG and its derivatives.

$$\mathrm{DS} = \frac{\Delta I}{\Delta T} = \frac{\left| I(\mathrm{Peak}) - I(\mathrm{Valley2}) \right|}{\left| T(\mathrm{Valley2}) - T(\mathrm{Peak}) \right|} \tag{6.12}$$

In these equations, *I(.)* identifies the amplitude of a point and *T(.)* indicates the time of an occurrence in the signal.

- **Estimation model:** The manually extracted features are applied to two tree-based ensemble regressors to estimate diastolic and systolic BPs (Figure 6.14). We can extend the variable importance in decision trees by using tree-based ensemble models. The purpose of an ensemble model is to combine the prediction of some base estimators to improve robustness [30].
- **Results:** We divided each record into three separate parts of training, validation, and testing sections claiming 60%, 15%, and 30% of cycles in each record, respectively. Table 6.2 shows the precision of the regression model based on extracted features. The results are presented based

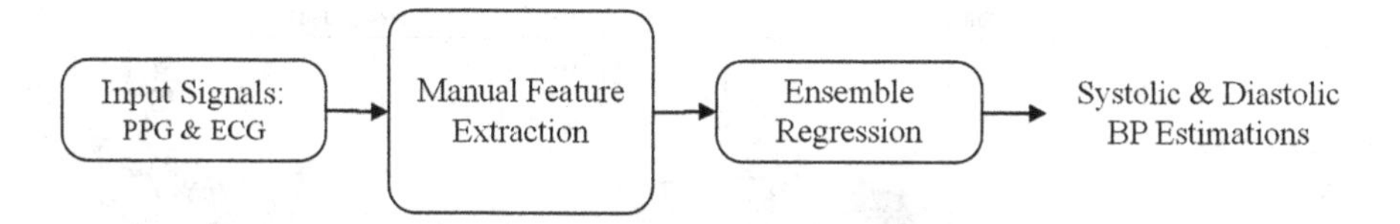

FIGURE 6.14 Block diagram representation of different steps of the proposed algorithm for BP estimation based on handcrafted features.

TABLE 6.2
Performance Comparison of the Two Algorithms

Method	Blood Pressure	RMSE (mmHg)	ME (mmHg)	STD (mmHg)
Manual features and Regression	Systolic	9.04	0.79	9.00
	Diastolic	4.12	−0.01	4.12
End-to-end method based on LSTM	Systolic	6.41	−0.61	6.38
	Diastolic	2.19	−0.11	3.17

on root-mean-square error, absolute error, and standard deviation of error. Figure 6.15 also depicts regression plots of the algorithm for systolic and diastolic BP estimations. Even though the reported errors in Table 6.2 for systolic BP are considerably higher than those of diastolic BP, the correlation coefficient (reported in Figure 6.15) between the estimated values and target values are higher for systolic BP. To interpret these seemingly contradictory statements, we should consider that the correlation coefficient that is defined in Equation (6.13) is based on relative variations, not absolute ones.

$$R(X,Y) = \frac{\operatorname{cov}(X,Y)}{\sigma_X \cdot \sigma_Y} \tag{6.13}$$

6.4.2 End-to-End Estimation Based on LSTM Networks

As we mentioned earlier, besides the feature engineering approach (for instance, the model in Section 6.4.1), we can propose models to extract features automatically or even without feature extraction and based on an end-to-end approach. Here, we introduce an end-to-end method based on long short-term memory to estimate diastolic and systolic BPs directly from waveforms after applying several preprocessing steps. More details and the implementation results are discussed in the following text:

- **Preprocessing steps:** Applied preprocessing steps are shown in Figure 6.16. The main difference between this method and the processing steps of the model based on the manual features is that we now divide signals into segments. The time interval of each segment is defined by the R-R interval in

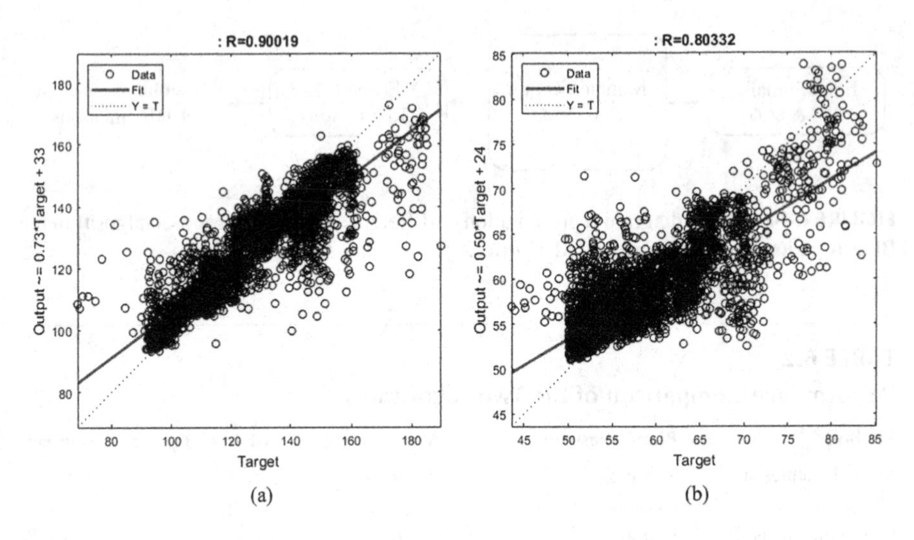

FIGURE 6.15 Regression plots of systolic and diastolic BP estimations for the proposed algorithm based on handcrafted features.

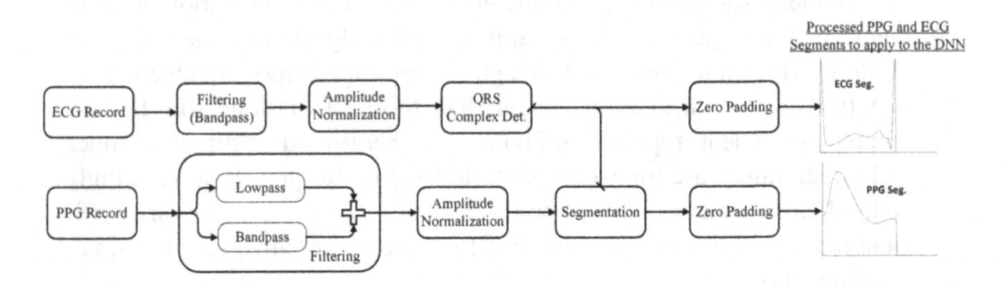

FIGURE 6.16 Preprocessing and signal segmentation steps to prepare data for the LSTM network in the end-to-end model.

the ECG signal. We also add zeros to the segments to adjust their length to 200 samples.

- **Estimation model:** The model is based on LSTM networks. As is shown in Figure 6.17, corresponding input segments of PPG and ECG signals are applied to the deep neural network. It encompasses 64 LSTM units. These recurrent neural networks can provide the representations of the current events based on the previous information stored by their feedback connections. They were invented to deal with the vanishing gradient problem in traditional recurrent neural networks [31]. The dropout layer tries to prevent overfitting during the learning procedure by randomly setting some input elements to zero with the given probability (0.2).
- **Results:** Like before, we divided each record into three separate parts of training, validation, and testing sections claiming 60%, 15%, and 30% of cycles in each record, respectively. Table 6.2 shows the precision of the

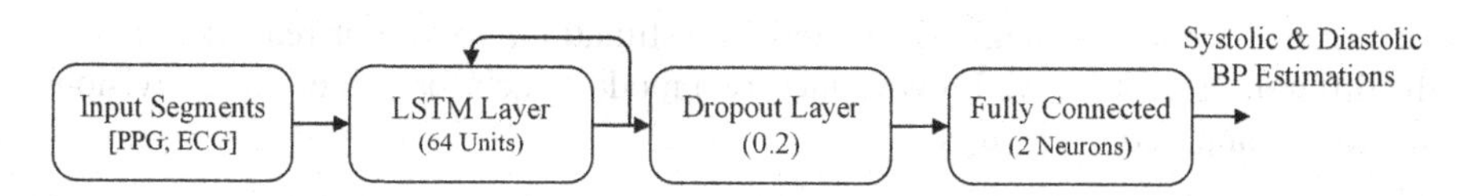

FIGURE 6.17 Proposed architecture for the LSTM network.

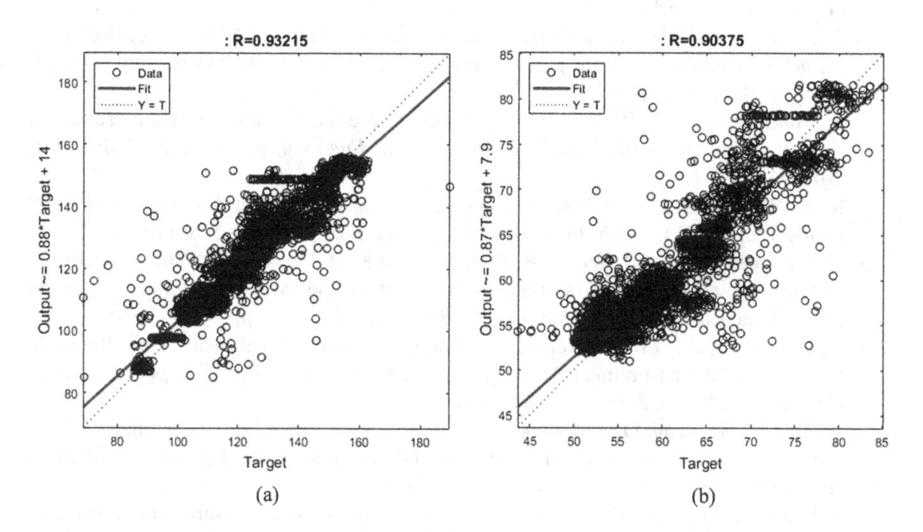

FIGURE 6.18 Regression plots of systolic and diastolic BP estimations for the proposed algorithm based on LSTM network.

regression model based on extracted features. Figure 6.18 also depicts regression plots of our model for systolic and diastolic BP estimations. *The results declare a better performance for this end-to-end model in comparison with the regression model based on manually extracted features.*

6.5 CONCLUSION

In this chapter, we revised fundamental issues related to noninvasive and cuff-less blood pressure monitoring based on PPG and ECG signals. At first, we investigated the physiological model of pressure pulse propagation in arteries to derive Bramwell-Hill and Moens-Korteweg equations describing the relationship between pulse wave velocity (PWV) and pulse transit time (PTT) with blood pressure.

Afterward, pulse arrival time (PAT) as another frequently used parameter instead of PTT is introduced. We also implemented an experiment based on some clinical data to compare the performance of these indicators in predicting BP. Our results confirm the claims made by some other researchers that "PAT is not an adequate surrogate of PTT as a marker of blood pressure" [12].

Then, we took one step further and categorized all proposed methods into two groups: methods based on handcrafted features and models merely based on artificial intelligence for feature engineering and BP estimation. To let our readers conceive the differences clearer, we implemented two models each for one of these divisions and then compared the results.

REFERENCES

1. "Disease control priorities in developing countries," *Choice Rev. Online*, 2006. doi:10.5860/choice.44-0343.
2. J. Esmaelpoor, M. H. Moradi, and A. Kadkhodamohammadi, "A multistage deep neural network model for blood pressure estimation using photoplethysmogram signals," *Comput. Biol. Med.*, p. 103719, 2020.
3. R. Mukkamala et al., "Toward ubiquitous blood pressure monitoring via pulse transit time: theory and practice," *IEEE Trans. Biomed. Eng.*, vol. 62, no. 8, pp. 1879–1901, 2015.
4. R. K. Webb et al., "The Australian incident monitoring study: An analysis of 2000 incident reports," *Anaesth. Intensive Care*, vol. 21, no. 5, pp. 520–528, 1993.
5. G. J. Langewouters, J. J. Settels, R. Roelandt, and K. H. Wesseling, "Why use Finapres or Portapres rather than intraarterial or intermittent non-invasive techniques of blood pressure measurement?," *J. Med. Eng. Technol.*, vol. 22, no. 1, pp. 37–43, 1998.
6. A. Benmira et al., "From Korotkoff and Marey to automatic non-invasive oscillometric blood pressure measurement: Does easiness come with reliability?," *Expert Rev. Med. Devices*, vol. 13, no. 2, pp. 179–189, 2016.
7. W.-H. Lin, H. Wang, O. W. Samuel, G. Liu, Z. Huang, and G. Li, "New photoplethysmogram indicators for improving cuffless and continuous blood pressure estimation accuracy," *Physiol. Meas.*, vol. 39, no. 2, p. 25005, 2018.
8. Y. Sawada et al., "Vascular unloading method for noninvasive measurement of instantaneous arterial pressure: Applicability in psychophysiological research," *Physiol. Meas.*, vol. 39, no. 2, pp. 709–714, 2018.
9. M. R. Nelson, J. Stepanek, M. Cevette, M. Covalciuc, R. T. Hurst, and A. J. Tajik, "Noninvasive measurement of central vascular pressures with arterial tonometry: Clinical revival of the pulse pressure waveform?," *Mayo Clin. Proc.*, vol. 85, no. 5, pp. 460–472, 2010.
10. J. Allen, "Photoplethysmography and its application in clinical physiological measurement," *Physiol. Meas.*, vol. 28, no. 3, p. R1, 2007.
11. L. S. Lilly, *Pathophysiology of Heart Disease: A Collaborative Project of Medical Students and Faculty*. Lippincott Williams & Wilkins, Philadelphia, PA, 2012.
12. G. Zhang, M. Gao, D. Xu, N. B. Olivier, and R. Mukkamala, "Pulse arrival time is not an adequate surrogate for pulse transit time as a marker of blood pressure," *J. Appl. Physiol.*, vol. 111, p. 1681, 2011.
13. J. E. Naschitz et al., "Pulse transit time by R-wave-gated infrared photoplethysmography: Review of the literature and personal experience," *J. Clin. Monit. Comput.*, vol. 18, no. 5–6, pp. 333–342, 2004.
14. M. Y.-M. Wong, C. C.-Y. Poon, and Y.-T. Zhang, "An evaluation of the cuffless blood pressure estimation based on pulse transit time technique: A half year study on normotensive subjects," *Cardiovasc. Eng.*, vol. 9, no. 1, pp. 32–38, 2009.
15. P. A. Lanfranchi and V. K. Somers, "Cardiovascular physiology: Autonomic control in health and in sleep disorders," In W. C. Dement, M. H. Kryger, and T. Roth (eds.) *Principles and Practice of Sleep Medicine*. Fifth Edition, Elsevier Inc., Amsterdam, 2010, pp. 226–236.

16. S. Kamalzadeh, *PTT-Based Method for Noninvasive Beat-to-Beat Estimation of Systolic and Diastolic Blood Pressure.* Master Thesis, Amirkabir University of Technology, Tehran, Iran, 2016.
17. H. Yin, Z.-H. Huang, and L. Qi, "The convergence of a Levenberg–Marquardt method for nonlinear inequalities," *Numer. Funct. Anal. Optim.*, vol. 29, no. 5–6, pp. 687–716, 2008.
18. R. A. Payne, C. N. Symeonides, D. J. Webb, and S. R. J. Maxwell, "Pulse transit time measured from the ECG: An unreliable marker of beat-to-beat blood pressure," *J. Appl. Physiol.*, vol. 100, no. 1, pp. 136–141, 2006.
19. J. Y. A. Foo, C. S. Lim, and P. Wang, "Evaluation of blood pressure changes using vascular transit time," *Physiol. Meas.*, vol. 27, no. 8, p. 685, 2006.
20. S. Feffer, "It's all about the features." [Online]. Available: https://reality.ai/it-is-all-about-the-features/.
21. S. Mottaghi, M. Moradi, and L. Roohisefat, "Cuffless blood pressure estimation during exercise stress test," *Int. J. Biosci. Biochem. Bioinforma.*, vol. 2, no. 6, p. 394, 2012.
22. M. Moghadam and M. H. Moradi, "Systolic and diastolic blood pressure estimation during exercise stress test using GK-MARS fuzzy function approach," in *2015 23rd Iranian Conference on Electrical Engineering*, 2015, pp. 109–114.
23. X.-R. Ding, Y.-T. Zhang, J. Liu, W.-X. Dai, and H. K. Tsang, "Continuous cuffless blood pressure estimation using pulse transit time and photoplethysmogram intensity ratio," *IEEE Trans. Biomed. Eng.*, vol. 63, no. 5, pp. 964–972, 2015.
24. M. Elgendi, "On the analysis of fingertip photoplethysmogram signals," *Curr. Cardiol. Rev.*, vol. 8, no. 1, pp. 14–25, 2012.
25. Y. Bengio, A. Courville, and P. Vincent, "Representation learning: A review and new perspectives," *IEEE Trans. Pattern Anal. Mach. Intell.*, vol. 35, no. 8, pp. 1798–1828, 2013.
26. J. Esmaelpoor, M. H. Moradi, and A. Kadkhodamohammadi. Cuffless blood pressure estimation methods: physiological model parameters vs. machine-learned features. Physiological Measurement. 2021 Mar 1.
27. M. S. Tanveer and M. K. Hasan, "Cuffless blood pressure estimation from electrocardiogram and photoplethysmogram using waveform based ANN-LSTM network," *Biomed. Signal Process. Control*, vol. 51, pp. 382–392, 2019.
28. A. G. Ramakrishnan, A. P. Prathosh, and T. V. Ananthapadmanabha, "Threshold-independent QRS detection using the dynamic plosion index," *IEEE Signal Process. Lett.*, vol. 21, no. 5, pp. 554–558, 2014.
29. J. S. Kim, K. K. Kim, H. J. Baek, and K. S. Park, "Effect of confounding factors on blood pressure estimation using pulse arrival time," *Physiol. Meas.*, vol. 29, no. 5, p. 615, 2008.
30. F. Pedregosa et al., "Scikit-learn: Machine Learning in {P}ython," *J. Mach. Learn. Res.*, vol. 12, pp. 2825–2830, 2011.
31. I. Goodfellow, Y. Bengio, and A. Courville, *Deep Learning.* MIT Press, Cambridge, MA, 2016.

7 Investigation of the Efficacy of Acupuncture Using Electromyographic Signals

Kim Ho Yeap, Wey Long Ng, and Humaira Nisar
Universiti Tunku Abdul Rahman

Veerendra Dakulagi
Guru Nanak Dev Engineering College

CONTENTS

7.1 INTRODUCTION

Acupuncture is an ancient therapeutic modality which has been practiced in China since thousands of years ago. According to traditional Chinese medicine (TCM), a form of interior bodily energy, which has been vaguely interpreted as *qi* in the literature, is generated in the internal organs and systems [1–3]. The *qi* is carried by the breath or air and circulates throughout the entire body, forming intricate interwoven paths known as the meridian system or *ching-lo* [1]. Physically, the meridians are perceived to be made up of groups of orderly arranged electrically polarized water molecules, which form water clusters with permanent electric dipole moment [2]. Acupuncture treatment is merely one of the possible therapies which manipulate the *qi* as it circulates the meridians to achieve curative effects [1]. The other examples which are based on this method are the cupping and moxibustion therapies, and the *tai-chi* and *qi-gong* exercises [4].

Despite its popular practice over millennia, the acupuncture treatment fails to gain worldwide acceptance within the mainstream orthodox clinical field [2]. Due to the plethora of confounding factors enshrouding this treatment, researchers have found it extremely difficult to definitively and convincingly verify the curative efficacy of the treatment [5]. In other words, a tangible and descriptive demonstrable mechanism is yet to be formulated to prove its scientific reality [1]. In fact, many believe that acupuncture may, at best, merely introduce psychogenetic effect to the patients. In [6], Tough examined the immediate effects of acupuncture on the electromyography (EMG) activity of the common wrist extensor muscles. Three experiments were carried out on 35 subjects – namely, genuine acupuncture, inappropriate acupuncture, and a no condition control. At the end of the study, he drew the conclusion that the acupuncture interventions did not register any meaningful change on the EMG activity. Farida et al. [7], on the other hand, showed that the therapy produced positive results. The authors examined the effect of acupuncture on the EMG activity from the bicep muscles. In the case study, two groups, with four subjects in each group, received stimulation from 5 kg load. The subjects in the first group were administered acupuncture while those in the second were not. The authors concluded that acupuncture therapy was capable of improving human stamina, particularly, on muscle exercises. Although both [6,7] attempted to correlate the effect of acupuncture with the EMG activity, it is apparent that their outcomes are in stark contrast. The actual curative efficacy of acupuncture therefore remains uncertain.

In order to probe further the efficacy of acupuncture therapy in treating muscle spasticity and flaccidity, we conducted an in-depth case study based on patients suffering from muscle impairment at different parts of the body. An EMG sensor was constructed from off-the-shelf components, and it was implemented to measure contraction of muscles before and after the treatment. In this chapter, the process of constructing the EMG circuit is first described in detail. This is then followed by the description of the case study. Analysis on the results and hypothesis on the underlying operational principal of acupuncture are discussed at the later sections of the chapter.

7.2 ELECTROMYOGRAPHY SENSOR

Electromyography (EMG) sensors are used to detect and examine the electrical signals generated by the movement of muscles or stimulation of nerve to the muscles. The electrical signal detected by the sensor during the neuromuscular activities is known as the electromyographic (EMG) signal. The contraction and relaxation of muscles are stimulated by impulses in the neurons to the muscle. The EMG signal can therefore be expressed in terms of a train of Motor Action Unit Potentials (MUAPs) which shows the muscle response to neural stimulation [8]. Mathematically, the EMG signal can be written as [8]

$$x(n) = \sum_{r=0}^{N-1} h(r)e(n-r) + w(n) \tag{7.1}$$

where $x(n)$ is the modeled EMG signal, $e(n)$ the point processed which represents the firing impulse, $h(r)$ the MUAPs, $w(n)$ the zero mean additive white Gaussian noise, and N denotes the number of motor unit firings. The electrodes of an EMG sensor can be used to detect the ionic flow across the muscle membranes that propagate through the tissues in order to generate the EMG signal [9]. Hence, the sensor can be used to measure the anatomical and physiological status of the muscles. Traditionally, EMG signals are used in biomedical science for identifying neuromuscular disorders. Nowadays, however, the applications of EMG signals have been expanded into the realm of biomedical engineering – it is also used for constructing EMG-based prosthetic, robotic and other useful systems.

According to [8], the quality of the signal detected by the EMG sensor is highly affected by two factors – the first is the signal-to-noise ratio (SNR), whereas the second is the distortion of the signal. The SNR is used to measure the magnitude of the EMG signals in comparison to the that of the noise. When detecting the EMG signal, electrical noise is very often coupled along. The electrical noise includes the inherent noise in electronic equipment, ambient noise, motion artefact, and the inherent instability of the EMG signal [8]. The EMG signal is picked up by electrodes. It then undergoes a series of amplifications, filtering, and rectification. At each process step, the signal may lose energy at different rates. Hence, beside noise contamination, the signal may also face the risk of being distorted. To put it simply, the following conditions have to be observed in order to optimize the detection of the EMG signal:

i. The magnitude of the EMG signal itself has to be optimal, while noise contamination has to be suppressed. This is to say, the higher is the SNR value, the better is the EMG signal detection.
ii. Signal distortion is to be minimized. Since EMG signal can be decomposed into a series of frequency-dependent components, the signal experiences distortion when each component attenuates differently. It is therefore important to ensure that the wave amplitudes of all frequency components sustain uniform losses. This is to say, the loss should be frequency-independent (or at least, close to independent), if not completely eliminated.

7.2.1 Materials and Components

The EMG sensor used in our case study is based on the design in [10]. The components involved in the construction of the EMG circuit include three TL072 integrated circuits (ICs), an INA106 integrated circuit, three surface EMG electrodes, two 9 V batteries, two 1 μF tantalum capacitors, a 0.01 and a 1 μF ceramic capacitors, a 100 kΩ trimmer potentiometer, two 1N4148 diodes and three 150 kΩ, two 1 MΩ, two 80.6 kΩ, six 10 kΩ and one 1 kΩ resistors. A microcontroller is used to process the output signal, so that it could be recorded for further analysis. In this section, the functions of the important components shall be briefly elaborated.

According to Jamal [11], the contraction of muscle of human body can be detected by using different types of EMG electrodes. EMG electrodes can be either invasive or noninvasive. The invasive types are intramuscular electrodes and can be further divided into needle electrodes and fine wire electrodes. The noninvasive types are surface electrodes. In general, the invasive electrodes provide higher accuracy and sensitivity. The signals detected using the invasive electrodes are also more stable. However, since the process involved pricking the electrodes into the skin, most volunteers were against using them. Hence, we resort to the noninvasive surface electrodes in our work here. The surface EMG electrodes are electrodes applied onto the surface of the skin. Hence, they do not impose discomfort to the patients. In order to let the current to flow through the surface EMG electrodes, a chemical equilibrium between the sensing surface and the skin of the body will be formed by electrolytic conduction [11]. Surface electrodes are, nevertheless, relatively sensitive to electrical noise. One has to be extremely precautious when using the electrodes for EMG detection.

The INA106 IC is a differential amplifier that consists of a precision operational amplifier (op-amp) and four on-chip metal film resistors, i.e., two 10 kΩ resistors connected to the input pins and another two 100 kΩ resistors connected to the sense and reference pins. The internal configuration of the chip is illustrated in Figure 7.1. INA106 produces accurate gain and relatively high common-mode rejection ratio (CMRR) of 86 dB which enables it to reject the noise of input signal [12]. Hence, it is employed at the first stage of the EMG circuit where the electrodes are connected directly to the inputs.

The TL072 IC consists of a low noise junction field effect transistor, JFET-input operational amplifier. The pin layout of the chip is depicted in Figure 7.2. As can be seen from the figure, the chip consists of four inputs and two outputs, which means it

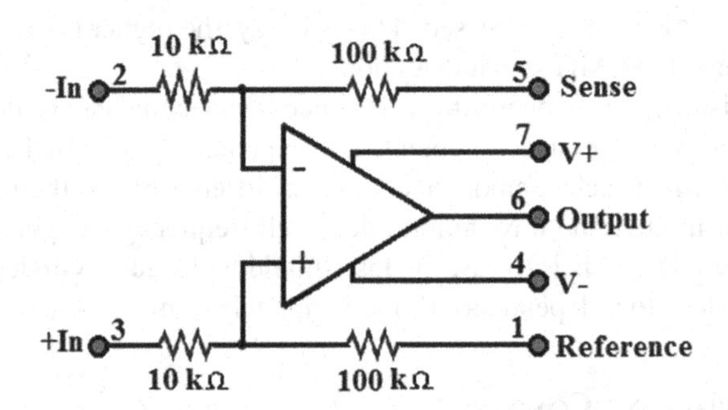

FIGURE 7.1 Pin layout of the INA106 IC.

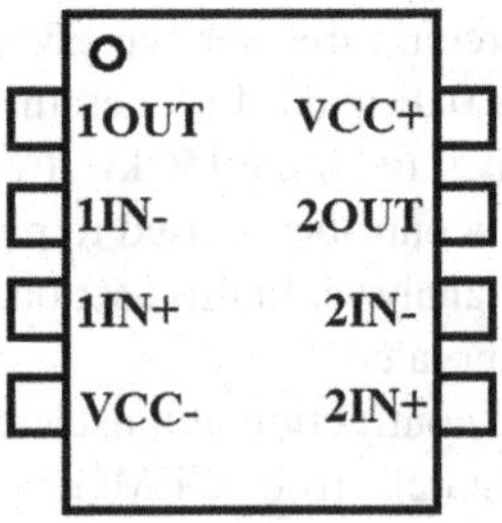

1OUT	VCC+
1IN-	2OUT
1IN+	2IN-
VCC-	2IN+

FIGURE 7.2 Pin layout of the TL072 IC.

is a two-channel op-amp. The TL072 op-amp has the advantages of low power consumption, low offset currents, low noise, high slew rate which is 13 V/μs, and relatively low total harmonic distortion which is 0.003% [12]. These advantages make it a suitable candidate for amplifying the weak EMG signals.

The microcontroller used for processing the EMG signal is Arduino Uno. The Arduino microcontroller is a free opensource platform widely used for developing and designing electronic based project. It is compatible with most of the available electronic devices in the market and is capable of transmitting and receiving data to and from the devices. According to [13], an Arduino can receive data from input devices such as sensors, antennas and potentiometers and transmit the data to output devices such as LEDs, speakers and motors. Therefore, Arduino Uno is used here as an interface to display the EMG signals at the computer. Figure 7.3 depicts the layout of the Arduino Uno board [14].

The Arduino Integrated Development Environment (IDE) is used to write and upload programs to Arduino Uno. As can be seen in Figure 7.4, the user interface of Arduino IDE is separated into three sections, namely, the command, coding, and message window areas. The command area comprises a list of function options. Here, the 'verify', 'upload', 'serial monitor', and 'serial plotter' functions are used to program the microcontroller. The 'verify' and 'upload' functions are used to compile and upload the code to the Arduino Uno board, while the 'serial monitor' and 'serial plotter' functions are used to display the output of the EMG signals. Programming is written at the coding area. Since a simplified version of the C++ language is used for programming, users with basic knowledge on C or C++ programming language should be able to pick up the skill with ease. There are two compulsory routines for every coding – namely the setup 'void setup ()' and loop 'void loop ()' routines. The setup routine is to initialize the program once the reset button on the Arduino Uno board is triggered. The loop routine, on the other hand, is used to notify the board to perform the task iteratively. The function of the message window area is to display

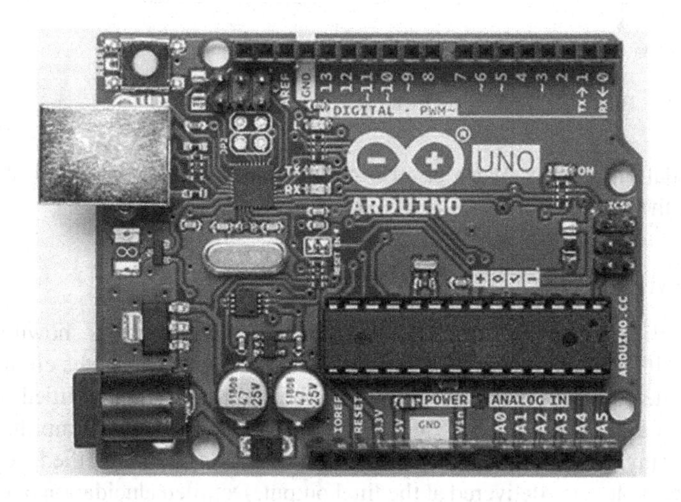

FIGURE 7.3 The layout of the Arduino Uno board [14].

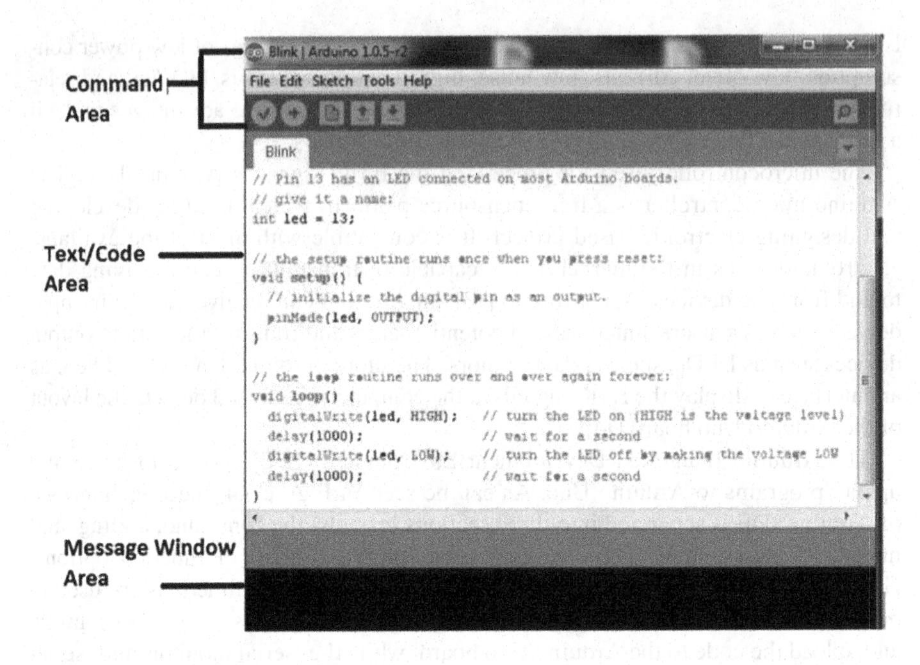

FIGURE 7.4 The Arduino IDE.

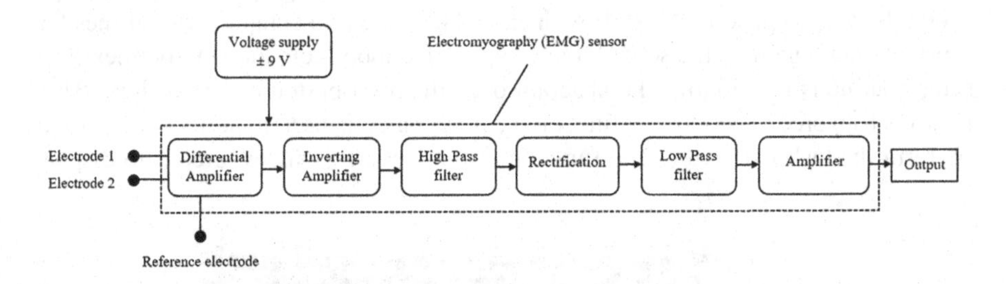

FIGURE 7.5 Block diagram of the EMG sensor.

the compilation process. Warning or error messages will be displayed in that area whenever the compiler comes across inaccurate syntaxes.

7.2.2 EMG Circuit

The block diagram of the EMG circuit is shown in Figure 7.5. As shown in the figure, the EMG signal has to undergo six stages of processes within the circuit. Firstly, the signal detected by the electrodes have to be compared and amplified by the differential op-amp. It has to subsequently go through two stages of amplification and signal filtering to optimize the SNR. The signal also has to be rectified, so that only positive DC voltage is delivered at the final output. Detailed elucidation of each stage is presented in this section.

As described at the early part of this section, EMG signals are highly susceptible to noise. Since charging and discharging a capacitor will contribute considerable electrical noise, power supplied from an IC regulator or a DC-to-DC converter is not suitable to be used as the source of the circuit. Instead, two 9 V dry cell batteries were used here. The schematic in Figure 7.6 illustrates the connection of the batteries to the EMG circuit.

Figure 7.7 depicts the circuit connection at the first stage of the EMG circuit. As can be seen from the figure, the electrodes are to be connected to the input pins of the INA106 differential amplifier. The signal at the second electrode is subtracted with that at the first electrode. This is to get rid of the common signal at both input signals, so that only clean signal is amplified at the output of the op-amp. The common signal is the ambient noise – the frequency of which resembles closely that of the nerve impulse [12]. The output amplifier gain A_1 can be computed based on (2) below:

$$A_1 = \frac{R_{\text{sense}} + R_1}{R_{\text{input}}} \tag{7.2}$$

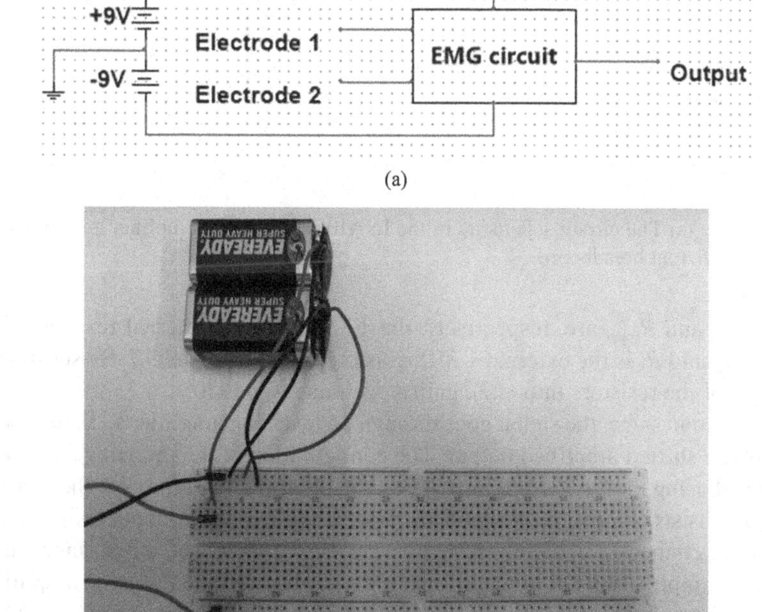

(a)

(b)

FIGURE 7.6 (a) The voltage supply circuit and (b) the connection of the voltage supply to a breadboard.

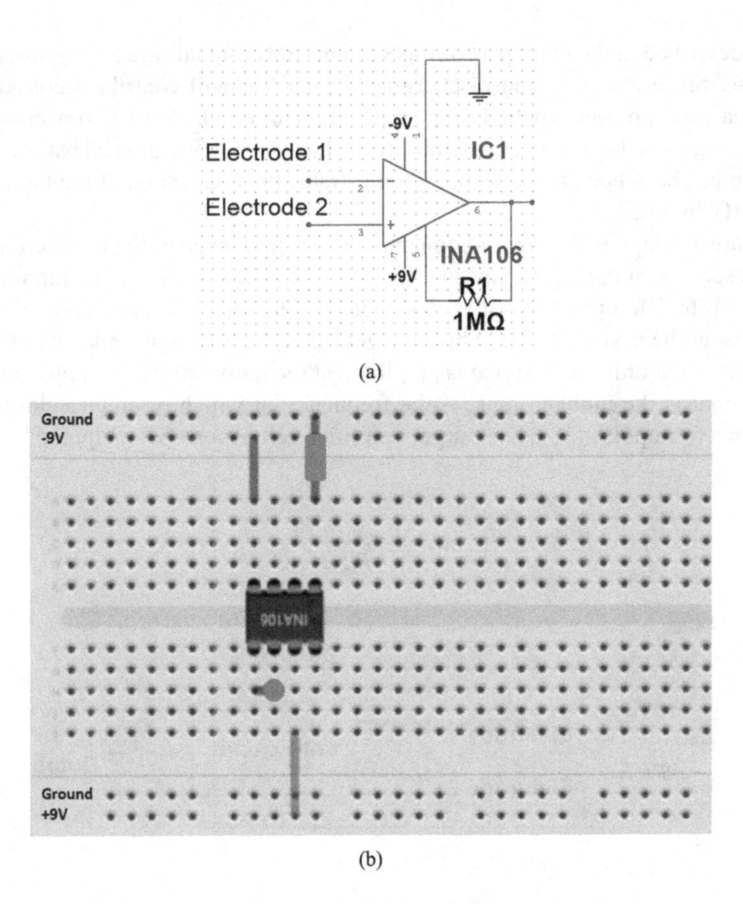

FIGURE 7.7 (a) The circuit schematic of the INA106 differential amplifier and (b) its connection on a virtual breadboard.

where R_{sense} and R_{input} are, respectively, the 100 and 10 kΩ internal resistors in the INA106 IC, and R_1 is the external 1 MΩ resistor shown in Figure 7.7. By substituting the values of the resistors into (7.2), gain A_1 is found to be 110.

In the second stage, the signal goes through an inverting amplifier so as to produce a 180° phase shifted amplified output. The configuration of the inverting amplifier is constructed using the TL072 op-amp. As can be observed in Figure 7.8, the inverting amplifier consists of a 150 kΩ R_f feedback resistor and a 10 kΩ R_{in} input resistor – both of which are connected to the inverting pin. The output signal at the first stage (i.e. the differential amplifier) is fed to the inverting pin. Gain A_2 of the inverting amplifier is 15 and can be found by substituting the values of the R_f and R_{in} into (7.3) below:

$$A_2 = -\frac{R_f}{R_i}. \tag{7.3}$$

The third stage of the EMG circuit constitutes a high pass filter. The output of the amplified signal in the second stage is connected to the capacitor in Figure 7.9. The

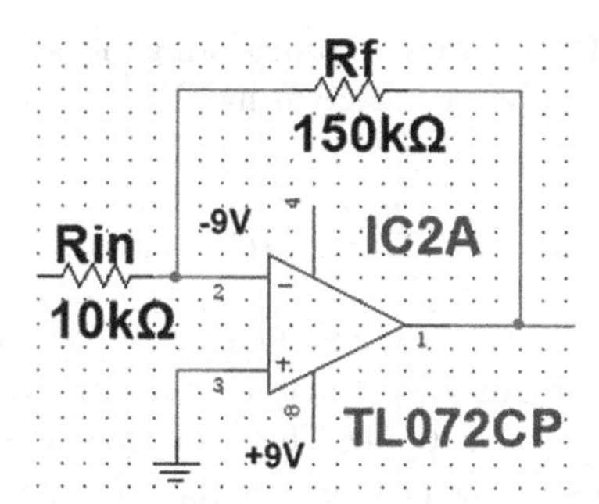

FIGURE 7.8 The circuit schematic of the inverting amplifier.

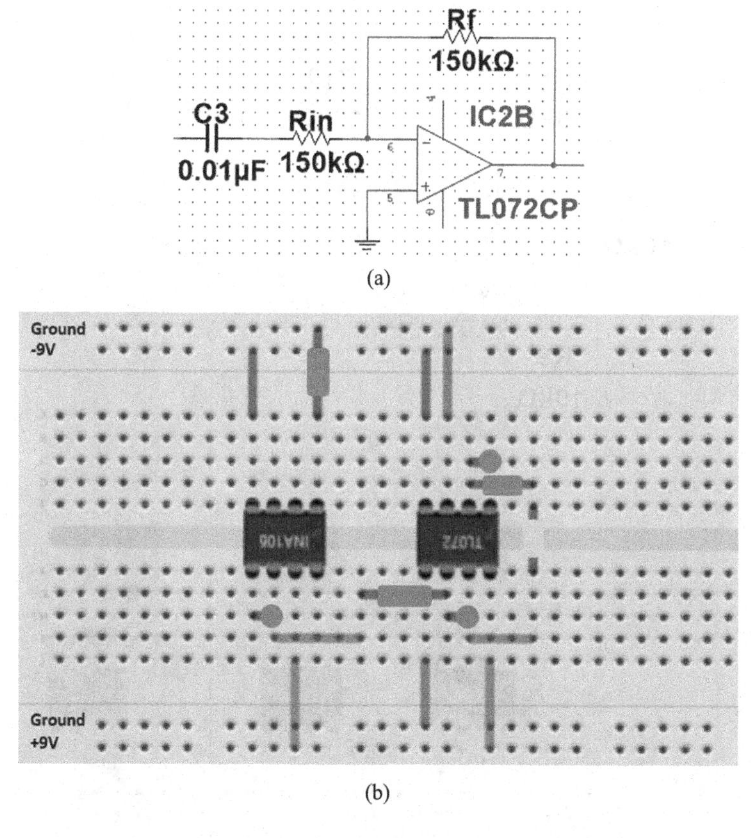

(a)

(b)

FIGURE 7.9 (a) The circuit schematic of a high-pass filter and (b) its connection to the differential and inverting amplifiers on a virtual breadboard.

function of the high-pass filter is to remove the noise created by motion artefact such as the movement of joints. As can be seen from the figure, two 150 kΩ resistors and a 0.01 μF capacitor are used in the circuit. The purpose of introducing the capacitor at the input pin is to block DC signal from propagating into the circuit [12]. The cut off frequency f_c of the filter can be calculated using (7.4)

$$f_c = \frac{1}{2\pi RC}. \tag{7.4}$$

where R and C are, respectively, the resistance and capacitance connected to the inverting input. Since noise created by motion artefact is typically below 10 Hz, the cut off frequency f_c is set to be at 106 Hz. This is to say, only signals with frequencies higher than 106 Hz are allowed to propagate to the subsequent stage.

In the fourth stage, the filtered signal goes through full wave rectification. As shown in Figure 7.10, the components involved in building the rectifier include four 10 kΩ resistors, two pn-junction diodes, and two op-amps. The rectifier converts

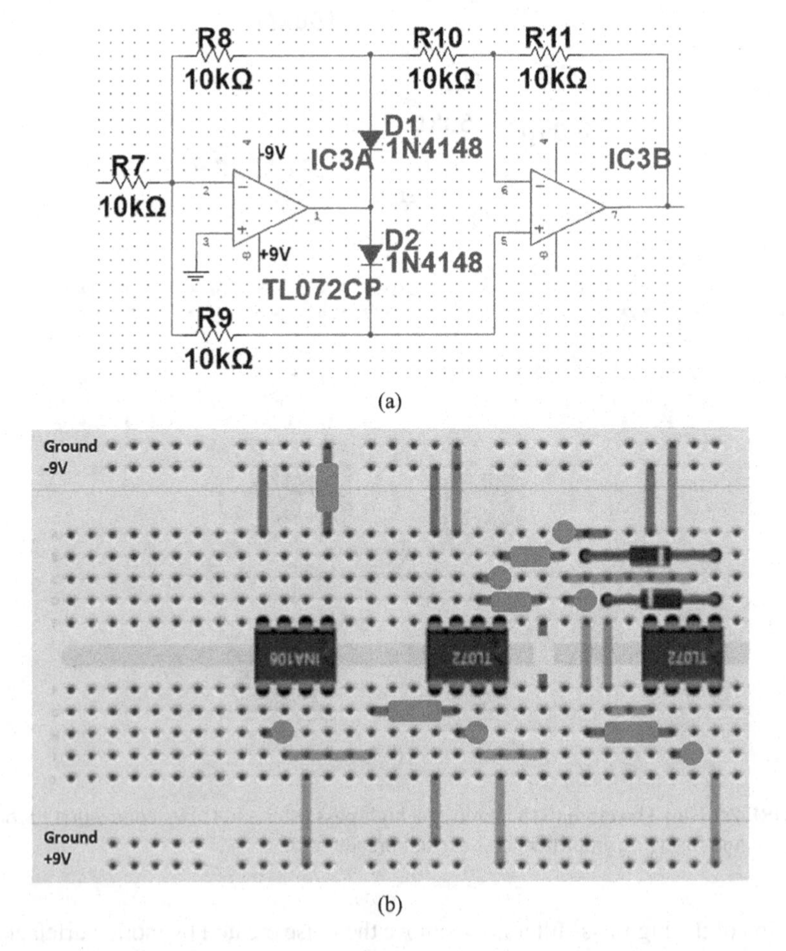

FIGURE 7.10 (a) The circuit schematic of a full wave rectifier and (b) its connection to the high pass filter and amplifiers on a virtual breadboard.

signals in the negative phase to the positive phase, i.e., the AC input signal is changed to DC signal at the output.

In the fifth process step, the rectified signal is fed to a low pass filter. The function of the low-pass filter is to remove the effect of aliasing high frequency components [12]. The filter at this stage is developed by connecting two passive components – a 1 μF capacitor and an 80.6 kΩ resistor – at the feedback loop and another 80.6 kΩ resistor to the inverting input. The schematic of the low pass filter is illustrated in Figure 7.11.

At the final stage, the EMG signal is amplified to a desirable detectable value. Most often than not, the EMG signal generated by the contraction of muscles is extremely weak. Hence, an amplifier with high gain is necessary to increase the output voltage to a reasonable magnitude. Here, the TL072 op-amp is again employed for this purpose. As can be seen in Figure 7.12, a 1 kΩ resistor and a 100 kΩ trimmer potentiometer are connected to the inverting input. The trimmer potentiometer is used to vary gain A_3 of the amplifier [12]. The gain is in direct proportion with the resistance of the potentiometer. Since the circuit configuration of this amplifier is similar to that in the second stage, gain A_3 can be computed by dividing the value of the feedback resistor with the 1 kΩ input resistor.

In a nutshell, the complete EMG circuit is constructed by combining the circuit networks from the first stage to the final stage, i.e., from Figures 7.6–7.12. Figure 7.13 illustrates the schematic of the overall EMG circuit and its components' connections on a virtual breadboard.

7.2.3 Signal and Data Acquisition

In order to analyze the efficacy of acupuncture, the data measured before and after the treatment is to be stored and analyzed. The Arduino Uno microcontroller acts like a circuit interface between the EMG sensor and the display (which is a computer in this case). The microcontroller records the EMG signal in digital form and display them onto the screen. Since Arduino Uno can only support analog input signal ranging from 0 to 5 V, care must be taken to ensure that the output signal amplified at the final stage

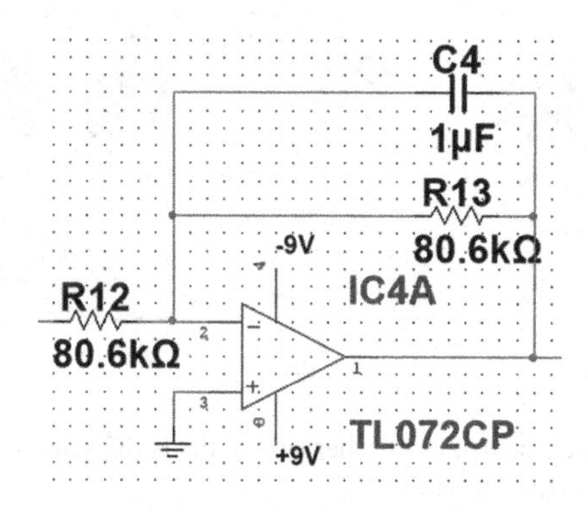

FIGURE 7.11 The circuit schematic of the low pass amplifier.

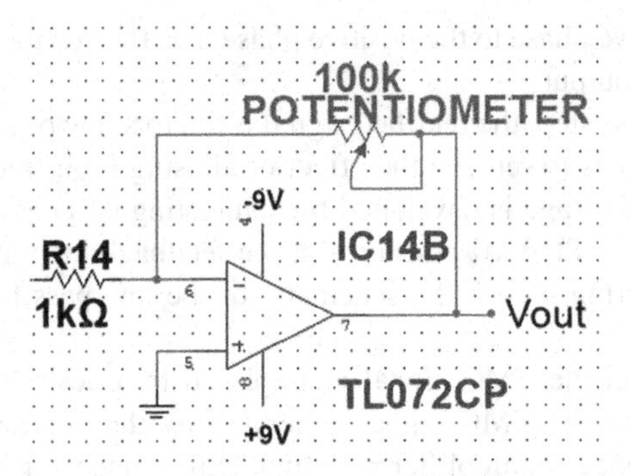

FIGURE 7.12 The circuit schematic of the inverting amplifier connected to the last stage of the EMG circuit.

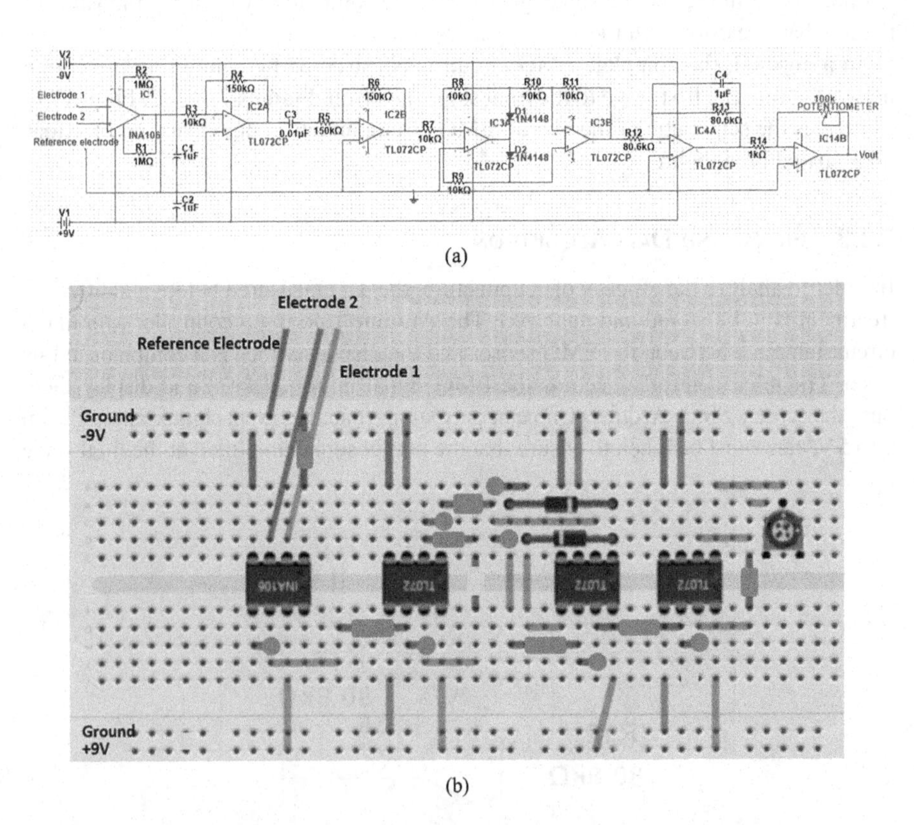

(a)

(b)

FIGURE 7.13 (a) The complete circuit schematic of the EMG sensor and (b) the connections of the components on a virtual breadboard.

of the EMG circuit is below 5 V. To perform data acquisition, the output signal from the EMG sensor is to be connected to the analog input pin of the Arduino Uno board and the ground wires of both devices are to be connected together, as shown in Figure 7.14. The output of the Arduino Uno board is to be connected to the USB port of a computer.

Once the hardware has been set up, the Arduino IDE is launched, and the code for displaying the result of the EMG signal is compiled and uploaded to the Arduino Uno board. A snapshot of the code used in this project is depicted in Figure 7.15

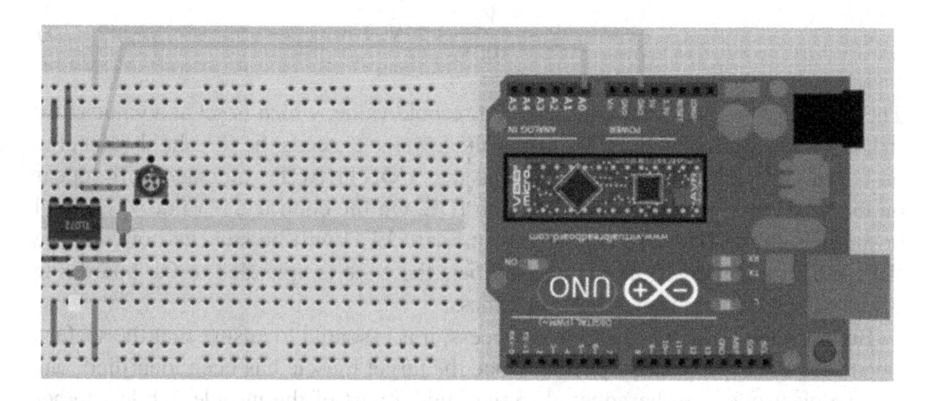

FIGURE 7.14 Connection of the EMG circuit to Arduino Uno on a virtual breadboard.

sketch_mar28a §

```
int arduinoLED = 13;   // Control the LED on the pin 13 of Arduino
int thresholdValue = 2.0; // Set a threshold value
void setup() {
  Serial.begin(9600); // Initialize serial communication at 9600 bits per second
  pinMode(arduinoLED, OUTPUT);  //Set the connected pin 13 as an output
}
void loop() {
  // Receive the output value from the EMG sensor and transmit to analog input A0
  int sensorValue = analogRead(A0);
  float voltage = sensorValue * (5.0/1023.0); //Convert the value received to voltage
  Serial.print(voltage);        //Display voltage value
  if(voltage > thresholdValue){
    //Trigger this when voltage value is larger than the threshold value
    Serial.println(" CONTRACT!");  //Display string
    digitalWrite(arduinoLED, HIGH); //Supply 5V to pin 13 of Arduino to turn on LED
  } else {
    //Trigger this when voltage value is lower than the threshold value
    Serial.println(" RELAX!"); //
    digitalWrite(arduinoLED, LOW); //Turn off the LED
  }
  delay(100); //Apply delay for the data acquisition
}
```

FIGURE 7.15 Arduino code for data acquisition.

(the complete Arduino code is listed in the Appendix). In the Arduino code, the analog input pin A0 is used to receive the output generated by the EMG sensor. Analog-to-digital conversion (ADC) is then performed so that the output value can be expressed in digital form V_d. Arduino Uno is equipped with a 10-bit analog to digital converter. This means that a 0 and 5 V operating voltage return the value of 0 and 1023, respectively. In order to express the digital value V_d in terms of voltage V_s, V_d which accounts a fraction of the total 1023 is multiplied by 5 V, i.e.

$$V_s = \frac{V_d}{1023} \times 5\text{ V}. \tag{7.5}$$

The voltage V_s is then compared with a threshold value, which is set at a value close to half of its amplitude, i.e., 2 V. If the voltage value exceeds the threshold value, the on-board LED will be switched on, and the 'CONTRACT!' message will appear on the serial monitor tool of the Arduino IDE. On the contrary, if value V_s is equal or lower than the threshold value, the on-board LED will be switched off and the 'RELAX!' message will be displayed. Once the code is uploaded to the board, the complete system is in immaculate readiness.

Before starting the measurement process, it is essential to ensure that the surface electrodes are appropriately placed. Once the target muscle has been identified, one surface electrode is to be adhered to the middle part of the muscle, while another electrode is to be adhered to the end of it. A third surface electrode which serves as the reference is to be adhered to the bony part which is in close proximity to the target muscle. It is to be noted that, the third reference electrode must be avoided from adhering to any parts with muscles since this will result in inaccuracy in the data acquiring process. An example of how the electrodes are adhered to measure the EMG signal from the bicep muscle is shown in Figure 7.16. Figures 7.17 and 7.18

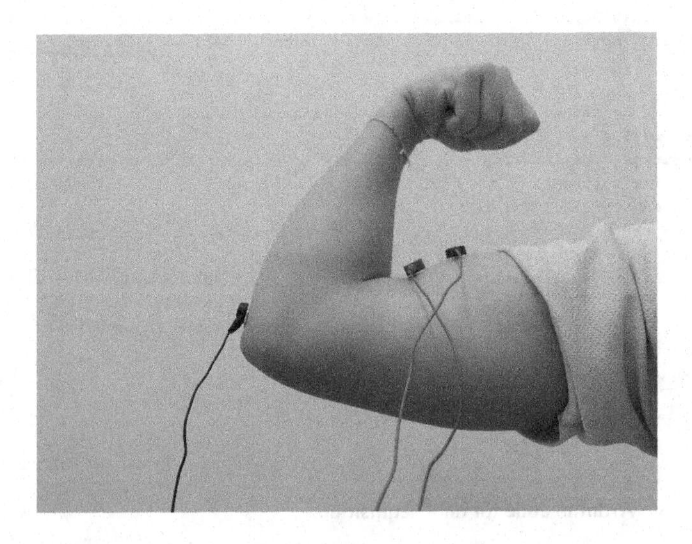

FIGURE 7.16 Placement of the surface electrodes on the bicep muscle.

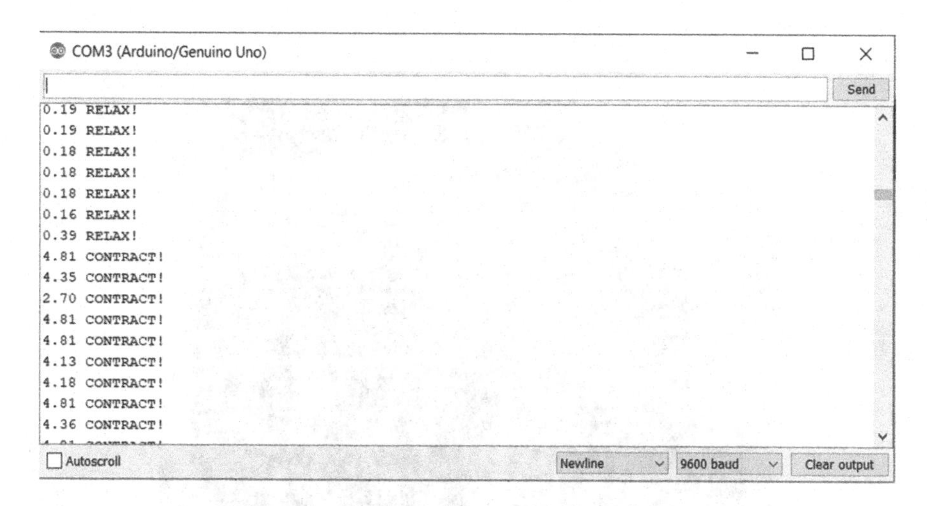

FIGURE 7.17 The voltage values generated during muscle contraction and the status of the muscles are displayed on the serial monitor of the Arduino IDE.

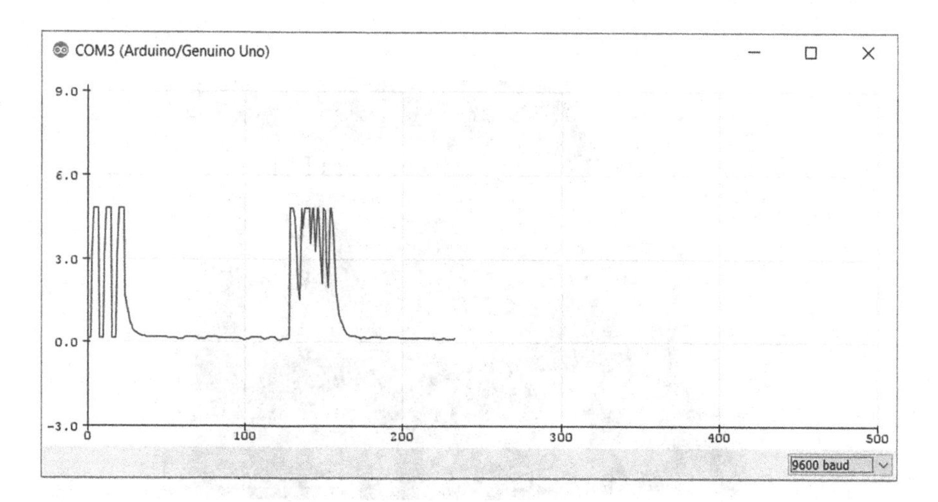

FIGURE 7.18 EMG signal generated by muscle contraction is displayed on the serial plotter of the Arduino IDE.

illustrate the display on the serial monitor and serial plotter when the bicep muscle is flexed and released. As can be seen from the figures, the serial monitor is capable of displaying the status of the muscle (i.e. either contracting or relaxing) and the voltage value of the EMG signal. Apart from the display on the serial monitor and serial plotter, the status of the muscle can also be observed from the Arduino Uno board. As shown respectively in Figures 7.19 and 7.20, the on-board LED will be switched on when the muscle is in contract condition and, it will be switched off otherwise.

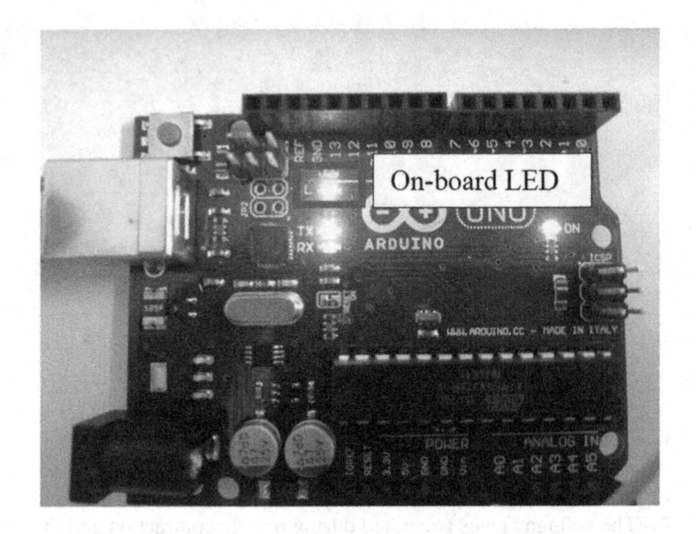

FIGURE 7.19 The on-board LED will be switched on when the muscle contracts.

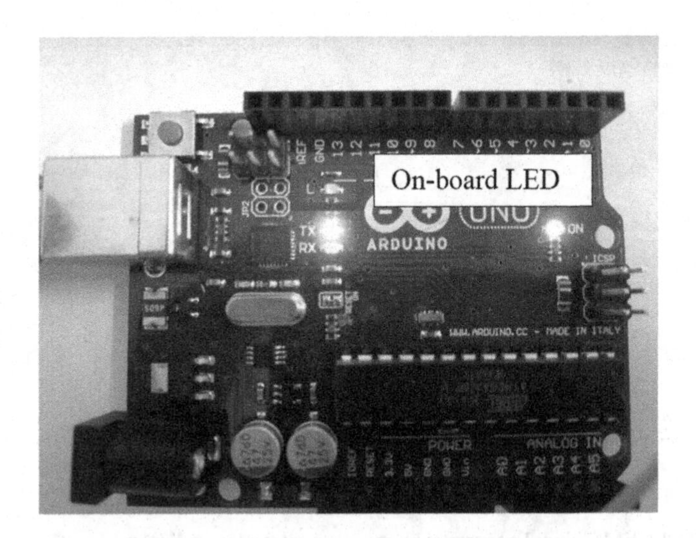

FIGURE 7.20 The on-board LED will be switched off when the muscle relaxes.

7.3 TEST PROCEDURES

Four volunteers had been involved in the acupuncture case study, with each of them suffering from muscle impairment at different parts of the bodies. The first volunteer suffered from neck pain, the second suffered from calf muscle cramp due to excessive exercises and the third and fourth suffered from thigh muscle pain. The patients were treated by an acupuncturist who has had more than 10 years of clinical experience.

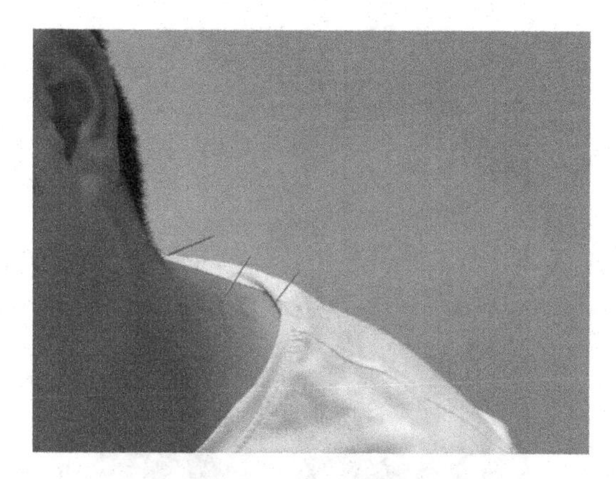

FIGURE 7.21 Acupuncture is administered on the first volunteer to remedy his neck pain.

The patients were rested on a treatment couch before the acupuncturist started carefully locating the areas of the injured muscles by palpation. According to Tsuei [1], each meridian is related to a specific organ. Hence, once the injured areas were identified, the meridians that went through those areas were traced. Acupuncture needles were subsequently inserted into the distal acupoints. Very often, when a needle was pricked, the acupuncturist would consult the patients if the needling sensation could be felt. According to the acupuncturist, once the needle reaches its intended depth and depending on the meridians being triggered, the patient should feel either a mild tingling sensation or a glitch of electric sensation. If the sensation is not felt immediately, it is elicited via needle rotation.

Since changes in the muscle length and movement may easily induce motion artefact, the EMG activity was measured during a 10-second, sub-maximal, isometric contraction. The reading at each second before and after the treatment was recorded. In order to minimize measurement errors, the EMG activity at each second was measured twice and the average was taken. Once the entire therapeutic process had finished, the EMG signals of the first three patients were measured immediately, while the fourth were measured 30 minutes afterward. Again, the EMG signal after the therapy was measured at each second for a consecutive duration of 10 seconds. Figures 7.21 and 7.24 illustrate the acupuncture therapies administered on the four patients, whereas Figures 7.25 shows the EMG measurement process performed after the therapy. Although the EMG activity was observed throughout the process (i.e. before, during, and after the therapy), only the results before and after the treatment were saved, compiled, and analyzed (Figures 7.22 and 7.23.).

7.4 RESULTS AND DISCUSSION

Figures 7.26–7.29 and 7.30–7.33 show, respectively, the EMG signals of the four volunteers before and after the acupuncture treatments. Clearly, the signals are constantly fluctuating since they are highly sensitive to electrical noise – in particular, motion artefact and the inherent instability of the signal. Hence, a variation within ±15% from its average value would be regarded as a normalcy and would not be

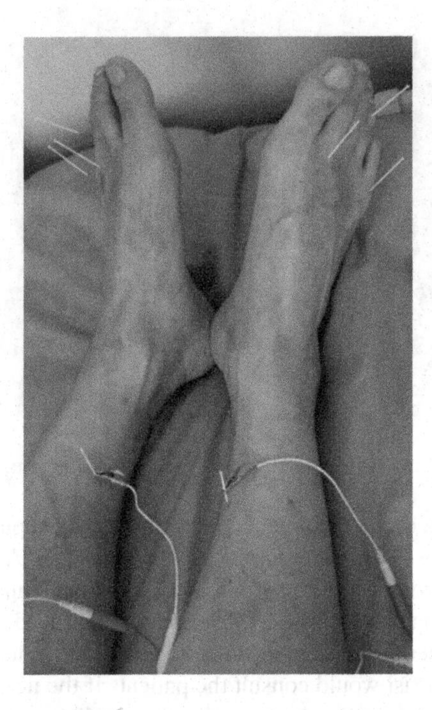

FIGURE 7.22 Acupuncture is administered on the second volunteer to remedy his calf muscle cramp.

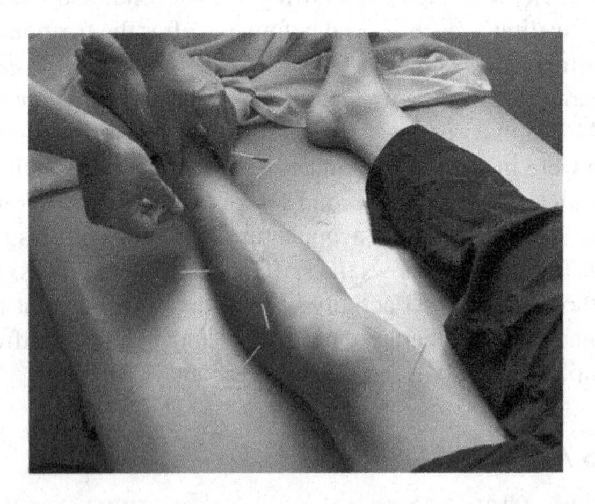

FIGURE 7.23 Acupuncture is administered on the third volunteer to remedy his thigh muscle impairment.

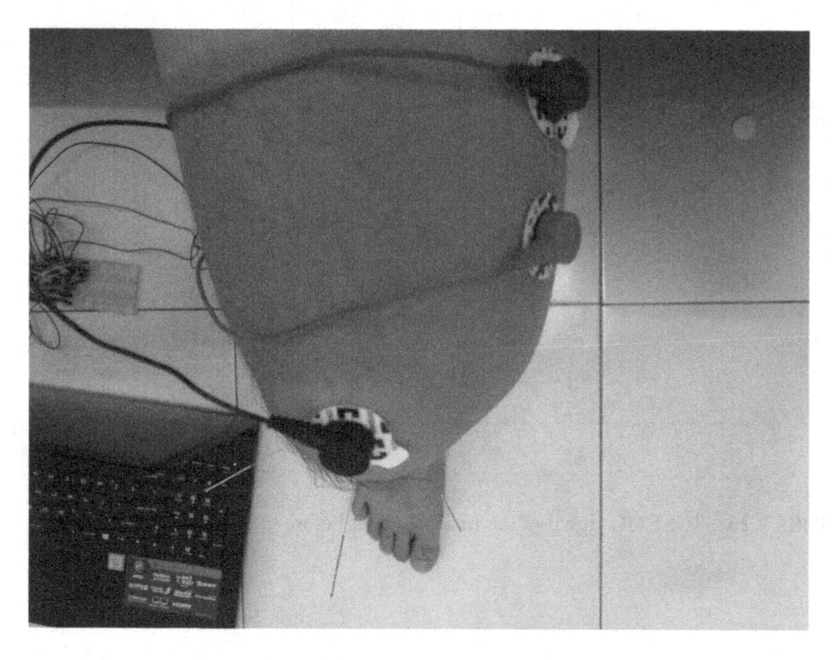

FIGURE 7.24 Acupuncture is administered on the fourth volunteer to remedy his thigh muscle impairment.

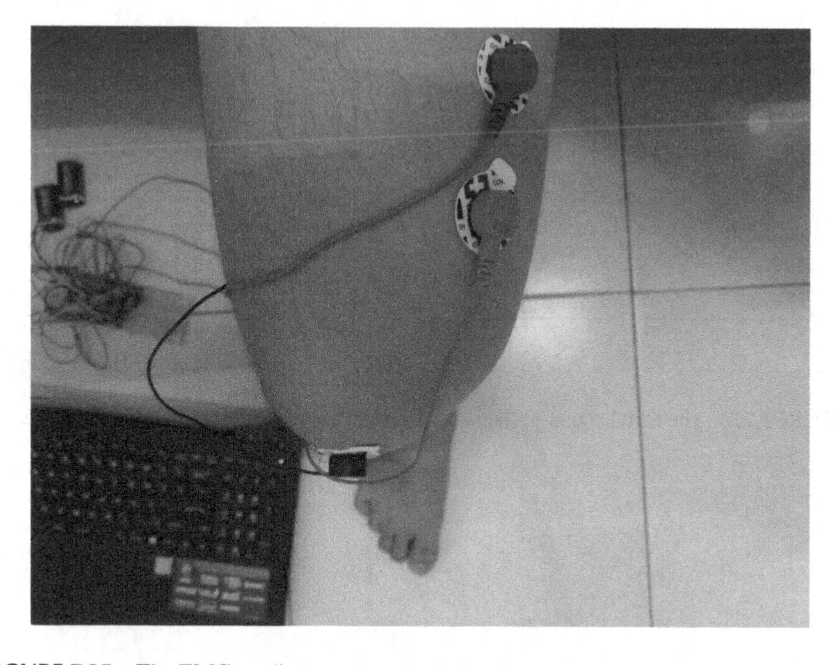

FIGURE 7.25 The EMG readings are acquired after the acupuncture treatment.

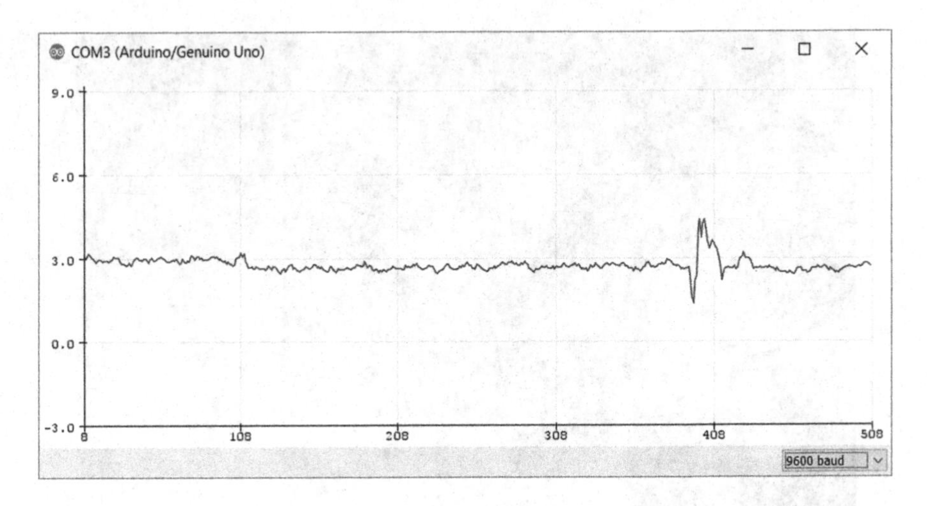

FIGURE 7.26 The EMG signal of the first volunteer before the acupuncture treatment.

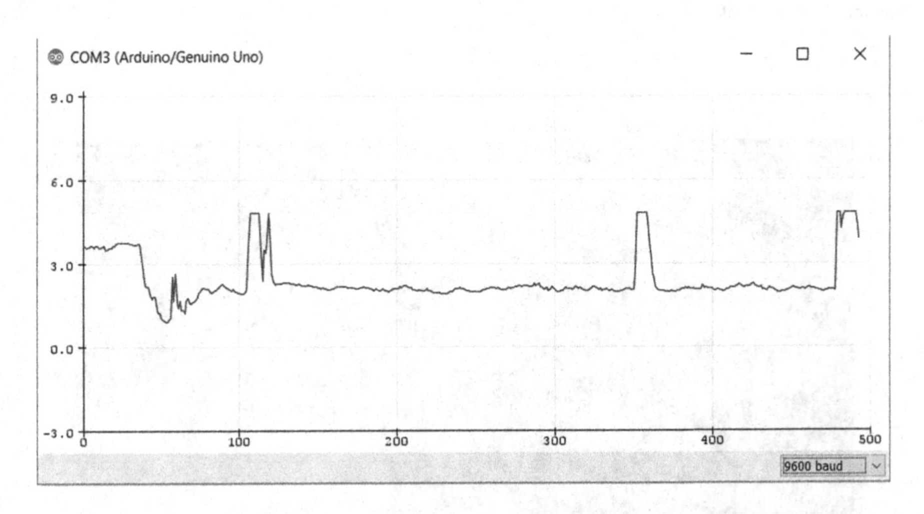

FIGURE 7.27 The EMG signal of the second volunteer before the acupuncture treatment.

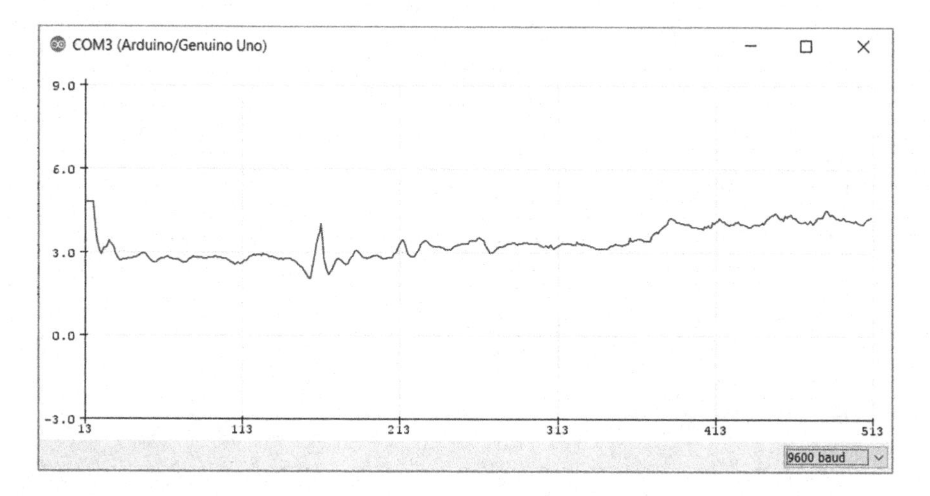

FIGURE 7.28 The EMG signal of the third volunteer before the acupuncture treatment.

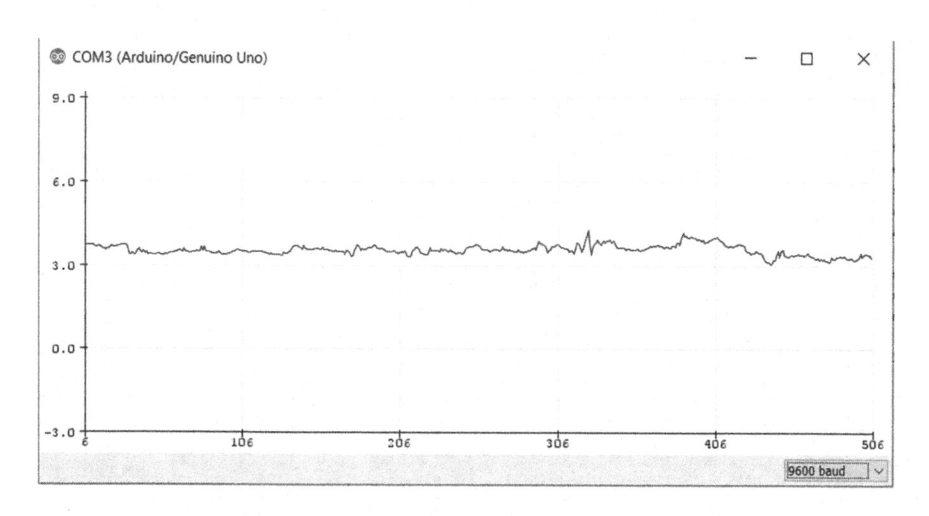

FIGURE 7.29 The EMG signal of the fourth volunteer before the acupuncture treatment.

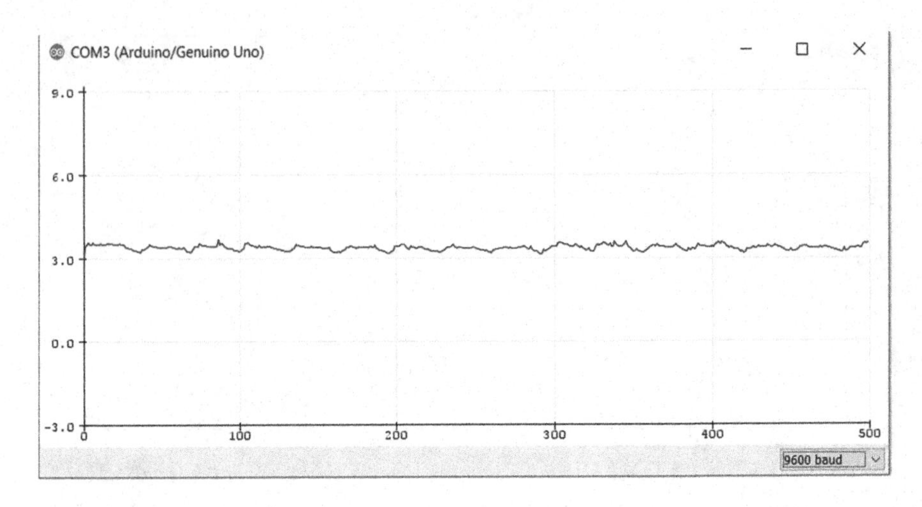

FIGURE 7.30 The EMG signal of the first volunteer after the acupuncture treatment.

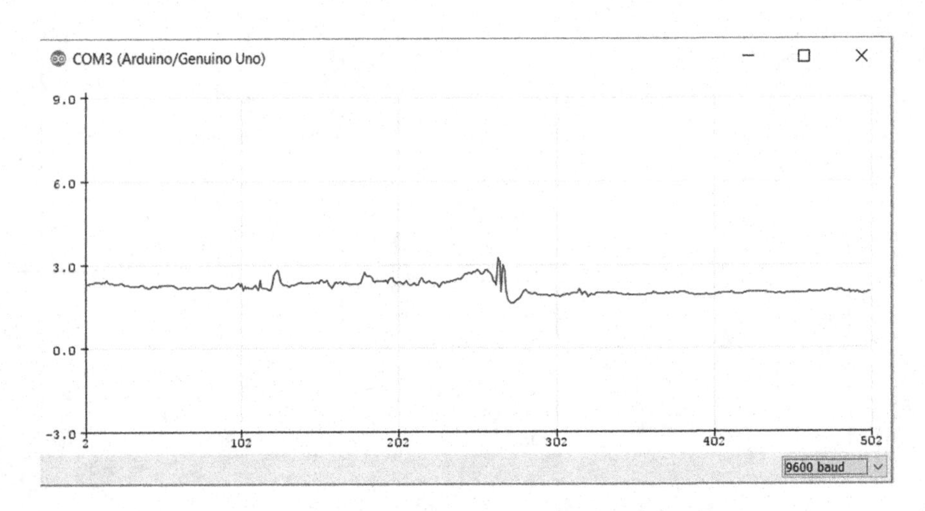

FIGURE 7.31 The EMG signal of the second volunteer after the acupuncture treatment.

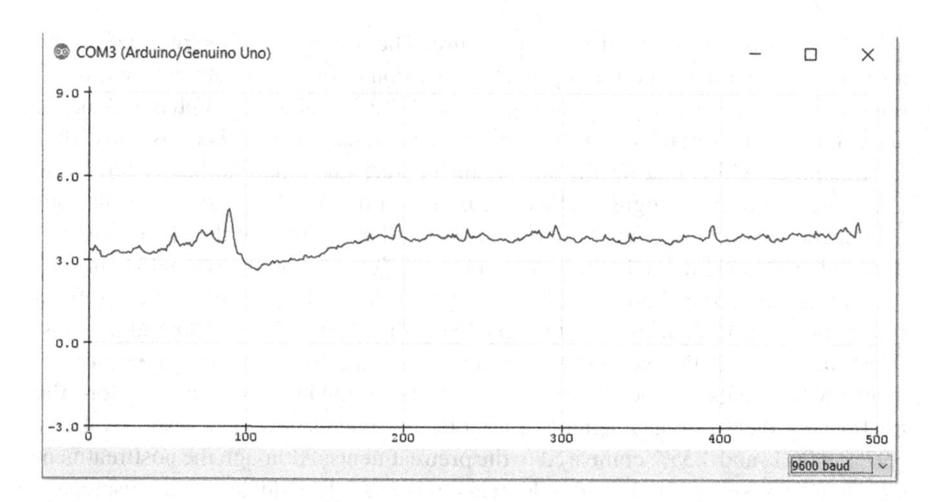

FIGURE 7.32 The EMG signal of the third volunteer after the acupuncture treatment.

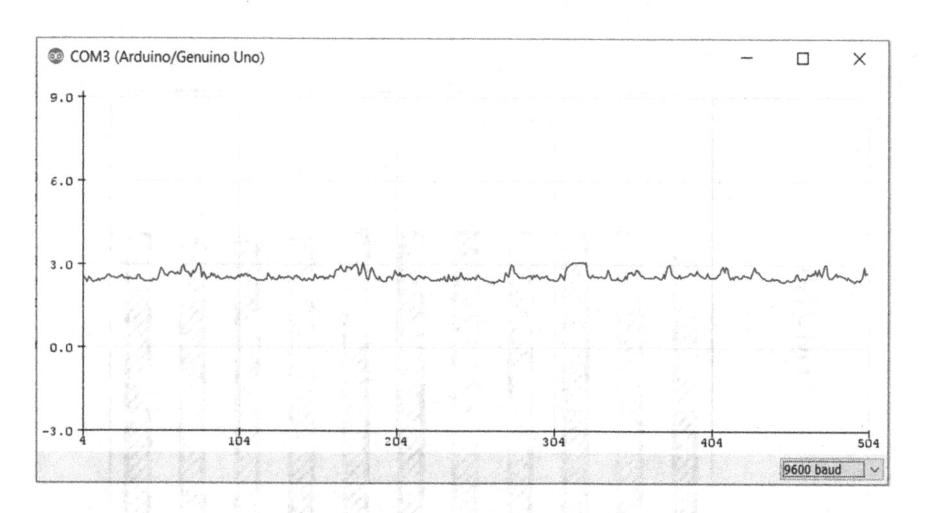

FIGURE 7.33 The EMG signal of the fourth volunteer after the acupuncture treatment.

considered as the after effect of acupuncture. The average EMG signal before the acupuncture treatment and the signal at each second after the treatment for a duration of 10 seconds are depicted in Figures 7.34–7.37. It is to be emphasized again, here, that the measurements for the first three volunteers were taken instantly after the treatment; while, that for the last volunteer were taken half an hour later. Upon close inspection on the figures, it can be observed that the EMG signal of the four volunteers before the acupuncture treatment are all above the 2 V threshold, with the third volunteer having the highest magnitude (i.e. 3.58 V) and the second having the lowest magnitude (i.e. 2.56 V). This is to say that their muscles were suffering from contractions due to injuries, and it is very likely that the third volunteer had the most severe injury, while the second the least severe. It can also be seen that the posttreatment EMG signals for the first three volunteers resemble closely those before the treatments – their average magnitudes after the treatments only vary, respectively, by 5.97%, 9.06%, and 4.55% compared to the pretreatments. Although the posttreatment signals for the second and third volunteers evince slight reductions, the discrepancies are still within the 15% range. Hence, the differences are very likely a result of electrical noise coupling effects. On the other hand, the average posttreatment magnitude for the fourth volunteer drops by 26.25%. The reduction rate is conspicuous and could be easily observed from Figure 7.37. Despite remaining above the threshold, it is apparent that the muscles of the fourth volunteer have manifested signs of relaxation after the treatment. The observation suggests strongly that acupuncture

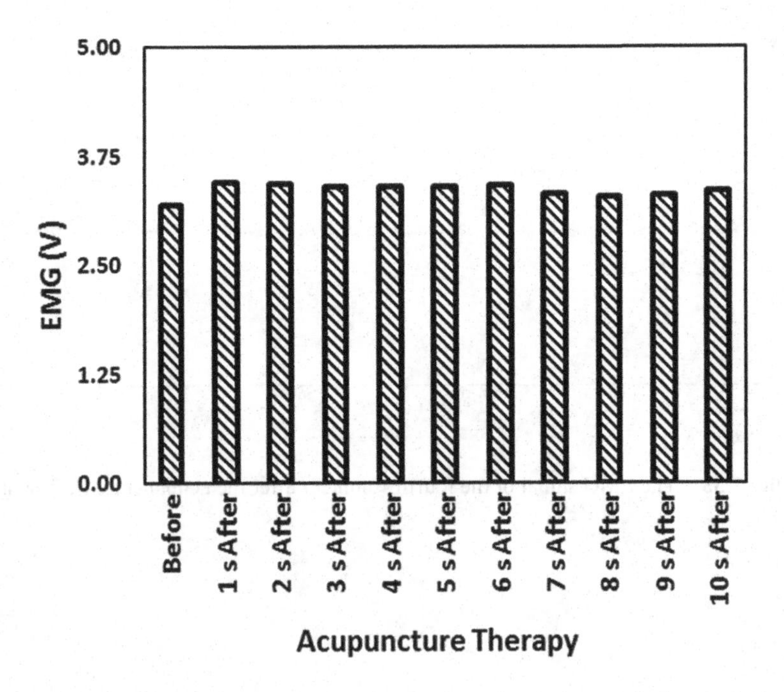

FIGURE 7.34 Comparison of the EMG signal of the first volunteer before and after the acupuncture treatment.

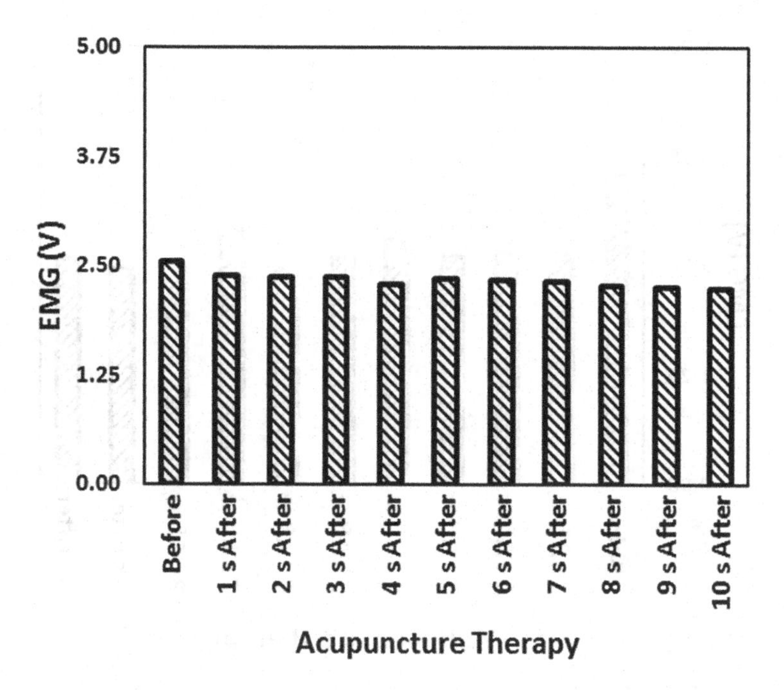

FIGURE 7.35 Comparison of the EMG signal of the second volunteer before and after the acupuncture treatment.

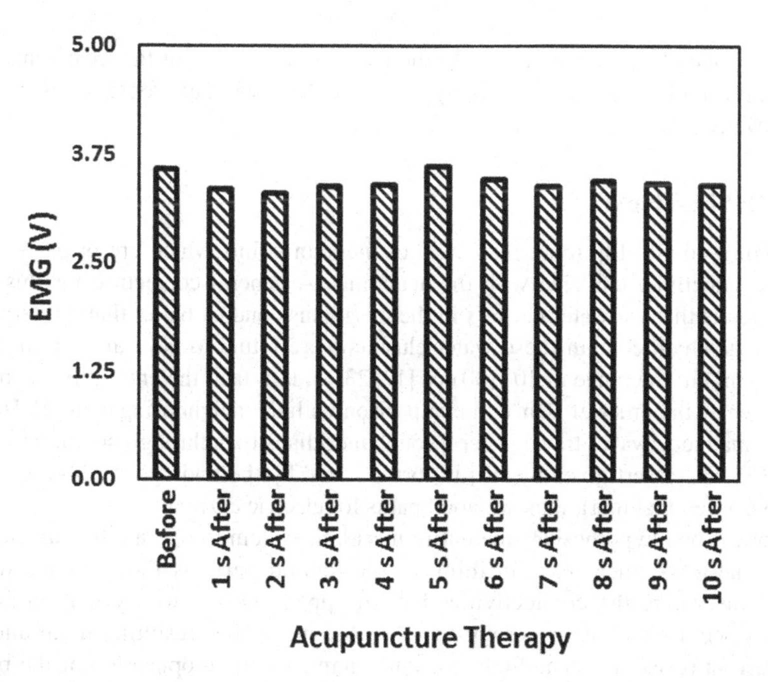

FIGURE 7.36 Comparison of the EMG signal of the third volunteer before and after the acupuncture treatment.

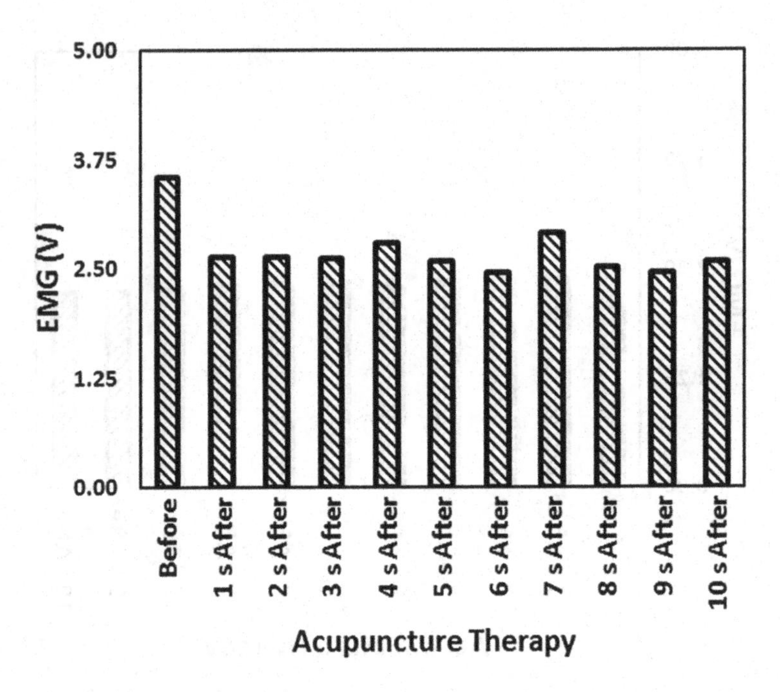

FIGURE 7.37 Comparison of the EMG signal of the fourth volunteer before and after the acupuncture treatment.

does provide effective medication to the patients. The effect of the treatment, however, may not be immediate and may, in fact, only slowly but progressively become noticeable.

7.5 HYPOTHESIS

According to [15–18], more than 90% of the skin points which are of particularly high conductivity coincide with the acupoints. A general conjecture for this phenomenon is that the water clusters in the meridians conduct better than proteins [2]. Solutions which contain these water clusters were found to have an electromotive force (emf) in the range of 10–100 mV [19–23] and, in fact, the emf at the acupoints is higher by the order of 10 mV in comparison with the neighboring skin [2]. Hence, electromagnetic waves travel faster through meridians than through nonmeridian tissue [15]. The assert given by [15] is corroborated by the findings in [24–26] which demonstrated that meridians are good paths for electric current.

Now, if one hypothesizes the entire meridian system to operate like an electric circuit network, then one can think of the injured parts as those related to the meridians where the conductivities have dropped. This is to say that an anomaly has occurred to the water clusters in those meridians, resulting in an unusual increase in resistance. The high resistance hampers the propagation of the polarized *qi*. When the improper distribution of the electrons (due to the unregulated *qi*) exceeds the intrinsic tolerance of a human body, one starts to feel uncomfortable or ill [27]. To allow sufficient amount of *qi* to flow through, it is apparent that alternate paths with much lower resistance are required. Most acupuncture needles are made of stainless steel; while some are made of silver – both of which are highly conducting materials. Inserting the acupuncture needles to the acupoints can be conceived as connecting parallel wires between the nodes with high resistance. A short-circuited path is therefore created at the abnormal meridians. Physically, this actually means that the needles are changing the constitutive properties of the body [28,29] within the region of the abnormal meridians. In other words, not only the conductivity but the permeability and permittivity which dictates, respectively, the magnetic and electric field densities at the meridians will be altered as well. It is to be noted, however, that this change is physiological and therefore the pace may be rather gradual. Once the constitutive properties of the meridians start to return to their healthy values, albeit not yet fully restored, the flow of *qi* would then be unclogged, and the imbalances in *qi* are regulated. The hypothesis is in congruence with the results observed in the case study conducted in this work. It is therefore safe to assert that acupuncture indeed provides curative efficacy, although the effect is not immediate.

7.6 CONCLUSION

In this chapter, the efficacy of acupuncture therapy has been investigated. An EMG sensor was built to assess the effect of the acupuncture treatment. The sensor consists of electrodes, amplifiers, filters, and a rectifier. To detect the muscle activity, the electrodes of the sensor were adhered to the skin of the volunteers. The output signal of the sensor subsequently went through an ADC process and was finally displayed at the serial monitor and the serial plot. The measurement results indicate that by helping to regulate the imbalances in *qi*, acupuncture produces remedy effect to the patients. The effect is, however, not immediately evident. Hence, the patients may only feel the remedy effect slowly but progressively.

Acknowledgement: This work was supported in part by the Universiti Tunku Abdul Rahman research fund (project: IPSR/RMC/UTARRF/2020-C1/Y03).

APPENDIX: CODE LISTING FOR EMG SENSOR TO EXTRACT DATA

```
int arduinoLED = 13; // Control the LED on the pin 13 of
Arduino
int thresholdValue = 2.5; // Set a threshold value
void setup() {
Serial.begin(9600); // Initialize serial communication at 9600
bits per second
pinMode(arduinoLED, OUTPUT); //Set the connected pin 13 as an
output
}
void loop() {
// Receive the output value from the EMG sensor and transmit
to analog input A0
int sensorValue = analogRead(A0);
```

```
float voltage = sensorValue * (5.0/1023.0); //Convert the
value received to voltage
Serial.print(voltage); //Display voltage value
if(voltage > thresholdValue){
//Trigger this when voltage value is larger than the threshold
value
Serial.println("CONTRACT!"); //Display string
digitalWrite(onboardLED, HIGH); //Turn on LED
} else {
//Trigger this when voltage value is lower than the threshold
value
Serial.println("RELAX!"); //Dislpay string
digitalWrite(onboardLED, LOW); //Turn off LED
}
delay(100) //Apply delay for the data acquisition
}
```

REFERENCES

1. Tsuei, J. J. 1996 The science of acupuncture-theory and practice, *IEEE Eng Med Biol Mag* **15**, 52–57.
2. Lo, S.-Y. 2002 Meridians in acupuncture and infrared imaging, *Med Hypotheses* **58**, 72–76.
3. de Camargo P. S., Lima C. R., Rezende M. L. A. E., Santos A. T. S., Hernandez J. W. R., and Silva A. M. 2018 The effect of auricular and systemic acupuncture on the electromyographic activity of the trapezius muscle with trigger points — A pilot study, *J Acupunct Meridian Stud* **11**, 18–24.
4. Yeung A., Chan J. S. M., Cheung J. C., and Zou L. 2018 Qigong and Tai-Chi for mood regulation, *Focus* **16**, 40–47.
5. Tsuei J. J., Lam F. M. K., and Chou P. 1996 Clinical applications of the EDST, *IEEE Eng Med Biol Mag* **15**, 67–75.
6. Tough L. 2006 Lack of effect of acupuncture on electromyo-graphic (EMG) activity – A randomised controlled trial in healthy volunteers, *Acupunct Med* **24**, 55–60.
7. Farida I. M., Ismail G., Susanti H., and Prasetio M. E. 2011 Observation of acupuncture stimulation on human stamina improvement using EMG. *2nd IEEE International Conference on Instrumentation Control and Automation*, pp. 71–76, Bandung, Indonesia.
8. Reaz M. B. I., Hussain M. S., and Mohd-Yasin F. 2006 Techniques of EMG signal analysis: Detection, processing, classification and applications, *Biol Proced Online* **8**, 11–35.
9. Webster J. G. 1990 *Encyclopedia of Medical Devices and Instrumentation*. John Wiley & Sons, Inc., Hoboken, NJ
10. Advancer Technologies. 2011. DIY Muscle Sensor / EMG Circuit for a Microcontroller. Instructables workshop. https://www.instructables.com/Muscle-EMG-Sensor-for-a-Microcontroller/ (accessed July 12, 2020).
11. Jamal M. Z. 2012 Signal acquisition using surface EMG and circuit design considerations for robotic prosthesis, *Comput Intell Electromyogr Anal. Perspect. Curr. Appl. Future Challenges* **18**, 427–448.
12. Desa H. M., Zuber M. S., Jailani R., and Tahir N. M. 2016 Development of EMG circuit for detection of leg movement. *IEEE Symposium on Computer Applications & Industrial Electronics*, pp. 46–51, Penang, Malaysia.

13. Margolis M., Jepson B., and Weldin N. R. 2020 *Arduino Cookbook: Recipes to Begin, Expand, and Enhance Your Projects.* O'Reilly Media, Newton, MA.
14. https://store.arduino.cc/usa/arduino-uno-rev3.
15. Chen K.-G. 1996 Electrical properties of meridians, *IEEE Eng Med Biol Mag* **15**, 58–63.
16. Zhu Z. 1981 Research advances in the electrical specificity of meridians and acupuncture points, *Am J Acupunct* **9**, 203.
17. Reichmanis M., Marino A. A., and Becker R. O. 1975 Electrical correlates of acupuncture points, *IEEE Trans Biomed Eng* **6**, 533–535.
18. Reichmanis M., Marino A. A., and Becker R. O. 1976 DC skin conductance variation at acupuncture loci, *Am J Chin Med* **4**, 69–72.
19. Holtzclaw B. J. 1998 New trends in thermometry for the patient in the ICU, *Crit Care Nurs Q* **21**, 12–25.
20. Jones B. F. 1998 A reappraisal of the use of infrared thermal image analysis in medicine, *IEEE Trans Med Imaging* **17**, 1019–1027.
21. Shevelev I. A. 1998 Functional imaging of the brain by infrared radiation (thermoencephaloscopy), *Progr Neurobiol* **56**, 269–305.
22. Ford R. G. and Ford K. T. 1997 Thermography in the diagnosis of headache: Seminars in neurology, *Semin Neurol* **17**, 343–349.
23. Sterns E. E., Zee B., SenGupta S., and Saunders F. W. 1996 Thermography: Its relation to pathologic characteristics, vascularity, proliferation rate, and survival of patients with invasive ductal carcinoma of the breast, *Cancer Interdisc Int J Am Cancer Soc* **77**, 1324–1328.
24. Niboyet J. 1958 Nouvelle constatations sur les proprietes electriques des ponts Chinois, *Bull Soc Acup* **30**, 7.
25. Darras J.-C., Vernejoul P. D., and Albarede P. 1992 Nuclear medicine and acupuncture: a study on the migration of radioactive tracers after injection at acupoints, *Am J Acupunct* **20**, 245–256.
26. Nakatani Y. 1956 An aspect of the study of Ryodoraku, *Clinic Chin Med* **3**, 54.
27. Chen K.-G. 1996 Applying quantum interference to EDST medicine testing, *IEEE Eng Med Biol Mag* **15**, 64–66.
28. Yeap K., Voon C., Hiraguri T., and Nisar H. 2019 A compact dual-band implantable antenna for medical telemetry, *Microwave Opt Technol Lett* **61**, 2105–2109.
29. Oh Z. X., Yeap K. H., Voon C. S., Lai K. C., and Teh P. C. 2020 A multiband antenna for biomedical telemetry and treatments, *J Phys Conf Ser*, **1502**, 012013.

8 Appliance Control System for Physically Challenged and Elderly Persons through Hand Gesture-Based Sign Language

G. Boopathi Raja
Velalar College of Engineering and Technology

CONTENTS

8.1 INTRODUCTION

Deafness is a physical challenge with difficulty of hearing, and such people's speech impediments can be severely limited. These people may still do few tasks more effectively even if they are hearing and/or speech impaired. The main barrier that separates these people from ordinary people is the way of communication. If it is possible for speaking-impaired people to communicate easily with common persons, then they have a chance to live comfort as the normal people do. The only possible way to communicate with others is sign language.

The term disability refers to the communication between people with an ailment such as cerebral paralysis, Down syndrome and wretchedness. Also, it may be due to individual and natural components, for example, negative mentalities, difficulty to reach transportation and public structures and restricted social backings [1].

8.1.1 Disability – A Public Health Issue

More than 1 billion people in the world are assessed to live with some type of disabilities. It corresponds to about 15% of the total population, with up to 190 million (3.8%) individuals with 15 years old and more than that having critical challenges in working, regularly requiring medical care administrations. The quantity of individuals living with inability is expanding to some degree because of ageing population and an expansion in chronic medical issue.

Disability is extremely different. While some medical issues related with disability bring about chronic weakness and broad medical care needs, others don't. The individuals with disability have similar general medical care needs as every other person and subsequently need admittance to standard medical service administrations. Article 25 of the UN Convention on the Rights of Persons with Disabilities (CRPD) fortifies the privilege of people with disability to achieve the best quality of medical care, without separation. Nonetheless, actually, a couple of nations offer sufficient quality types of assistance for individuals with disability [1,2].

The few countries collected the information to empower disaggregation by disability in the living area. This turned out to be evident during the COVID-19 pandemic where nations neglected to incorporate disability reliably in their reaction to control the pandemic. This left individuals with disability presented to three expanded dangers with pulverizing results: the dangers of contracting COVID-19, creating extreme manifestations from COVID-19 or dying from the sickness, just as having illness during and after the pandemic, regardless of whether they are contaminated with COVID-19.

8.1.2 Disability Statistics in India

One of the disability statistics reported the statement of UNESCO that 90% of kids with disabilities in agricultural-based nations have lesser chance to go to class. In the OECD nations, physically challenged students in higher education stay under-spoke to, despite the fact that their numbers are on the large quantity [3].

In 1991, Brazilian census released a survey that the disability rate was just 1%–2%. However, in the 2001 statistics, it was reported as a 14.5% rate. Comparative bounces in the deliberate pace of disability have happened in Turkey with 12.3% and Nicaragua with 10.1%.

People with handicaps are bound to be survivors of viciousness or assault, as per a 2004 British investigation, and more averse to get police mediation, legitimate security or preventive consideration. Ladies and young ladies with handicaps are especially helpless against misuse. A review in Orissa, India, discovered that practically the entirety of the ladies and young ladies with handicaps were beaten at home, 25% of ladies with scholarly inabilities had been assaulted and 6% of ladies with incapacities had been coercively disinfected. Exploration shows that brutality against kids with handicaps happens at yearly rates in any event 1.7 occasions more noteworthy than for their companions without inabilities [3].

Census 2001 has reported that more than 20 million people in India were experiencing any one disability. It was approximately equal to 2.1% of the entire population. In that, 12.6 million were male and 9.3 million are female. It was 57%–58% of males and 42%–43% of females. The disability rate is nothing but the number of impaired per 100,000 persons. The disability rate in India was 2130. The disability rate of male alone was 2369, and 1874 for female [4]. Table 8.1 shows the type of disabilities with disability population along with percentage (Figure 8.1).

The information has been collected about the five types of disabilities. The disability in seeing was 48.5% arising as the top class. The disability in movement was 27.9%, 10.3% of people were affected by mental disorder, speech impairing was in 7.5% and 5.8% of people with disability in hearing. The crippled by sex follow a comparative example aside from that the extent of impaired females is higher in the category of seeing and hearing disability.

The highest number of disabled people has been reported in Uttar Pradesh with 3.6 million. Critical quantities of disabilities have additionally been accounted from states like Bihar with 1.9 million, West Bengal with 1.8 million and Tamil Nadu and Maharashtra with 1.6 million each. Tamil Nadu is the main state that has a higher number of disabled females than males. Among the states, Arunachal Pradesh has reported with the highest number of disabilities in males of about 66.6% and least number of females disabled.

TABLE 8.1
Type of Disability versus Disability Percentage

Types of Disability	Population	Percentage (%)
In seeing	10,634,881	1.0
In movement	6,105,477	0.6
Mental	2,263,821	0.2
In speech	1,640,868	0.2
In hearing	1,261,722	0.1

Source: Census of India 2001.

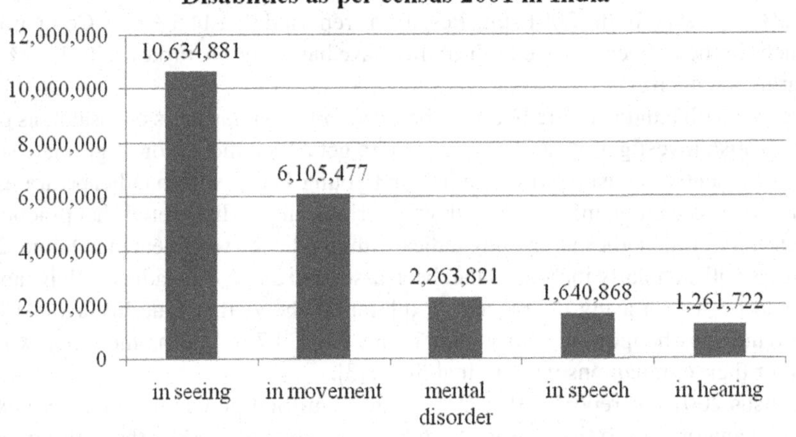

FIGURE 8.1 Disabilities in India as per 2001 census.

The National Statistical Office (NSO) comes under the Ministry of Statistics and Program Implementation. As a part of the 76th round of National Sample Survey (NSS), it has led a survey on the disabilities during July to December 2018.

The review report of NSO has discussed that the consolidated range of people with disability in the entire population was around 2.2% during July to December 2018 in India. Before this, NSO conducted the review on a similar subject in the 58th round conducted from July to December 2002. In this review, the level of people with disabilities in the total population of India was around 2.2%. It includes 2.3% in rural areas and 2% in metropolitan areas. Pervasiveness of disability was found maximum for males than females. That is, the disability rate for male was 2.4%, while it was 1.9% for females.

The fundamental goal of the survey was to find the factors of occurrence and pervasiveness of disability, cause, onset age and facilities accessible to those people. They are in trouble looked by them in getting to/utilizing public structure/public vehicle, course of action of ordinary guardian, cash-based costs identifying with disability, and so on.

The survey reported that 52.2% of people with disability of 7 years old or more were educated. Among people with disabilities of 15 years old or more, 19.3% had the highest education qualification. Around 10.1% of people with disabilities from age 3 to 35 went to preschool education program. Also, it reported that around 62.9% of people with disabilities from 3 to 35 years underwent school education.

Around 3.7% of the people with disabilities live alone without family support, while 62.1% of people with disabilities had guardians. About 21.8% received help from government, and another 1.8% received support from various associations other than government. It also cleared that 22.8% of people with disabilities had the certificate of disability. The unemployment rate of people with disabilities with age more than 15 years was around 4.2% [5].

8.1.3 Barriers to Healthcare

People with disabilities experience a scope of obstructions when they endeavor to get to medical services including the accompanying:

- **Prohibitive expenses**: People with disabilities do not get genuinely necessary medical care in low-pay nations due to two primary reasons such as affordability of medical services and transportation. Simply half portion of individuals with handicap can't bear the cost of medical care compared with about 33% of individuals without disability.
- **Limited accessibility of services**: There is an absence of appropriate services for individuals with disabilities. Numerous investigations uncover high neglected requirements for medical care among individuals with disability because of inaccessibility of administrations, particularly in provincial and far-off regions.
- **Physical boundaries**: Uneven access to hospitals, primary health centers, inaccessible clinical hardware, helpless signage, restricted entryways, inner advances, lacking washroom offices and unavailable stopping zones make obstructions to medical care offices. For instance, women with versatility challenges are regularly unfit to get to breast and cervical disease screening since assessment tables are not adjustable to height.
- **Inadequate knowledge and training to medical service providers**: Individuals with disabilities were more than twice as liable to report discovering medical service supplier skills deficient to address their issues, multiple times bound to report being dealt with gravely and almost multiple times bound to report being denied care.

This report consists of an introductory part, and the overall organization of the rest of the chapter is as follows. Section 8.2 elaborates about the several literature studies reviewed corresponding to the proposed work. Sections 8.3 and 8.4 present the details about device-based and visual-based techniques. Section 8.5 discusses the existing techniques. The glove-based framework and the camera-based framework were introduced in Sections 8.6 and 8.7, respectively. The chapter ended with proper conclusion and future scope.

This chapter consists of introduction about gesture recognition techniques, objective, theme and organization of the project. The following chapter discusses about the surveyed chapters with its existing techniques and procedure to design a proposed system.

8.2 LITERATURE SURVEY

In this chapter, the literature available within the preview of the objectives of the present study is reviewed. The existing system has voice-input communication. This system has user interface and speech synthesis circuit. But this system is suitable only for deaf people. Users need to speak with user interface which is provided in this system. This speech signal goes under further processing to acquire more information from the input. The gadget can be designed to empower the client to make either straightforward or complex messages utilizing a mix of a generally small arrangement of input words. But this method is difficult to implement and requires complex design and accurate analysis equipment.

For deaf people, the sign language technique is very popular, and it supports to communicate with ordinary people. This helps them get little attention from ordinary people. As ordinary people, we often overlook the importance of sign language, unless there are deaf loved ones. One of the best ways to communicate with the deaf is to use sign-language translation tools. But the use of sign language interpreters may be expensive. The cost-effective way is needed so that they can communicate normally.

Therefore, several research studies were carried out to identify the better solution for deaf people to communicate more easily with the common person. The development of this is a system of recognition of sign language. The purpose of this framework is to recognize sign language. It translates it into desired language by text or speech. But, designing the system was much costly, complicated in design and difficult to use for everyday use. The past researchers found a better solution, that is, sign-language recognition systems using data gloves. However, the cost gloves and bulletproof material makes everyone as luxurious product. With that in mind, the researchers further made a clean impression of improved sign language recognition (SLR) programs. However, there are difficulties, especially in tracking hand movements.

From the image acquisition stage to segmentation stage, the SLR technique suffers with lot of challenges. Investigators are still finding the better solution to get an image. The collection of images using the camera complicates the preprocessing phase of the image. The use of an active sensor device was much expensive. Some challenges may arise in the present research studies based on image classification. The wide selection of observation methods makes it difficult for researchers to focus on one particular path. The selection of one focus method often creates another method that could be a better SLR suit, not test. Experimental alternatives prevent researchers from developing one method to its full potential [6].

The only medium used in communication between a hearing-impaired community and the general public is Sign Language. The SLR program, which is required for SLR, has been widely studied for years. The studies are based on a variety of input sensors, touch detection and feature extraction and differentiation methods. This chapter aims to analyze and compare the techniques preferred in the SLR programs and the classification methods that have been used and proposes the most promising approach to future research. Due to recent advances in segregation methods, many recent proposed activities contribute significantly to segregation approaches, such as the hybrid approach and Deep Learning. This work focuses on the classification methods used in the previous SLR system. According to our review, the methods designed for HMM have been extensively tested in previous research, including its modification. Advanced Learning as a Convolutional Neural Network has become popular over the past 5 years. Hybrid CNN-HMM and in-depth learning methods have shown promising results and provide opportunities for further testing. However, excess and high computational requirements still prevent their detection [7,8].

The computerized gesture-based communication provided efficient services for the individual with hard of hearing since it conquers the communication gap that exists among them and the rest of the community. Gesture is one of the important forms in SLR. It provides the significant function in improving the recognition of gesture-based communication. Video databases are important for programmed or computer-based recognition of crises from communication via gestures to support the deaf communities. In the fields of Hand Gesture Recognition (HGR) and SLR, this information base is more essential and valuable for researchers to do research [9]. Likewise, vector- and feature-based classification of emergency gestures has been done, and the base grouping execution shows that the database can be utilized as a benchmarking dataset for creating novel and improved methods for perceiving the hand gestures of crisis words in Indian sign language.

The recognition of reasonable body movements that incorporate the changes in position of face, head, arms, fingers, hands or body made for the need of exchanging data or interfacing with nature is known as gesture recognition. This work is viewed as valuable for applications dependent on a smart and effective interface of human and computer. In particular, the recognition of activity applies to a wide scope of PCs, for example, those including interactions with kids, gesture-based communication acknowledgment, monitoring of physical activity or occasions including individuals with disabilities or the elder aged peoples, clinical or enthusiastic injury or exposure, extortion in visual, video chat communication, distance education and monitoring and resting status.

The use of a variety of visual or auditory gadgets to follow development was required in the implementation of computer-based detection. For recognizing body movements, it is necessary to use current visual channel, the most preferred way to detect body movements. Visual recording gadgets are generally introduced in a fixed position. The activity recognition is limited to a closed space. The wearable gadgets utilized for visual acuity incorporate a lens of camera and a wrist mounted gadget with an infrared phantom (IR) camera. The monitoring of finger movements is a specific and essential task in visual activity [10]. It is utilized in gesture-based communication and in augmented simulation and on robots. Nerve gadgets, for example, gloves with sensors and electromyogram (EMG) gloves, are additionally used to record the movements of finger accurately. The ring is made of another wearable item that is raised to identify the touch of a finger. The word development of touch-handling care of gadgets is additionally an intriguing theme.

This chapter means to examine the SLR system utilized by specialists. In this chapter, we will talk about the idea of Sign Language application. This chapter will examine the gadget utilized for acquisition of information, for example, information from beginning examination or self-produced information, the location technique as of late utilized by analysts and the release of past exploration.

In everyday life, it is a difficult task to communicate and control the electronic appliances through wired medium. The remote-controlled appliances require an electronic control device to be carried by the individual in order to control the appliance. This method is not reliable as there is a chance of losing the control device, and each appliance requires a different remote controller to be used. However, the control signals produced by the remote are limited and often require line of sight communication. Hence, it is difficult to use in environments like manufacturing units, military bases, etc. [11,12].

8.3 PREFERABLE TECHNIQUES

8.3.1 Device-Based Techniques

Gadget-based strategies include the type of template or layout. For example, the status and the position of hand were determined by a glove or glove-based system designed along with flex sensors and position trackers [13,14].

8.3.2 Visual-Based Techniques

Visual-based methods use efficient camera that must have the capability to track the movements continuously, whereby the customer wears gloves with explicit shadings or markers demonstrating individual elements of the hands, exceptionally the fingers. It is necessary to record the movement of a person continuously with the help of a high-resolution camera along with the position of the hand as the customer signs. The hand shape, position as well as direction of the hand or fingers are analyzed, and valid gestures are recognized and/or recovered from the image captured from the camera [15–17].

8.3.3 Device- versus Visual-Based Techniques

Components of the device-based technique are quite compact and relatively cheap. There are two major limitations in this technique. Firstly, the data retrieved are only as accurate as the individual devices sent for measurement and are subjected to various forms of noise (optical or magnetic for the tracking devices). Secondly, the person must wear a glove and is restricted by wires returning to a receiver. This situation could be improved by utilizing wireless technology imposing only the glove itself. As opposed to the device-based technique, the visual-based technique does not require useful data immediately. Also, two cameras are required if 3D information is desired, and this compounds the processing exponentially. With the degree of processing required comes the problem of storage and delay, and hence, this technique would not easily be realized as a portable, real-time system.

8.4 EXISTING SYSTEM

The visual-based system requires a camera to capture the image of the gesture to convert the sign language into corresponding symbol or alphabet [18,19]. It requires a complex designing technique and is of high cost. Controlling electronic equipment using a remote device requires an electronic system to be carried by the person. However, this also requires line of sight communication between the controlling device and the electronic appliances.

8.5 PROPOSED METHODOLOGY

8.5.1 Data Glove-Based System

The proposed system uses a hand glove technology to communicate with the electronic appliances using the language used by the dumb people for communication with the normal people which is generally called the sign language. It includes the movement of fingers and the hands to create gestures which correspond to words or characters in the sign language. An electronic glove is a simple, easy-to-use device which can be used as a normal glove to be fitted to the hand [20,21].

The flex sensors and the accelerometer sensor were used in the design of electronic gloves. For each and every hand motion, there is a corresponding sign which is captured by the sensors relating to the hand sign regulator. The role of hand sign regulator or controller is to continuously verify the matching between hand gestures with images stored in database. The gadget interprets letters in order as well as meaningful words from high-quality motions. The translation of larger gestures must be done by the proposed gadget based on movement of single hand. Hence, corresponding signals can be produced for each particular hand gesture. Hence, this method can be used in all environments and also for physically disabled and dumb people for communication with electronic appliances as well as people.

8.5.1.1 Objective

This chapter proposes a method to convert the hand signs into an electronic command. This is done with the help of embedded technology. This technology also facilitates communication between two persons who cannot converse directly. One person using sign language while the other unable to understand it needs something in between which can perform translation between the two different modes of communication they know. Speaking impaired people, that is, dumb individuals, rely upon the communication based on gesture-based translator. However, they cannot rely upon mediators consistently in life essentially. It is due to the significant expenses and the trouble in determining and booking qualified interpreters or translators. This framework can support the disabled people in empowering their personal satisfaction fundamentally. This strategy can be utilized to control gadgets.

8.5.1.2 Theme

The procedure discussed in this work is to effectively recognize the hand sign, with more accuracy was done by designing a device using glove technology. The data glove used in the proposed framework consists of two main parts. They are flex sensors and an accelerometer. It is necessary to design a sensor glove with sensor in order to improve accuracy. The work has been improved by capturing the direction of hand movements by the inclusion of two or more accelerometers once the gesture is made. It may extend the capability of framework to translate larger gestures.

8.5.1.3 Summary

In a gesture-based communication, sign is nothing but the particular hand movement with a prescribed shape made out of them. Additionally, facial expressions are also included simultaneously along with hand gestures. The drawback of vision-based strategies incorporates complex calculations for data preparing.

Another challenge associated with this approach is the preparation of video and image incorporates shifting lighting conditions, foundations and field of view constraints and impediment. The insight concerning framework description is clarified in the accompanying section.

8.5.1.4 System Description

The primary objective of this theme is to encourage individuals by methods for a glove-based dumb communication translator (or) interpreter framework. Each glove consists of approximately 5–6 flex sensors and 1 or 2 accelerometers. For every particular signal, the flex sensor creates a corresponding variation in resistance, and accelerometer quantifies the direction of hand. The processing of these hand motions was done by suitable microprocessor or microcontroller. The glove incorporates two methods of activity preparing mode to make benefit to each client and an operational unit. The concatenation of letters to frame words is also performed by the microcontroller. Moreover, the framework also incorporates a transfer control block which makes an interpretation of the coordinated motions into control signals.

Gesture recognition is also known as motion acknowledgment. This technique suggests a method by which data is collected from the various parts of the human body, typically the head, fingers or hand. It may be analyzed to decide attributes, for example, direction, hand shape and speed of motion being performed.

The gadget-based procedures work in two different types of modes. These are listed as follows:

1. Learning mode
2. Operational mode.

8.5.1.5 Learning Mode

In this mode, it is necessary to store database with a set of recognized hand gesture images in the framework. The customer should make offers to use gestures of all the letters in the database sets. An LED is utilized to check whether the framework is available to the task or busy with other activity. At that time, the customer should make sign for the letters in order that are being shown on LCD. In this cycle, the customer will twist his fingers in a particular way to make the motion that will make the diverse flex sensors in various fingers to twist by specific points which might be the same or unique in relation to one another relying upon the signals to be made.

It leads to modify the resistance value of the flex sensors. Thus, the resistance will increase if the flex sensors are bent. This adjustment in resistance will be changed over into voltage by associating the flex sensors in a potential divider circuit. Along these lines, the analog voltage from each flex sensors will be given to the ADC ports of the microcontroller. This simple voltage will be changed over into computerized structure by ADC in the microcontroller.

8.5.1.6 Operational Mode

In this mode, the framework will recognize the gestures made by the clients. Also, it will find the alphabets from the database made during the learning mode to show it on the LCD.

8.5.1.7 System Architecture

The block diagram of the glove-based hand gesture recognition framework is shown in Figure 8.2. The framework has numerous modules. They are flex sensors, accelerometer sensor, microcontroller, ZigBee module, LCD display, relay module and power supply.

Figure 8.3 shows the block diagram of the transmitter section used in glove-based hand gesture recognition system. The entire transmitter section is placed along with person with disability. The transmitter section consists of Data Glove, Raspberry Pi 2/3 and Zigbee module. The data glove comprises two submodules. They are

a. Flex sensors
b. Accelerometer sensors.

The receiver part of the glove-based hand gesture recognition framework is shown in Figure 8.4. It consists of Raspberry pi processor, zigbee module, LCD display and driver circuit. Raspberry pi processor analyzes the signal received from the transmitter section through zigbee Tx/Rx unit. The decision is taken by the receiver side

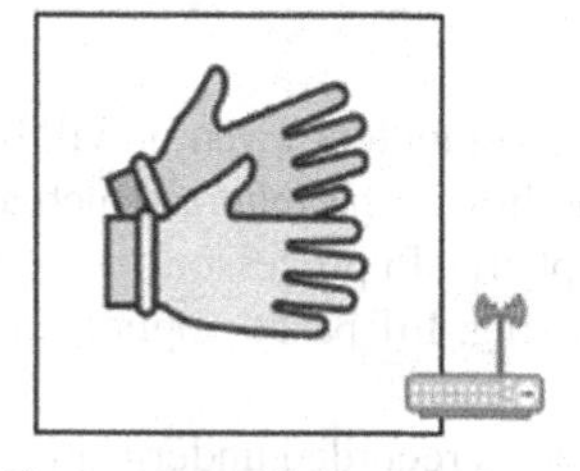

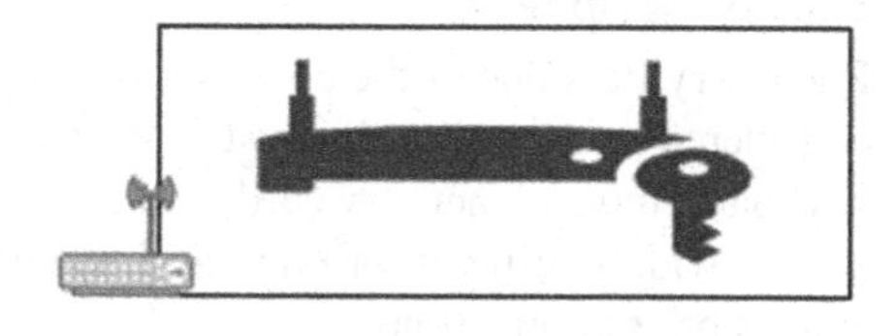

FIGURE 8.2 Block diagram for glove-based hand gesture recognition system.

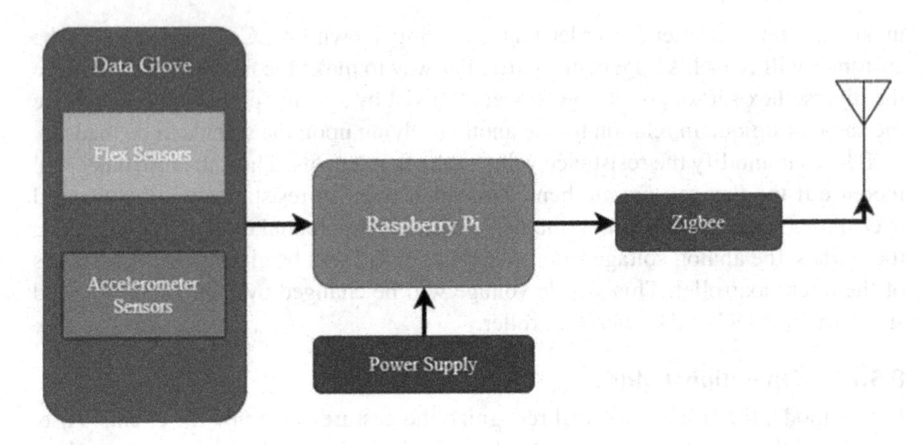

FIGURE 8.3 Transmitter section of glove-based framework.

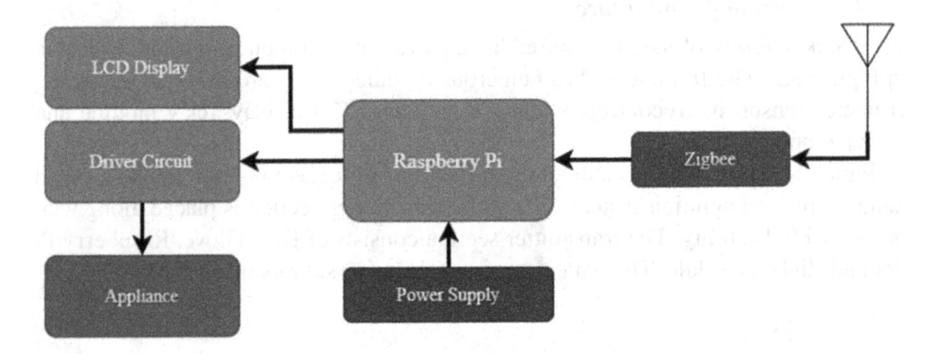

FIGURE 8.4 Receiver section of glove-based framework.

processor based on the finger position of the person. The recognized sign is converted into a suitable form and sent to the corresponding driver circuit to make the appliances either ON or OFF. It is one of the most preferable ways to control the home appliances without direct contact.

8.5.1.8 Raspberry Pi

Raspberry Pi is one of the compact and tiny single board computers. Even, it will be considered as a smaller than usual PC by interfacing additional peripherals such as keyboard, mouse, memory card, and camera to the Raspberry Pi processor.

It is widely utilized for ongoing Image/Video processing, IoT-based applications and robotics applications.

There are various renditions of raspberry pi accessible as recorded underneath:

- Raspberry Pi 1 Model A
- Raspberry Pi 1 Model A+
- Raspberry Pi 1 Model B

- Raspberry Pi 1 Model B+
- Raspberry Pi 2 Model B
- Raspberry Pi 3 Model B
- Raspberry Pi Zero.

8.5.1.9 Data Glove

There are two different categories of data gloves available. They are flex sensor and accelerometer sensor. The response of the accelerometer sensor is perceived by the tilt area module. The response produced by the flex sensors and the overall proposal of the hand are recognized by the recognition unit. The recognition of motion or gesture is performed by the microcontroller.

8.5.1.10 Flex Sensor

Flex sensors consist of resistive carbon parts. The sensor produces responses as resistance corresponded to the span if there arises an occurrence of bent. The change in the resistance is generally around 10 kΩ. An unflexed sensor has a resistance of about 10 kΩ, and when twisted, the resistance increased to 30 kΩ at 90°. The sensor is about ¼ inch wide and 4.5 inches long. Figure 8.5 shows the structure of flex sensor.

The sensor is incorporated in gadget having a voltage divider network. Voltage divider is utilized to find the output voltage across two resistors associated in series as shown in Figure 8.6.

The resistor and flex create a voltage divider which partitions the input voltage by a proportion controlled by the variable and fixed resistors. In this module, any one microcontroller is preferred, and five analog pins of that microcontroller are

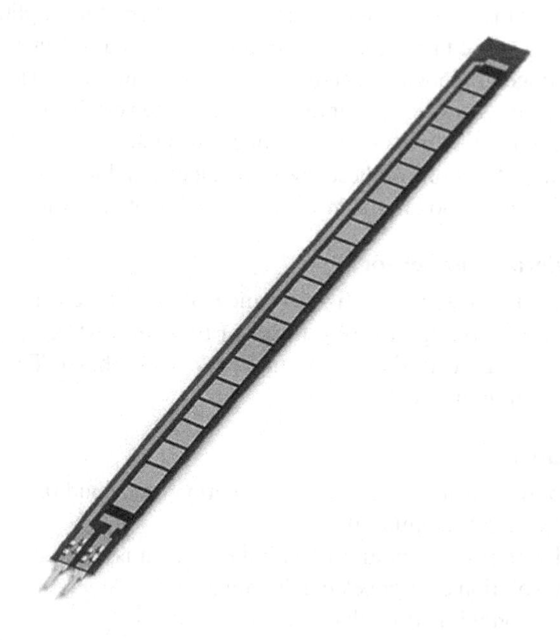

FIGURE 8.5 Flex sensor.

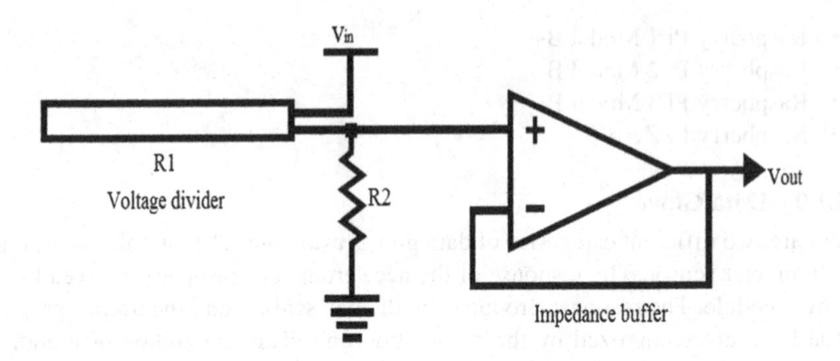

FIGURE 8.6 Equivalent circuit of flex sensor.

associated with the flex sensors. The inbuilt analog to digital converters of the microcontroller change over the analog output of the flex sensor into an understandable form by the preferred microcontroller.

The bend sensors were managed individually by the preferred microcontroller. The response of the principal bend sensor was monitored by microcontroller and ascertains its sufficiency. After the calculation of each bend sensor, the output was stored by microcontroller, and afterward, it moves toward the second bend sensor and computes its amplitude in the comparative way. The amplitude of the bend sensors can be calculated continuously one by one. The amplitudes of five bend sensors have been calculated, and then the microcontroller moves toward the following stage of the module, for example, gesture recognition. Gesture detection or sign recognition is the main part of this module.

The amplitude of the obtained signal can be calculated by the amplitude calculation module. It may be acquired from the bend sensors at a standard stretch. Indeed, even a little bend of the finger is recognized at this phase of the framework. Hence, the bowing of the figure has endless degrees of curves, and the framework is touchy to the bowing of the finger. Presently, the twisting of each finger is quantized into ten levels. At any stage, the finger must be at one of these levels, and it can undoubtedly be resolved how much the finger is bowed. So far, the individual twisting of each finger is caught.

8.5.1.11 Accelerometer Sensor

Accelerometer in the gesture vocalized framework is utilized as a tilt sensor, in which it checks the inclining or tilting factor of the hand. ADXL 345 is a computerized accelerometer used to decide the inclining of the hand. The accelerometer ADXL 345 is shown in Figure 8.7.

8.5.1.12 Features

- Ultralow power: as low as 23 μA in estimation mode and 0.1 μA in backup mode at VS = 2.5 V (common)
- Power utilization scales naturally with data transmission
- Supports resolution as user selectable range
- Fixed resolution with 10-bit data rate
- Activity/inertia checking

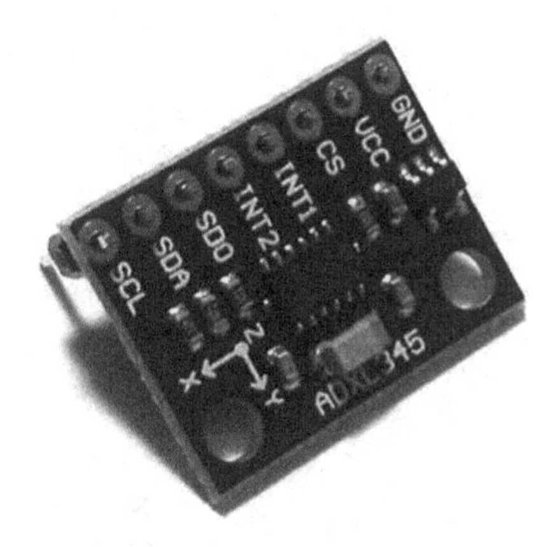

FIGURE 8.7 Accelerometer sensor.

- Supply voltage range: 2.0–3.6 V
- I/O voltage range: 1.7 V to 2.5 V
- SPI (3- and 4-wire) and I2C digital interfaces
- Flexible interrupt modes mapping to either interrupt pin
- Measurement ranges selectable by means of sequential order
- Bandwidth selectable by means of sequential order
- Wide temperature range (−40°C to +85°C)
- 10,000 g shock survival.

8.5.1.13 General Description

The ADXL345 is one of the popular accelerometers. It is tiny, thin, ultra-low power, 3-axis accelerometer with high-resolution estimation at up to ±16 g. The digital output is arranged as the complement of 16-bit rows. It is available through either a SPI (3- or 4-wire) or I2C advanced interface. The ADXL345 is appropriate for cell phone applications. Its high goal empowers estimation of tendency changes under 1.0°.

A few uncommon detecting capacities are given. The detection of active and idle case is necessary to recognize the presence or absence of movement by contrasting the quickening on any axis with predefined threshold values. Tap detecting recognizes single and twofold taps toward any path. Free-fall detecting distinguishes if the gadget is falling. These capacities can be planned separately to both of two interrupt output terminals. A coordinated memory management framework with a 32-level first in, first out (FIFO) buffer can be utilized to store information to limit the processor action and the overall power utilization. The intelligent motion-based power management was enhanced by low power modes with suitable threshold sensing and active acceleration measurement at minimal power dissipation. The ADXL345 is provided in a compact, tiny, 3 mm × 5 mm × 1 mm, 14-lead, plastic bundle.

8.5.1.14 System Flow

When the system starts to function, the movement of the hand is recognized by the sensor fixed on the hand, and the data are collected. The data are then passed to the

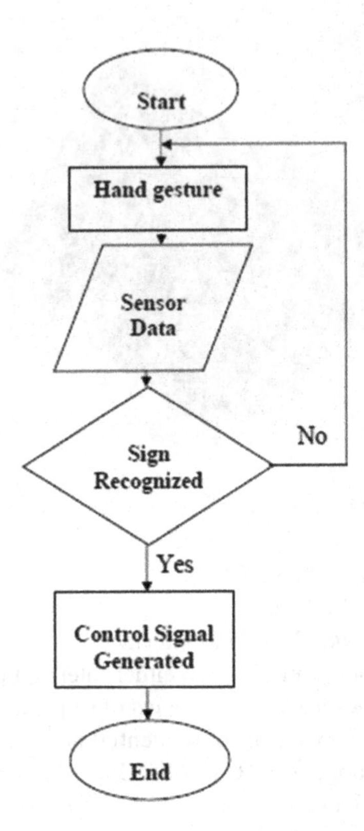

FIGURE 8.8 Flowchart for recognition process in glove-based system.

controller in order to verify it with the predefined values. If both values are the same, the control signal is produced, otherwise the procedure gets started again. Figure 8.8 shows the flowchart for recognition process in glove-based system.

8.5.1.15 System Functionality

The position and direction of the hand are procured from the data glove once the power is turned on. It consists of five flex sensors on the fingers (thumb, list, middle, ring and pinky) and one accelerometer of three yields (X, Y and Z positions). The slanting of the palm can be captured by the accelerometer where flex sensors can evaluate the touch of the five fingers when making a sign. During that point, when the customer plays out a movement/letter, signals coming from the sensors are strengthened by methods for a committed improvement circuit to each flag. Subsequently, the microcontroller collects this information, which may change the simple signals over to digitized qualities through its ADC pins.

These characteristics are coordinated into a clear state grid: five characteristics for the flex sensors and one for each center point of the accelerometer. In this way, each letter in the American Sign Language (ASL) will have a specific computerized level for the five fingers and the three rotations of the accelerometer. Each level is addressed by an incentive some place in the scope of 0 and 255-a stretch of time three

TABLE 8.2
Look-Up Table of Digital Levels for Fingers and Accelerometer Axis Outputs

Letter	Thumb	Index	Middle	Ring	Pinky	X,Y,Z Positions
A	12	15	18	12	12	18
B	23	23	28	23	23	23
C	35	38	35	33	35	35
D	46	48	41	41	46	43
E	51	53	53	56	56	53
F	64	64	61	69	69	64
G	79	74	76	79	74	76
H	84	81	87	87	81	84
I	94	92	94	97	92	94
J	104	102	104	107	102	104
K	112	112	115	115	117	117
L	122	125	127	122	127	125
M	133	135	133	138	135	133
N	143	148	143	148	143	145
O	151	153	157	155	158	151
P	163	168	165	168	163	163
Q	174	171	176	177	177	174
R	184	183	189	186	189	182
S	191	194	193	195	197	199
T	201	206	209	209	202	204
U	215	217	219	212	215	217
V	225	227	223	221	223	225
W	237	232	237	235	235	237
X	241	243	241	243	244	243
Y	247	246	248	247	248	248
Z	253	253	252	252	254	254

levels should be idea about in case the customer couldn't keep his hand reliable. The relating modernized levels are given in Table 8.2.

8.5.2 Camera-Based System

Figure 8.9 shows the block diagram of Appliance Control System using hand gesture-based sign language. The proposed technique is based on image processing techniques.

The working of the proposed system is categorized into three phases. They are

I. Capturing input hand gesture
II. Gesture recognition
III. Appliances control.

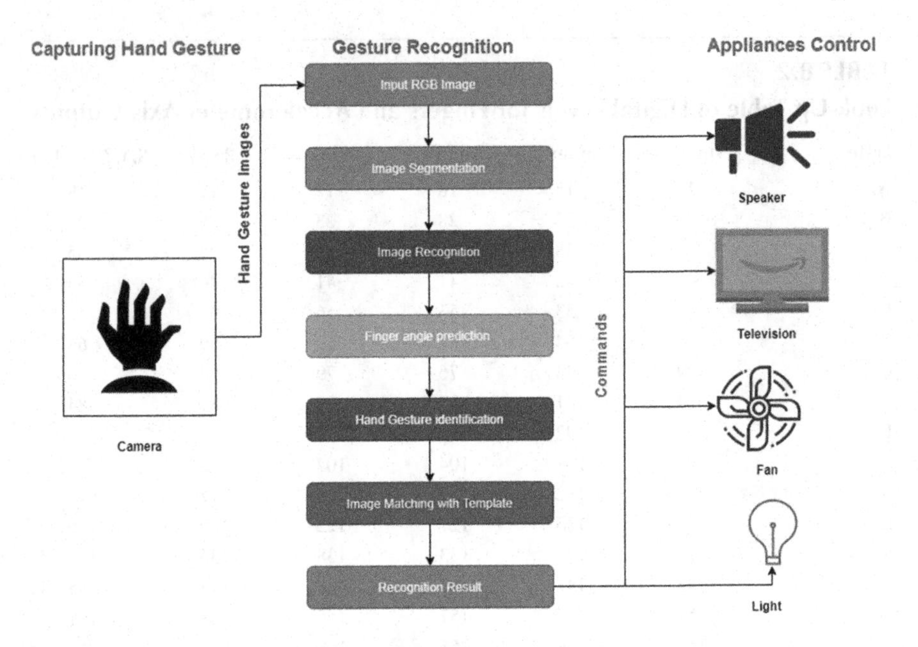

FIGURE 8.9 Block diagram of camera-based system.

8.5.2.1 Phase I – Capturing Input Hand Gesture

This is the first step in this appliance control system. The suitable high-resolution camera is placed in front of physically challenged and/or elderly person. The specification and range of resolution of the camera may be decided based on the application. Once the framework was switched ON, the camera was kept as focusing the corresponding person, and it continuously captures the gesture images of that person in a smaller periodic time interval usually within 2 seconds.

Once the capturing of gesture image is done, immediately it forwards the images to processing.

8.5.2.2 Phase II – Recognition of Input Hand Gesture

This is the second phase to be performed after the capturing of each input hand gesture. Figure 8.10 shows the flowchart of recognition process used in camera-based hand gesture recognition system.

The recognition of input hand gesture consists of following steps. They are

- Input RGB image
- Image segmentation
- Image recognition
- Finger angle prediction
- Hand gesture identification

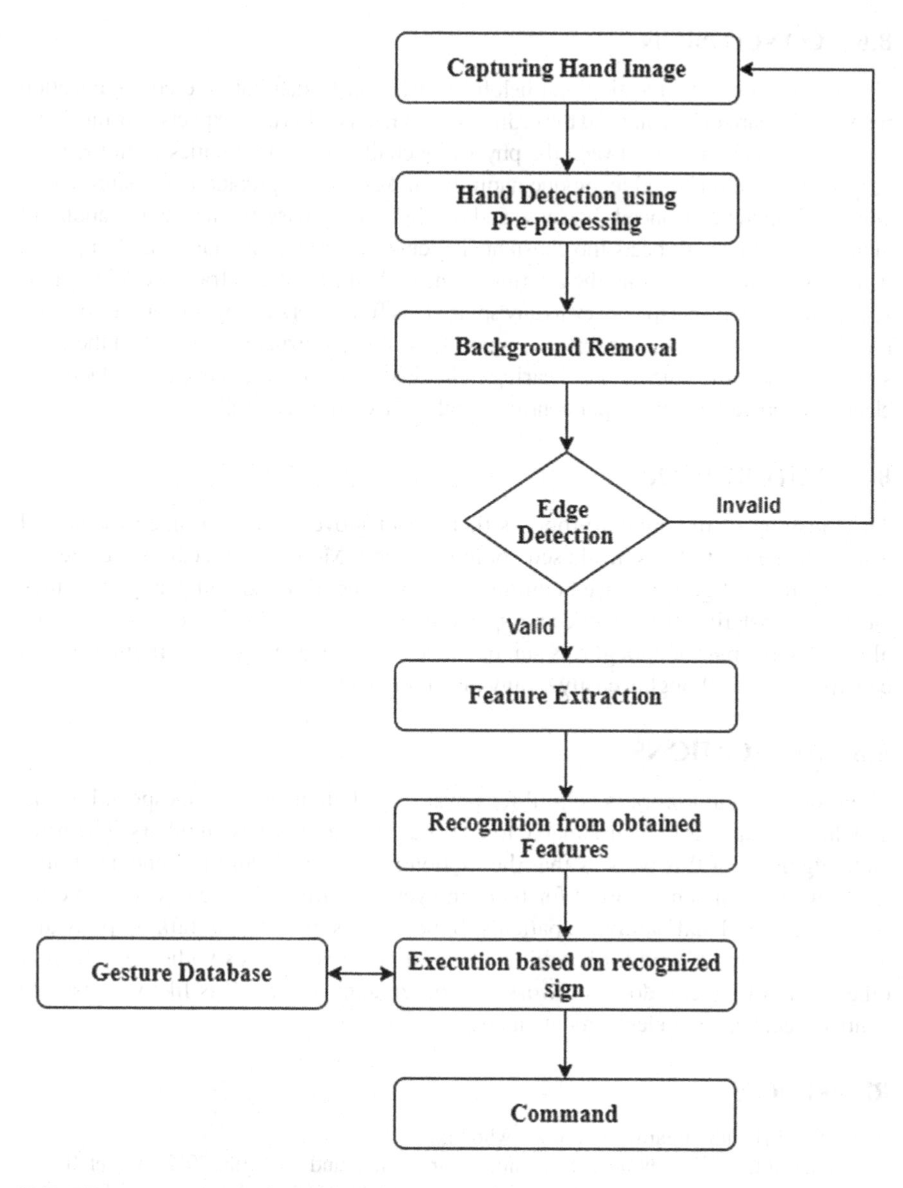

FIGURE 8.10 Flow diagram of camera-based system.

- Image matching with template
- Recognition output.

8.5.2.3 Phase III – Appliance Control

This is the final phase in the proposed framework. In this phase, microcontroller or microprocessor plays a major role. Based on the response obtained from second phase, control unit decides the controllability of each appliance.

8.6 CONCLUSION

Gesture-based communication is a helpful instrument to facilitate the communication between the hard of hearing and the ordinary individuals. This task expects to bring down the communication gap between the physically challenged communities from the ordinary world. The proposed technique naturally makes an interpretation of gesture-based communication to advanced showcase and fulfills them by passing on contemplations all alone. The framework beats the constant challenges of stupid individuals and improves their way of life. Contrasting the existing framework, the proposed framework is conservative and conceivable to convey to any spots. This framework changes over the communication via gestures and converts them into some content structure showed on the LCD screen, to encourage the hard of hearing individuals also and to control the gadgets and electrical apparatuses by proper control signals delivered by controller.

8.7 FUTURE SCOPE

The finishing of this model proposes that sensor gloves can be utilized for partial acknowledgement of gesture-based communication. More sensors can be utilized to perceive the full gesture-based communication. A helpful and compact gadget may work in translating framework and speakers. Also, the collection of body sensors along with the pair of data gloves can be made so that hearing and speak impartment can convey their thoughts easily to anyone at anyplace.

8.8 APPLICATIONS

The proposed framework is helpful for physically challenged people especially deaf and dump people as they are unable to communicate properly with others. The principle highlight of this work is that the motion recognizer is an independent framework, which is much required for them in everyday life. It is likewise valuable for speech impaired and paralyzed patients. In both cases, they do not talk properly and are furthermore utilized for handling essential home appliances without the help of others. Even they can do some work in modern applications. It is likewise used to control electrical and electronic gadgets.

REFERENCES

1. World Health Organization. www.who.int.
2. Amarjot, S., K. Devinder, S. Phani, K. Srikrishna and A. Niraj, 2012, An intelligent multi-gesture spotting robot to assist persons with disabilities, *International Journal of Computer Theory and Engineering*, Vol. 24, No. 2, pp. 122–125.
3. https://www.disabled-world.com/disability/statistics/
4. https://censusindia.gov.in/Census_And_You/disabled_population.aspx.
5. NSO survey for July-December 2018, The Economic Times. https://m.economictimes.com/news/economy/indiators/indias-2-2-population-suffereing-from-disability-nso-survey-for-july-dec-2018/amp-articleshow/72202650.cms.
6. Suharjito, R.A., F. Wiryana, M.C. Ariesta and G.P. Kusuma, 2017, Sign language recognition application systems for deaf-mute people: a review based on input-process-output, *2nd International Conference on Computer Science and Computational Intelligence 2017*, Procedia Computer Science 116, 441–448.

7. Adithya, V. and R. Rajesh, 2020, Hand gestures for emergency situations: A video dataset based on words from Indian sign language, *Data in Brief*, Vol. 31, pp. 1–7.
8. Yewale, S. and Y. Bharne, 2011, Hand gesture recognition using different algorithms based on artificial neural network, *IEEE Transactios on Computer Vision and Pattern Recognition*, Vol. 2, No. 8, pp. 287–292.
9. Mezari, A. and I. Maglogiannis, 2018, An easily customized gesture recognizer for assisted living using commodity mobile devices, *Hindawi Journal of Healthcare Engineering*, Vol. 2018, pp. 1–12.
10. Suharjito, M.C.A., F. Wiryana and G.P. Kusuma, 2018, A survey of hand gesture recognition methods in sign language recognition, *Pertanika Journal of Science and Technology*, Vol. 26, pp. 1659–1675.
11. Alois, F., R. Stefan, H. Clemens and R. Martin, 2007, Orientation sensing for gesture-based interaction with smart artifacts, *IEEE Transactions on Audio, Speech, and Language Processing*, Vol. 28, No. 8, pp. 1434–1520.
12. Jean, C. and B. Peter, 2004, Recognition of arm gestures using multiple orientation sensors: gesture classification, *IEEE Intelligent Transportation Systems Conference on Electronics*, Vol. 13, No. 1, pp. 334–520.
13. Tongrod, N., S. Lokavee and T. Kercharoen, 2011, Gestural system based on multi-functional sensors and zigBee networks for squad communication, *IEEE Defense Science Research Conference and Expo*, Vol. 2, No. 4, pp. 1–4.
14. Charthad, J., M.J. Weber, T.C. Chang, and A. Arbabian, 2015, A mm-sized implantable medical device (IMD) with ultrasonic power transfer and a hybrid bi-directional data link, *IEEE Journal of Solid-State Circuits*, Vol. 50, No. 8, pp. 1741–1753.
15. Flores, H., C.M.B. Siloy, C. Oppus and L. Agustin, 2014, User oriented finger-gesture glove controller with hand movement virtualization using flex sensor and a digital Accelerometer, *IEEE Humanoid, Nanotechnology, Information Technology, Communication and Control, Environment and Management*, Vol. 4, No. 24, pp. 5–8.
16. Ravikiran, J., M. Kavi, M. Suhas, R. Dheeraj, S. Sudheender and V. Nitin, 2009, Finger detection for sign language recognition, *Proceedings of the International Multi Conference of Engineers and Computer Scientists*, Vol. 39, No. 12, pp. 334–62.
17. Boopathi Raja, G. 2021, *Fingerprint based Smart Medical Emergency First Aid Kit using IOT, Electronic Devices, Circuits, and Systems for Biomedical Applications*, 1st edition, Academic Press, Cambridge, MA.
18. Joyeeta, S. and D. Karen, 2013, Indian sign language recognition using Eigen value weighted Euclidean distance based classification technique, *International Journal of Advanced Computer Science and Applications*, Vol. 4, No. 2, pp. 434–820.
19. Subha, R. and K. Balakrishnan, 2010, Indian sign language recognition system to aid deaf – dumb people, *IEEE International Conference on Computing Communication and Networking Technologies*, Vol. 20, No. 13, pp. 136–145.
20. Cheok, M.J., Z. Omar, and M.H. Jaward, 2017, A review of hand gesture and sign language recognition techniques, *International Journal of Machine Learning and Cybernetics*, Vol. 10, pp. 131–153. Springer.
21. Ahmed, M.A., B.B. Zaidan, A.A. Zaidan, M.M. Salih and M.M. bin Lakulu, 2018, A Review on Systems-Based Sensory Gloves for Sign Language Recognition State of the Art between 2007 and 2017, Sensors.

9 Computer-Aided Drug Designing – Modality of Diagnostic System

Shalini Ramesh
Thiagarajar College

Sugumari Vallinayagam, Karthikeyan Rajendran, and Sasireka Rajendran
Mepco Schlenk Engineering College

Vinoth Rathinam
P.S.R. Engineering College

Sneka Ramesh
Thiagarajar College

CONTENTS

9.1 INTRODUCTION

Drug discovery is the method of new remedial entities that can be recognized, using a mixture of computing techniques, practical, translational, and scientific models. This drug discovery is a very costly, extended, complex, and effective process with a great attrition. Drug designing is the incorporated discipline and a creative process of identifying new medications according to the information of a biological target. This process involves the interaction and binding of the molecular target. The present drug development involves the recognition of molecules, medicinal chemistry, screening hits, maximization of those compounds to enlarge the affinity, efficacy, oral bio-availability, sensitivity, and metabolic constancy (to enhance the half-life). Once a compound accomplishes all of these necessities, then it will initiate the process of drug development previous to clinical trials and identify a new drug. The important features of an "ideal" compound are as follows:

i. Must be secure and efficient
ii. Should be taken orally
iii. Bioavailability
iv. Metabolically constant and with a high half-life
v. Nonhazardous with negligible or no side effects
vi. Should have discerning supply to target tissues.

Nowadays, target and lead molecules are designed with the help of computational tools [1]. They can probably protect the pharmaceutical sectors, government, and institutional laboratories from continuing the "wrong" leads. The design process of a drug is given in Figure 9.1. Drug designing is often a computer process that is referred to as computer-aided drug design.

Computer-aided drug design (CADD) is an evolving cascade comprising a broad range of theoretical and computational knowledge that are part of modern drug

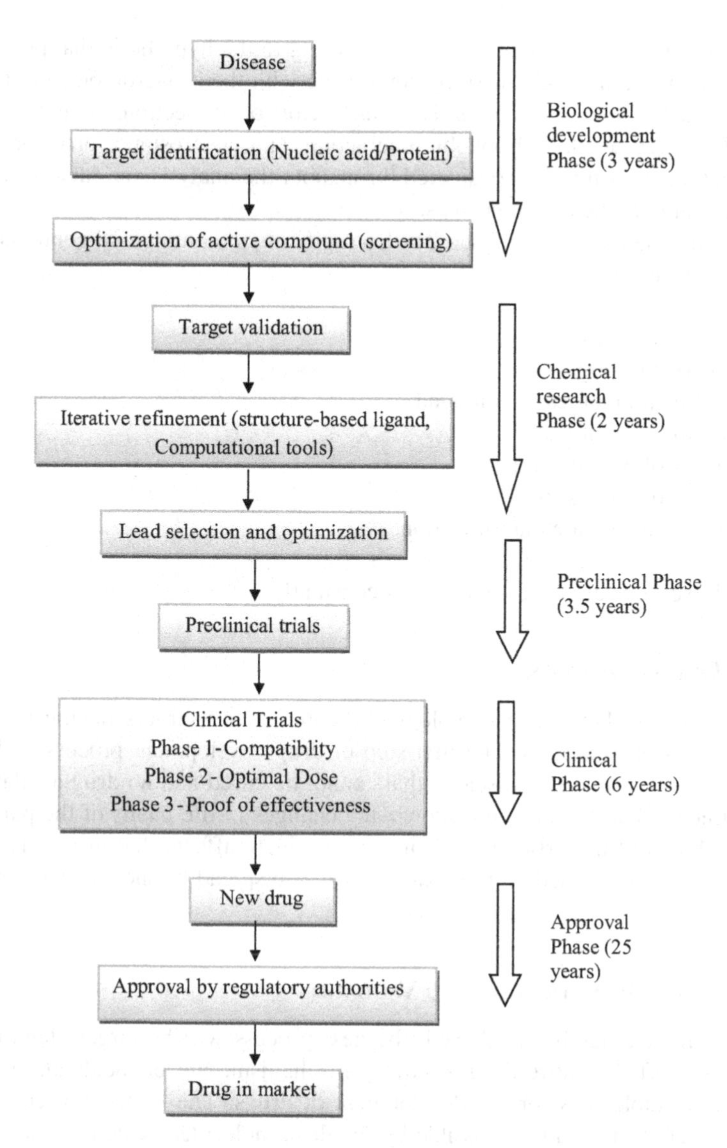

FIGURE 9.1 Phases of drug discovery.

discovery and development. Computer-aided drug design (CADD) offers enormous tools and methods that help in different stages of drug design process which drop the cost of research and expansion time of the compound. The cost benefit of using computing techniques in the lead maximization stages of drug development is considerable, and it takes normally 10–15 years to introduce into the market [2]. The time invested by the pharmacological research is heavy during the various phases of drug development, starting from therapeutic target identification, candidate drug development, drug optimization through preclinical and extensive clinical experiments to assess the efficiency and safety of newly developed drugs [3]. Computational tools of drug designing and development are according to the hypothesis that pharmacologically active compounds serve by connecting with their macromolecular targets, primarily nucleic acids or proteins. The main factors of connections are exterior molecules, hydrogen bond, hydrophobic interaction, and electrostatic force formation. These factors are primarily considered throughout the analysis and identification of interaction among the two molecules.

The maintenance of drug discovery from process to commercial contains seven fundamental steps:

- Selection of disease
- Selection of target
- Identification of lead compound
- Optimization of lead
- Testing of preclinical trial
- Testing of clinical trial
- Pharmacogenomic maximization.

The final five steps are necessary to pass constantly.

9.1.1 Disease Selection

The medical, biochemical and biological databases and servers having the information of various diseases. The first step of drug development process is disease selection. There are lots of diseases that cannot be cured and no drug available for the treatment. Diseases have not shown any changes in life habits of the particular people, who lived in particular locality but it widely affects that group. The drug discovery is started based on the abandons disease spread in one particular region/group [4].

9.1.2 Target Identification and Validation

Once the disease has been selected, the next process will be target identification which boots off the entire drug discovery mechanism. Nucleic acids and proteins act as target molecules for the development of drugs. The target molecule needs to be safe, efficacious and accessible by the drug molecule. Mode of action of the lead compound to be evaluated by the efficacy of the lead molecule interaction with the active site of detected drug target [5,6]. The obvious next step is identifying the small molecules which lead to have an effect against targets, and this process is hit identification. These hit approaches can be identified by virtual screening or high-throughput screening.

9.1.3 Lead Optimization

After a molecular target (nucleic acid/protein) structure has been approved, the next step is to find molecules known as leads that are at very low to a low-to-moderate level and have preferred outcome on the target. Leads relatively attach to target configuration and have rigorous side effects with view to produce a preclinical drug candidate [7,8]. The specialist combination in metabolism of drug development, computational chemistry and other areas can afford unique approaching into this late step of the process. Once a lead compound is found during optimization process, the process initiates with the preclinical research to conclude the efficiency and safety of the compound. Researchers resolve the following about the drug:

- Absorption, metabolization and delivery
- Mechanisms
- Dosage and route of administration
- Potential benefits
- Gender effects and ethnicity groups
- Association with other treatments
- Side effects
- Efficiency compared to related drugs.

9.1.4 Preclinical Trials

Preclinical test is a test of the novel drug on nonhuman matter for effectiveness, efficiency, safety, hazardous and pharmacokinetic (PK) information [9,10]. These experiments are performed by scientists at laboratory conditions and human with unlimited dosages.

9.1.5 Clinical Trails

- **Phase 1 –** Drug tested with 20–100 healthy volunteers or people with the disease/condition. It takes several months; mostly, 70% drugs pass to the next phase.
- **Phase 2 –** Drug tested up to several hundreds of people with the disease/condition. It takes several months to 2 years; mostly, 33% drugs pass to the next phase.
- **Phase 3 –** Drug tested with thousands of volunteers who have the disease or condition. It takes several years; mostly, 33% drugs pass to the next phase. Drugs once approved by FDA are introduced into the market.

The drug for testing can be derived from natural sources (plants, animals and microbes) and by chemical production. These compounds can be eliminated as perspectives due to absence or low action, complexity of synthesis, existence of hazardous or carcinogenicity, inadequate competence, etc. As an outcome, only one of 100,000 drug substances may be established to the market, and one standard amount of novel drug rises up to 800 million dollars. The dropping of cost and time intensity of the final phases of compound testing is not likely due to severe state standard on their recognition. The major efforts to raising the competence of growth of drugs are directed to phases of drug discovery and maximization of ligands, and *in silico* technique can assist in reorganization of drug targets through bioinformatics tools. They can also be used to examine the target

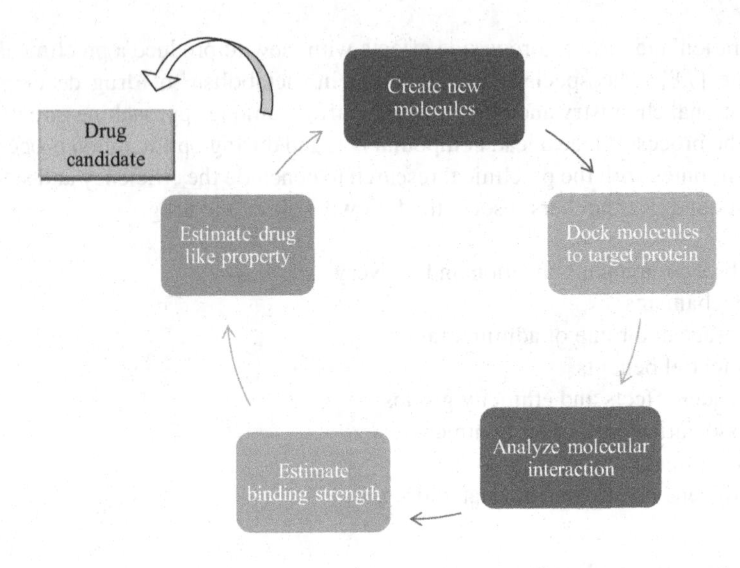

FIGURE 9.2 Principle of drug design via CADD.

structure for potential binding region or binding sites, produce the candidate molecules, dock these molecules with the target compound, check for their likeness, position them based on their binding affinities and further maximization of the molecule to enhance binding characteristic. The major use of computational technique is to infuse in every phase of drug designing, and today it develops the core of (a) structure-based drug design [11,12] and (b) ligand-based drug design [13,14]. The principle of CADD is shown in Figure 9.2.

9.2 WORKING OF COMPUTER-AIDED DRUG DESIGNING (CADD)

The basic workflow (Figure 9.3) of computer-aided drug designing is collectively used within analytical techniques to discover new lead compounds and also direct iterative ligand maximization. The process initiates with the detection of biological target molecules to which ligand binds and directs to antimicrobial mechanism. In structure-based drug designing (SBDD), the 3D structure of the target molecule can be identified by NMR spectroscopy or X-ray crystallography or using homology modelling. Ligand-based drug designing (LBDD) is mainly processed in the lack of the 3D structure of the target molecule where information is on conversion of the lead compound to enhance the action can be attained. Computer-aided drug-designing (CADD) methods are used to design the compounds which is subjected to biological assay and chemical synthesis. The researchers are continually developing and executing new CADD methods with elevated levels of speed and accuracy [15,16].

9.3 FACTORS AFFECTING DRUG-DESIGNING PROCESS

There are several factors affecting the development of drug discovery; the important ones are as follows:

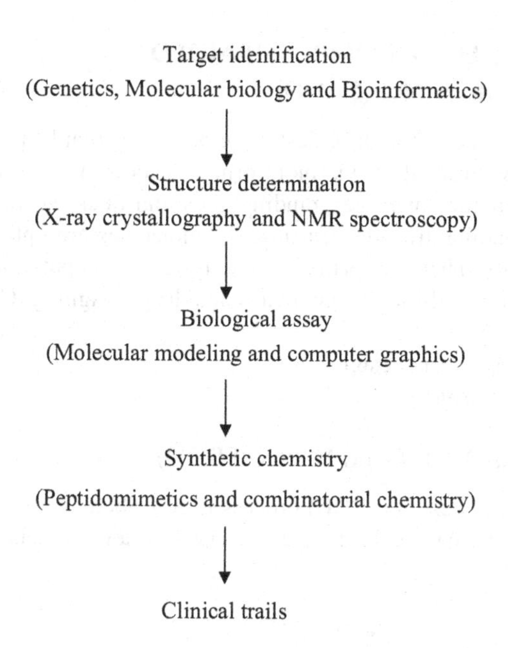

FIGURE 9.3 Workflow of *Insilico* to *Invitro* research

a. **Medicinal objective:** The main objective is to develop new drug through drug development process, for example, it is easy to develop the antacid using this technique but is more difficult to develop specific proton pump inhibitor. This may affect the likelihood of success or failure in new drug development.
b. **Ability of Medicinal chemist:** On basis of knowledge, the researchers will develop the new drugs (chemistry of lead molecule and biology diseased state).
c. **Screening facilities:** Rapid mass screening is mainly successfully as it depends on evaluation of a large number of compounds and is easy to detect potentially useful drugs within short life span.
d. **Drug development facility:** The major field like biology, chemistry and pharmacy needs to develop new drugs.
e. **Cost of new drug:** There are main three factors for cost drug development:
   i. Number of compounds synthesized: Only 5000–10,000 drugs reach the market
   ii. Nature of the lead molecule: Production cost will be high for lead molecule which is prepared by an expensive route.
   iii. Standards required for new drugs: The drug is approved by authorities to release into the market.

Due to all these factors, the drug discovery process is undergoing a complete overhaul to be cost-effective and to meet the supply and demand fundamentals [17–19].

9.4 APPROACHES OF COMPUTER-AIDED DRUG DESIGNING (CADD)

In silico method is one of the drug-designing processes that help in identifying target molecule to synthesis drug via bioinformatics tools. This method can be used to analyze the structure of target, binding sites and docking molecules and rank them based on bonding affinities; further, the molecules are optimized to improve the binding capacity. There are primarily two types of computational approaches in drug-designing process through computer-aided drug designing (CADD):

1. Structure-based drug design
2. Ligand-based drug design.

9.4.1 Structure-Based Drug Design (SBDD)

Structure-based drug design (SBDD) process is described as one of the most inventive and iterative approaches in drug discovery and development. The structure of

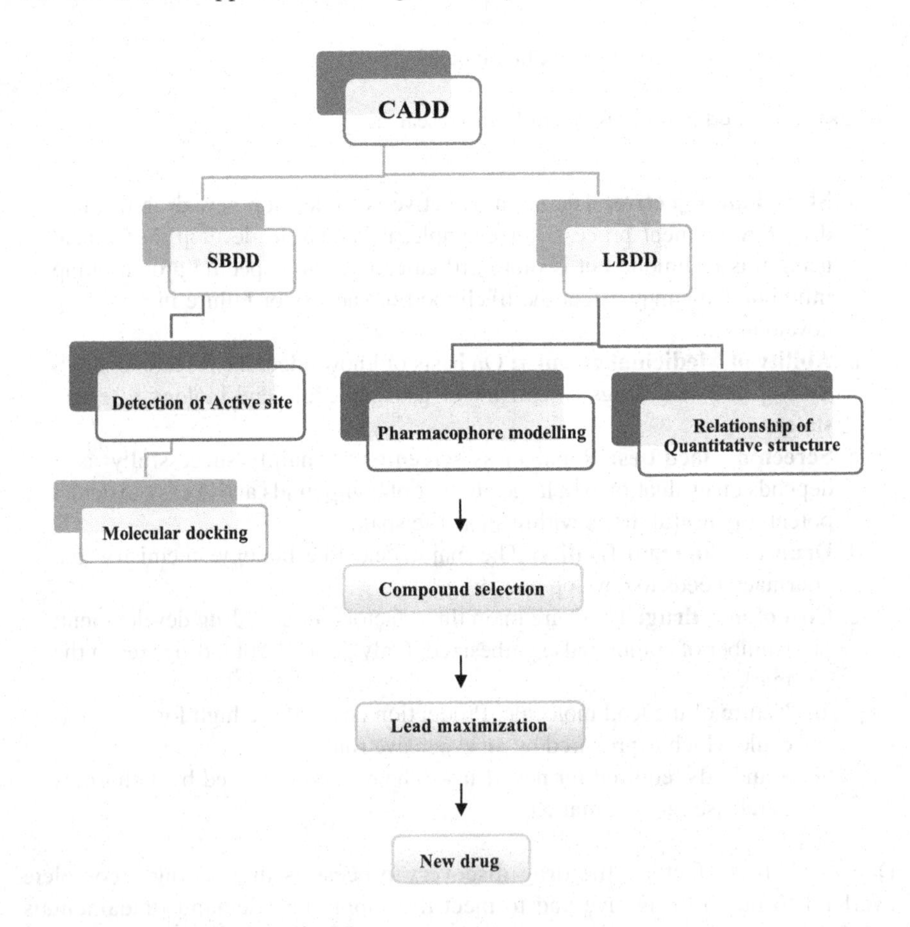

FIGURE 9.4 Workflow for CADD.

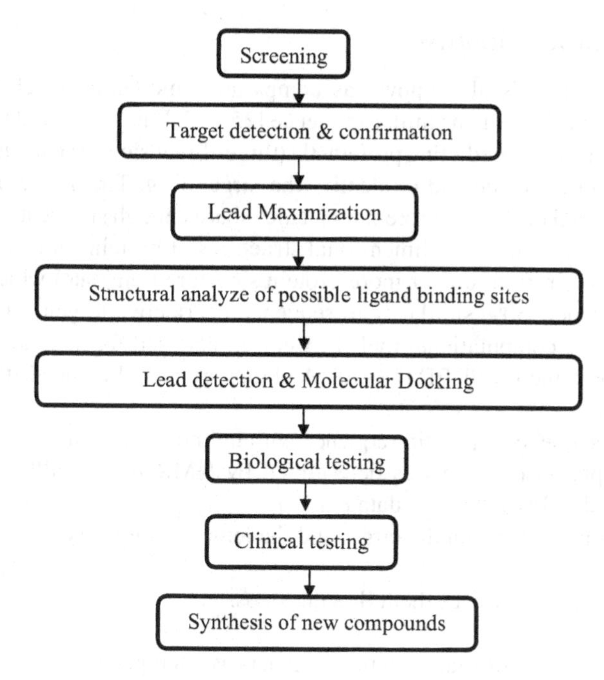

FIGURE 9.5 Steps involved in SBDD.

target protein molecule was known and requires three dimensional structures (3D) of target molecule, preferentially target protein complexes among a ligand, where affinity, joining mode and confirmation of a ligand joining can be determined. This bio-affinity of compounds is calculated next to the process of molecular docking in order to intend a novel drug molecule which illustrates improved interaction with protein [20–22]. A series of methods have been developed to design greater affinity of inhibitor in structure-based drug designing either via effective screening or synthesis of ligand molecule. Current advances in computing tools for lead discovery contain different commercially available software for structure-based drug designing is iterative design, selectivity, *de novo* drug design and evaluation of ligand-binding affinities.

Structure-based drug designing (SBDD) undergoes several stages cycles (Figure 9.5) before the maximized lead achieves into clinical trials. The initial stage of SBDD is separation, purification and configuration resolve of the target protein, and methods include NMR, X-ray crystallography and homology modeling. The drugs are positioned on the basis of interaction which includes electrostatic, hydrophobic and steric interaction of molecules that interact with binding site of target molecule. The second stage of SBDD is configuration resolution of target protein with the outcome of optimistic lead of the primary cycle [23,24]. After several stages like lead synthesis, further lead optimization through composite structure of protein among lead molecule, these optimized compounds show high addition in binding affinity and compound specificity. The compounds are tested in assays using information to guide SBDD.

9.4.2 Homology Modeling

Homology modeling is also known as comparative modeling which predicts the structure of protein based on similar sequence [25–27]. It is considered to be the best computational tool for predicting protein 3D (three-dimensional) structure that determines the target molecule and to identify the target drug. This modeling works on the principle based on "if two protein molecules share enough similarity of sequence, they are very similar in three dimensional structures of protein". It identifies the 3D structure of protein from one or more protein structure (template) which resembles the query sequence, 30% similarity in sequence is effective to generate the model. There are several computational tools or web servers used for homology modeling, e.g., MODELER and PSIPRED [28–30]. A homology modeling needs three inputs:

1. "Target sequence" (protein sequence with unknown structure)
2. 3D template (structure was determined by NMR or crystallography and published in PDB "protein data bank")
3. An alignment between the target and the template sequence.

Homology modeling involves the following steps:

1. Identification of similar protein which acts as a template
2. Alignment of template and target molecules
3. Copy of aligned regions
4. Framework of target structure
5. Refining of target molecule and evaluation.

9.4.2.1 Template Recognition

This process involves the identification of homologous or similar sequence in protein structure database which act as template for homology modeling. This template can be searched in tools like BLAST and FASTA but better search in PSI-BLAST or protein threading.

9.4.2.2 Target Alignment

The second step involves alignment of template and target sequence; the highest similarity of sequence is selected as template. The better tool for the target and template alignment is Praline and T-coffee, etc.

9.4.2.3 Construction of Target Molecule

The step involves building an outline structure of the target protein molecule consisting of main chain atoms. If two sequences are identical, the side chains are copied, whereas if it differs, backbone molecule is copied.

9.4.2.4 Optimization

This step includes addition of protein molecules and optimizes the side chain; the method was achieved by SCWRL (side chain placement with a rotamer library) and a UNIX program which shows better results.

9.4.2.5 Model Optimization

This method is to optimize the energy level of the molecule. The irregular form of structure is corrected by the energy minimization process; the alternative best method for optimization is molecular dynamics stimulation, e.g., GROMOS (UNIX program).

9.4.2.6 Evaluation

The final process of homology modeling is evaluation of the target molecule. The process is to increase the stability of target and consistent with physicochemical properties. The process is repeated until accurate molecule is obtained.

Uses of homology modeling:

- The novel functions of protein molecule
- This homology is used for structure-based drug design
- Mainly used for analysis of protein interaction, antigenic behavior and function of protein
- Provides a useful structural model for generating a hypothesis of protein function (Figure 9.6).

9.4.3 Ligand-Based Drug Design

The ligand-based drug discovery (LBDD) is an indirect approach that involves in examining of ligand molecules to interrelate with a desired target. The three-dimensional structure of intended protein was unknown, but the binding of ligand to desired target site was known. This ligand-based techniques are mainly used for pharmacophore approach and quantitative-structure activity relationships (QSARs) [31,32]. There are two fundamental approaches of ligand-based drug design.

i. Based on chemical similarity, the compound was selected to known active sites using some similarity measure

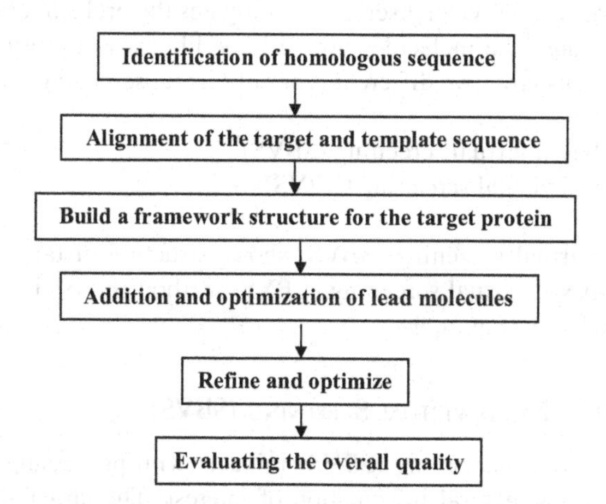

FIGURE 9.6 Steps involved in homology modeling.

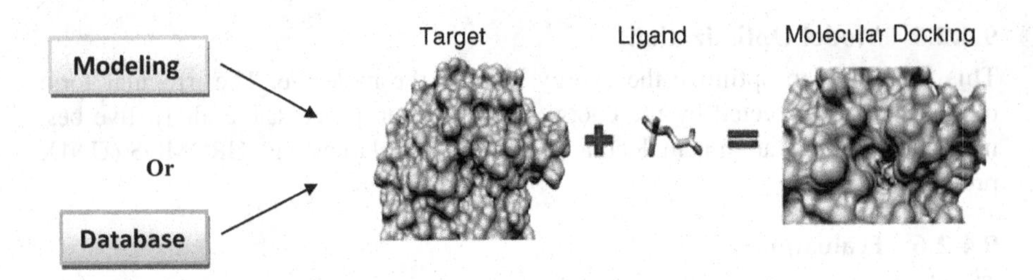

FIGURE 9.7 Steps involved in LBDD.

ii. The quantitative structure activity relationship (QSAR) approach predicts the biological activity from the chemical structure.

Ligand-based drug-designing process is based on the principle of similar property which states that molecules that have similar properties are structurally similar. Ligand-based drug-designing approaches in contrast to structure-based drug-designing approaches can also be applied for unknown structure of the biological target (Figure 9.7).

9.5 VIRTUAL SCREENING

Virtual screening is one of the computational tools to find the bioactive compounds using known target protein molecule or active ligand compound. It is the best alternative screening technique mainly due to cost effectiveness and is used to find appropriate hit verification through filter. The virtual screening is used to

- Screen all large molecules of databases
- Complement high throughput screening for drug designing and development.

This technique depends on the amount of information regarding target molecules [33–35]. To a large extent, virtual screening mitigates the problem of drug discovery and synthesis because the molecules utilize large libraries of presynthesized compounds. There are usually two different types of virtual screening that include

a. Structure-based virtual screening (SBVS)
b. Ligand-based virtual screening (LBVS).

Structure-based virtual screening (SBVS) shows structure of target protein active site, and ligand-based virtual screening (LBVS) method shows similar active compound from data bases (Figure 9.8).

9.5.1 Structure-Based Virtual Screening (SBVS)

Structure-based virtual screening (SBVS) initiates with processing the 3D (three-dimensional) target structural information of interest. The target structure can be determined by NMR, X-ray, homology modeling, neutron scattering spectroscopy

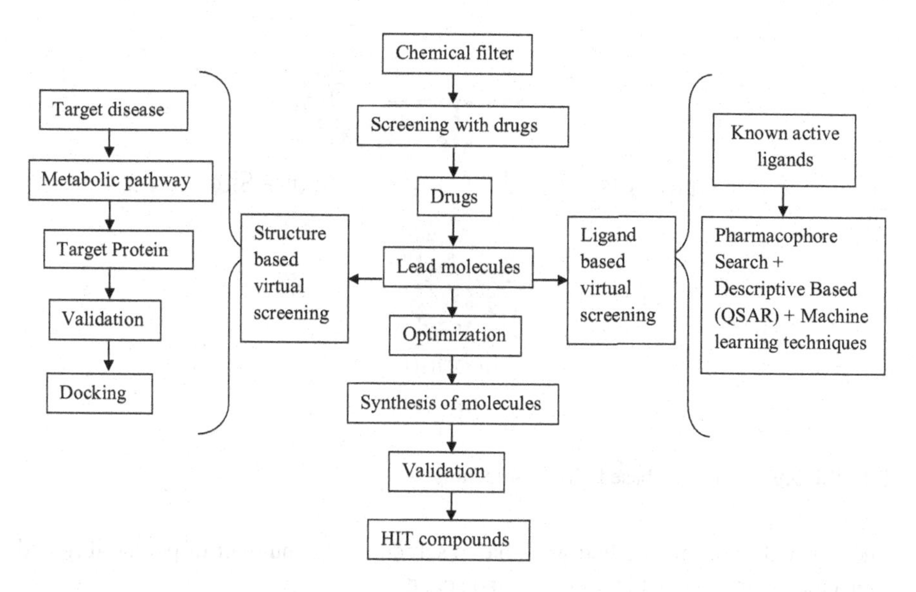

FIGURE 9.8 Schematic diagram of virtual screening.

or Molecular Dynamics (MD) simulations. The biological target was examined in SBVS like drug ability in receptor, binding site and relevant protein structure, etc. SBVS docking plays an important role; the compound is virtually docked into the target binding site using docking program. The aim of docking is to predict ligand-protein complex structure and explore conformational changes in binding site of protein molecule. Scoring of molecules happens mainly to find approximate free energy in binding site of protein and docking pose in ligand. The scoring and docking of selected compounds which are post processing is examined by binding sites, chemical moieties, metabolic liabilities and desired physicochemical properties. The selected compounds further carried out for experimental assaying process (Figure 9.9).

9.5.2 Ligand Based Virtual Screening (LBVS)

Ligand-based virtual screening (LBVS) is one of the virtual screening methods where the active ligand molecule was known. It only chosen when there is no 3D (three-dimensional) structure of target protein was not available. This ligand based virtual screening involves two essential elements:

1. Scoring method
2. Efficient similarity measure.

This LBVS includes pharmacophore which generates a pattern of distance between molecular properties like hydrogen bond and aromatic system it calculates the similarity value of corresponding patterns. The scoring and ranking value of ligand-based virtual screening is effectively differentiating the active compounds from inactive

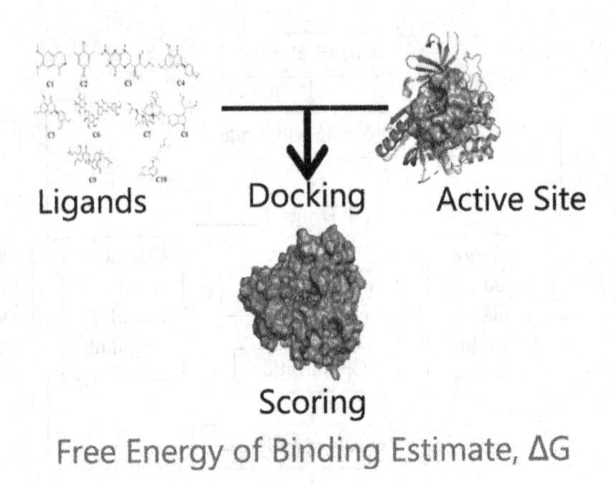

FIGURE 9.9 Structure-based virtual screening.

ones. In addition, this method was able to screen a large number of potential ligand molecules with reasonable accuracy and speed.

Our advantages:

- To create LBVS software tools
- Pharmacophore modeling, machine learning and 2D/3D QSAR
- Database contains over 10 million compounds (Figure 9.10).

9.6 MOLECULAR DOCKING

Molecular docking is an *in silico* method of computational techniques which predicts the ligand molecules inside the binding site of their target protein (receptor). The molecular docking plays an essential mechanism in the rational design of drug designing, and it determines the complex structure produced by interaction between two or more ligand molecules with the receptor which is applied in virtual screening to optimize the lead compounds. Method of molecular docking is searching of the algorithm, scoring functions and analyzing conformational changes in the ligand molecules. This molecular docking consists of three main goals that are interconnected [36–38].

- Prediction of binding pose (confirmation of a ligand molecule within target site)
- Bioaffinity
- Virtual screening.

These molecules can be docked in three different ways:

1. Rigid docking (both target molecule and ligands are treated as rigid entities)
2. Flexible docking (both ligand and target protein are flexible)
3. Flexible ligand docking (ligand is flexible and the target is rigid).

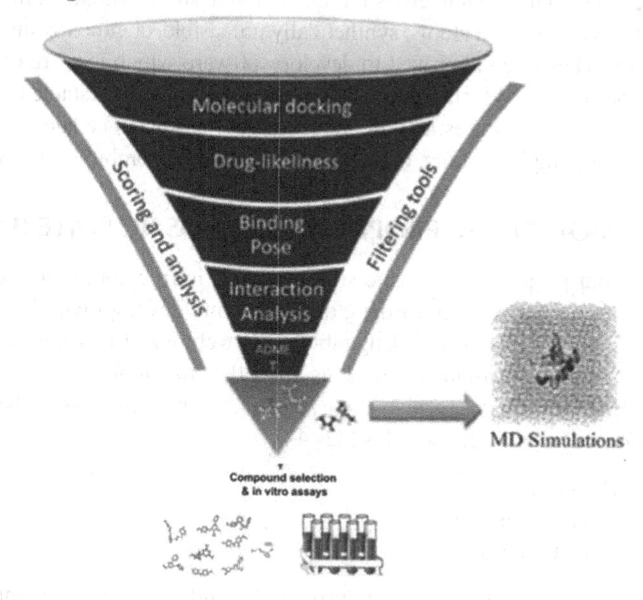

FIGURE 9.10 Structure based and Ligand based Virtual screening.

Different types of molecular docking

- Protein-ligand docking
- Protein-protein docking
- Protein-nucleic acid docking
- Antibody-antigen docking
- Protein-peptide docking
- Protein-carbohydrate docking
- Protein-lipid docking.

There are different kinds of molecular docking programs developed recently that include AutoDock, FlexX, Surflex, ICM, Glide, Gold and LigandFit, which have been used for many computer-based drug discovery projects [39–41]. The algorithm search and scoring function plays an important role in protein-ligand interaction. The responsibility of the algorithm is to search different poses of conformation of ligand molecule within the target protein, whereas scoring function estimates the bioaffinity and identifies the receptor; this scoring helps to determine the physicochemical properties of molecules and interaction of thermodynamics.

9.7 CHALLENGES IN COMPUTER-AIDED DRUG DESIGN

CADD is an interdisciplinary knowledge of various fields such as biology, chemistry and computation; this is the major challenge of CADD. The processing and accuracy of target molecule plays an important role in computation. The accuracy of ligand receptor interaction is most significant challenge in computer-aided drug designing. The next challenges of CADD are numerous numbers of undesired structures; they nearly have combinations of different atoms, synthetically unfeasible, chemically unstable and with high toxicity. They have improved to develop software which is more user-friendly and has fast computational techniques. These recent findings have stable chemical compounds and refinement features and are synthetically feasible. The success of computer-aided drug designing is docking, de-nova designing and thrombin inhibitor, etc. (Figure 9.11).

9.8 MOLECULAR PROPERTY DIAGNOSTIC SUITE (MPDS)

Molecular property diagnostic suite (MPDS) is free source tool chemo-informatics web portal mainly used for drug discovery and development. It is a software tool to set the rational diagnoses (druggable); this web portal is designed for enormous diseases such as TB, diabetes mellitus and other metabolic diseases. The main aim of the MPDS tool is to appraise and evaluate the drug likeness of the target compound. MPDS contains three modules [42–44]:

1. Data libraries
2. Data processing
3. Data analysis.

These tools are designed and interrelated to aid drug development for particular diseases. Some tools are specific to disease, whereas others are nonspecific. Molecular property diagnostic suite (MPDS) is a web server. Updated version of the server has the disease specific database with huge value. This suite incorporate with chemo-informatics, analogue-based drug discovery approaches, bioinformatics and

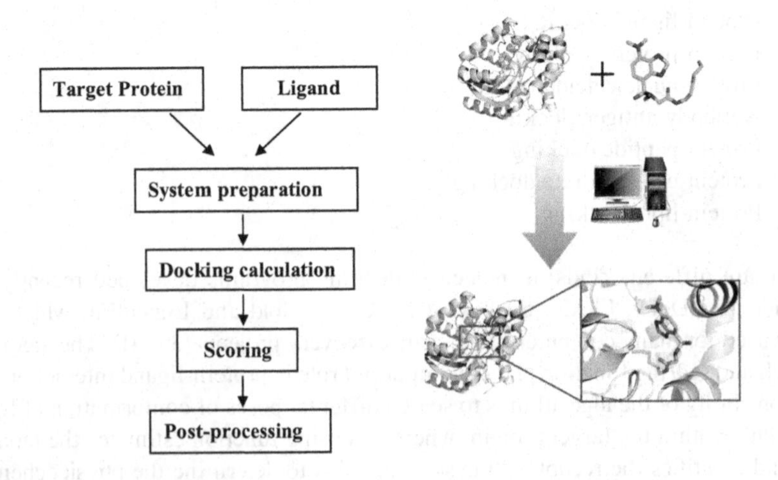

FIGURE 9.11 Post docking analysis in Virtual screening.

molecular modeling. Data library contains vast information about chemical space of the molecule, and this MPDS contains specific molecules' information produced from public domain databases, and each molecule contains unique ID which provides the complete details for molecules. The MPDS tool is used to diagnose diabetes mellitus (MPDSDM) (https://mpds-diabetes.in/) that provides drug targets, biomarkers, genes and literature details, etc.; the purpose of this web portal is to explore the drugs for diabetes. The current research is in developing web portal for specific diseases like tuberculosis (MPDSTB), and the primary goal is to incorporate all the literature, computing tools and data information which include chemo-informatics and computational biology in a particular platform that is openly available. This MPDSTB targets the mycobacterium tuberculosis (Figure 9.12).

9.8.1 Salient Features of the MPDS Tool for Tuberculosis

1. A disease-specific web-portal that provides all information about disease in the case of tuberculosis
2. Computer-aided drug design, chemo-informatics and other computer tools are available in single portal

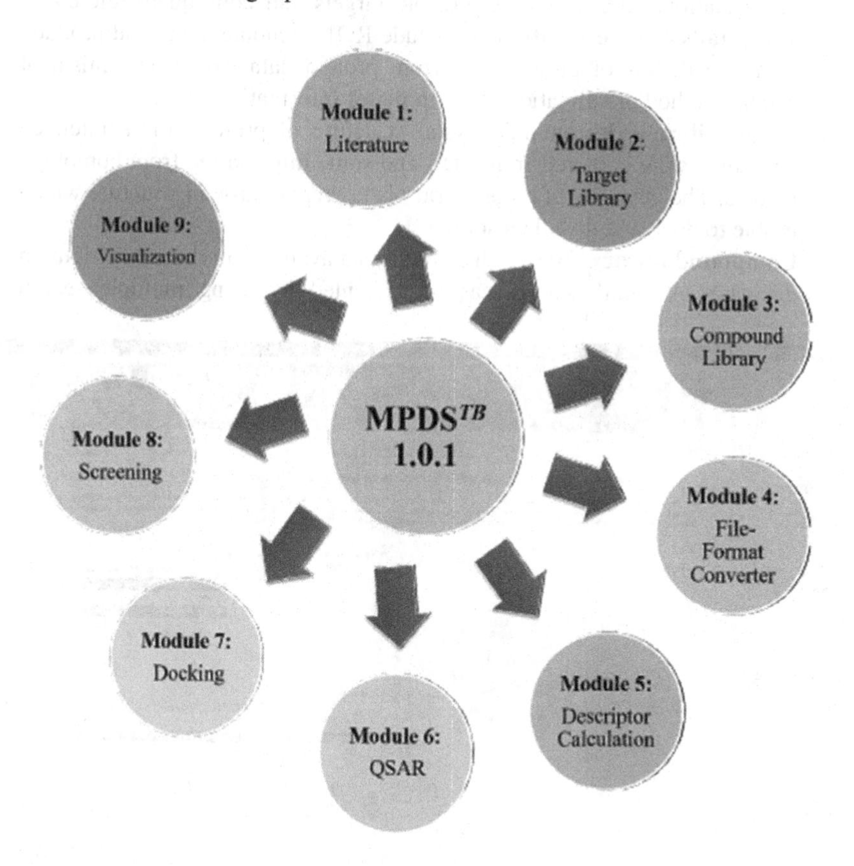

FIGURE 9.12 MPDS tool.

3. Every compound has a specific ID number
4. MPDS card provides IUPAC name, two-dimensional chemical structure and remarks, and it is possible to create additional pages for query molecule (Figure 9.13).

9.9 STRUCTURE OF MPDSTB

This molecular property diagnostic suite is structured into

- Data library
- Data processing
- Data analysis.

These MPDS tools are processed for tuberculosis and diabetes mellitus (Figure 9.14).

9.9.1 DATA LIBRARY

1. **Literature**: This provides information about target protein, gene information and other approved drugs from FDA (information from FDA – identification, pharmacology, possible targets and consequent reference). The details of genetics afforded include RvID, genome name and product, complete details of protein data from protein data bank, mechanism of action, method of validation, drug/inhibitor information, etc.
2. **Target library**: It contains crystal structure of protein; these intended structures were gathered from PDB and some information from homology models. The objective of target library is to prepare protein structure which is able to dock and give data source.
3. **Compound library**: To search a compound available in the public domain database. A small search was implemented by using multiple search

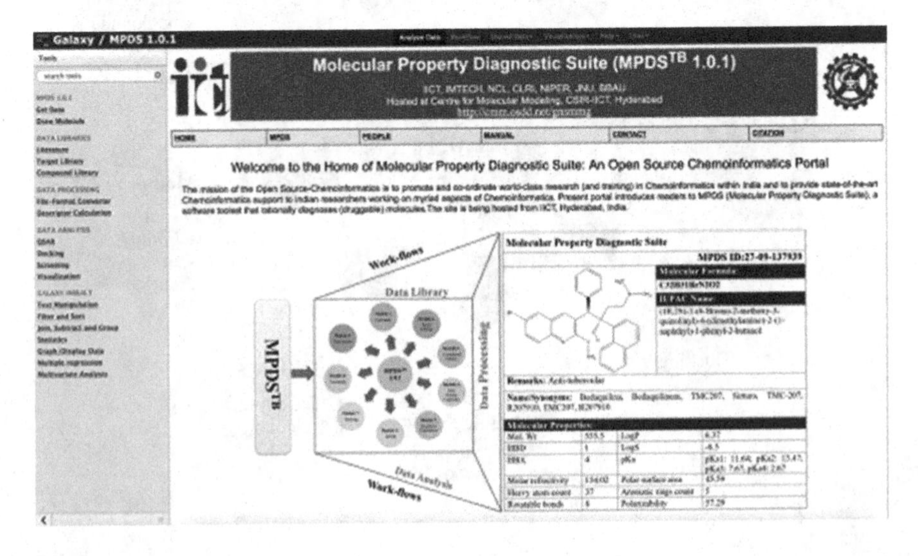

FIGURE 9.13 Web portal of MPDS.

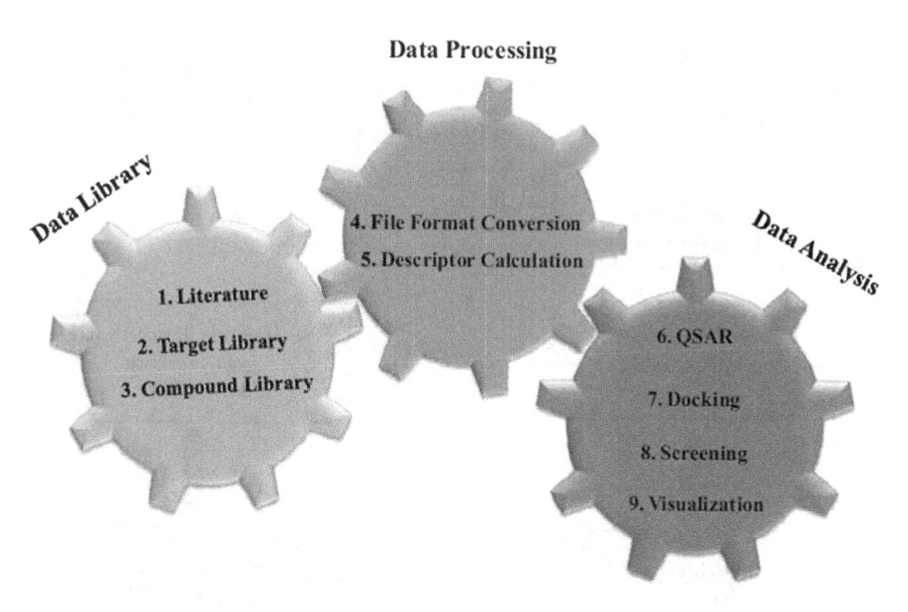

FIGURE 9.14 Structure of MPDS.

strategies that help for identification of novel anti-TB compounds or diabetes mellitus.

9.9.2 Data Processing

1. **File format conversion**: Main requirement of this system is to connect a link between two analyses of tools which can be easily read. This file format is used to represent the chemical structure, and this open source is able to convert the workflow of the system. A variety of tools necessitate for particular input file formats (mol2, mol, sdf, SMILES, etc.) and will generate output in another accurate format (mol2, sdf, mol, and PDB). These files generate 2D or 3D formats according to the hybridization of atoms.
2. **Descriptor calculation**: The main two descriptor tools are chemistry Development Kit and PaDEL, which incorporate MPDSTB and MPDSDM. These are used to calculate various compounds and their properties. The descriptor tool for input is sdf and supplies output in CSV design.

9.9.3 Data Analysis

There are two techniques of data mining, quantitative structure activity relationships (QSAR) and SVM which are included in MPDSTB:

1. QSAR – It is based on genetic algorithms which help for developing QSAR models. The construct of QSAR model is one of the quantitative structure activity relationship tools used for descriptor format of molecule with all recognized actions and assists the user to fill the name and column which

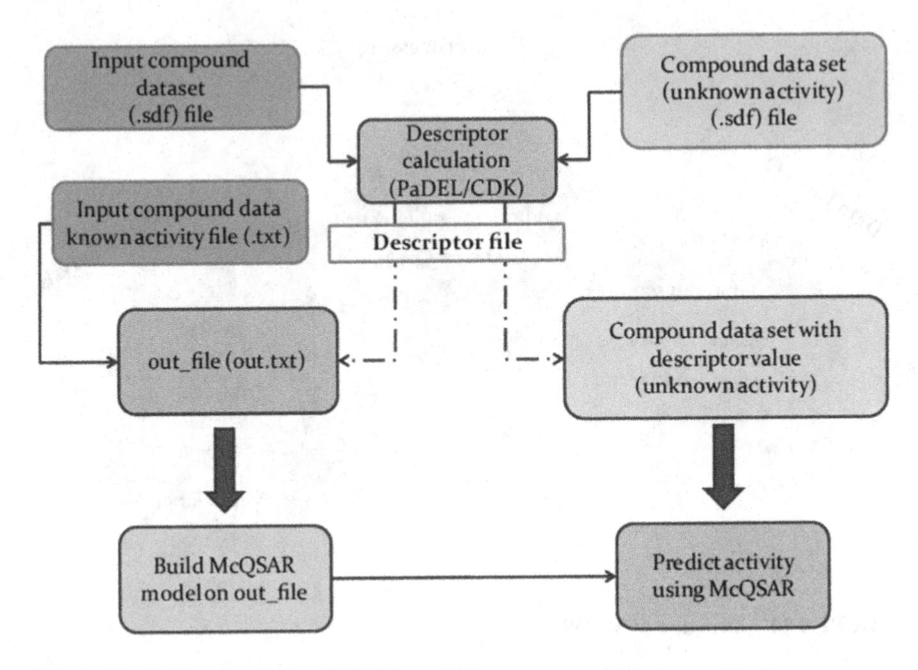

FIGURE 9.15 Data analysis of QSAR model.

has to predict. In order to remove all undesired characteristics, the user has set six separate options. This option involves the exclude sparse conformers and descriptors, reject correlated descriptors, exclude identical conformers, exclude inactive compounds and exclude descriptors with zeros. McQSAR can predict the tool which is formerly mentioned. This QSAR admits the two input files:

2. Hold the compound descriptors whose activity required to be identified
3. Subsequent is a model format formed by the 'Build QSAR Model' tool (Figure 9.15).
4. Molecular docking – It includes energy minimization process and visualization. The best tool for ligand optimization phenix eLBOW.

9.9.4 Screening

It is a prioritization of molecules for drug-like characteristics using DruLiTo tool, detection of toxicophoric set in a molecule and Biopharmaceutical Classification System (BCS) (Figure 9.16).

9.9.5 Visualization

This is to visualize the interaction between protein-ligand with a tool called Jmol and the Ligplot.

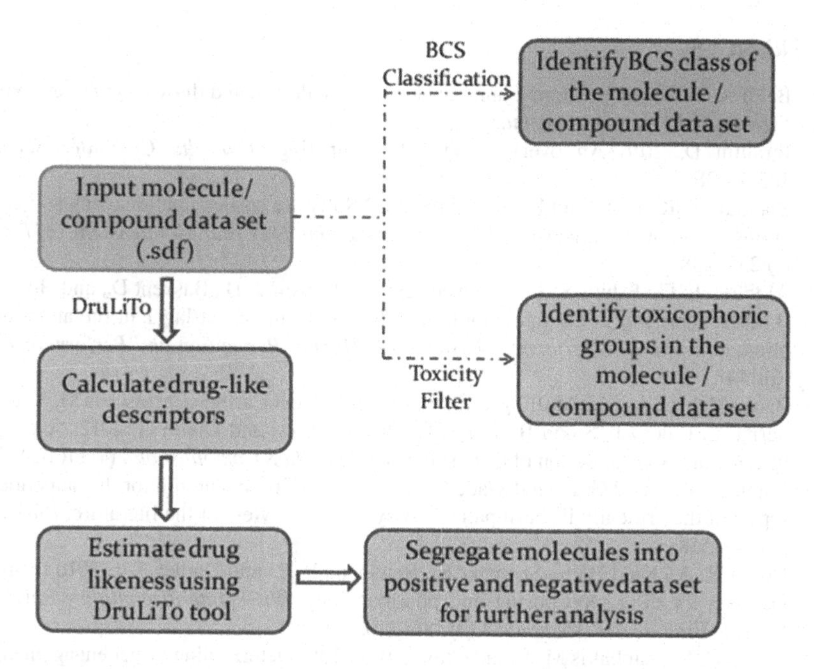

FIGURE 9.16 Workflow of compound screening using DruLiTo tool.

9.10 APPLICATION OF COMPUTER-AIDED DRUG DESIGNING

- Easy identification of binding site, docking molecule and ranking the bioaffinites and optimization of molecule
- Applied in research field and development
- Used for pharmacokinetic and ADMET prediction
- It is a cost-effective and automatic process
- Reduce biological and synthetic testing
- Rapid and time-consuming process
- Eliminate the undesirable compounds
- Least chance of failure at last stage.

9.11 CONCLUSION

The success of a computer-aided drug-designing tool for developing new drugs in the precedent few years exhibited the utility in the mechanism of drug development. This will enhance the available tools and techniques to assist in the drug discovery process. This promotes valuable details about intended molecule, lead compound and optimization, and latest development like QASR; other database provides the ligand-interaction and inhibitor. This CADD is effective than conventional techniques which give better results. Definitely, CADD will enhance the excellence of research in future and aid the numerous drug developments.

REFERENCES

1. Baldi A. 2010 Computational approaches for drug design and discovery: An overview. *Systematic Reviews in Pharmacy* 1 (1):99.
2. Ibrahim D. 2016 An overview of soft computing. *Procedia Computer Science* 102:34–38.
3. Ziauddin S. K. T., Zaman K., and Zia S. 2012 Software cost estimation using soft computing techniques. *Advances in Information Technology and Management (AITM)* 2 (1):233–238.
4. Akyürek E. G., Eshuis S. A., Nieuwenstein M. R., Saija J. D., Başkent D., and Hommel B. 2012 Temporal target integration underlies performance at lag 1 in the attentional blink. *Journal of Experimental Psychology: Human Perception and Performance* 38 (6):1448.
5. Bauer-Mehren A., Van Mullingen E. M., Avillach P., del Carmen Carrascosa M., Garcia-Serna R., Piñero J., Singh B., Lopes P., Oliveira J. L., and Diallo G. 2012 Automatic filtering and substantiation of drug safety signals. *PLoS Comput Biol* 8 (4):e1002457.
6. Mann E. A., Wood G. L., and Wade C. E. 2011 Use of procalcitonin for the detection of sepsis in the critically ill burn patient: A systematic review of the literature. *Burns* 37 (4):549–558.
7. Hodos R. A., Kidd B. A., Shameer K., Readhead B. P., and Dudley J. T. 2016 In silico methods for drug repurposing and pharmacology. *Wiley Interdisciplinary Reviews: Systems Biology and Medicine* 8 (3):186–210.
8. Simon G. M., Niphakis M. J., and Cravatt B. F. 2013 Determining target engagement in living systems. *Nature Chemical Biology* 9 (4):200–205.
9. Vugmeyster Y., Xu X., Theil F.-P., Khawli L. A., and Leach M. W. 2012 Pharmacokinetics and toxicology of therapeutic proteins: Advances and challenges. *World Journal of Biological Chemistry* 3 (4):73.
10. Fortun P., West J., Chalkley L., Shonde A., and Hawkey C. 2008 Recall of informed consent information by healthy volunteers in clinical trials. *QJM: An International Journal of Medicine* 101 (8):625–629.
11. Blundell T. L. 1996 Structure-based drug design. *Nature* 384 (6604 Suppl):23.
12. Ferreira L. G., Dos Santos R. N., Oliva G., and Andricopulo A. D. 2015 Molecular docking and structure-based drug design strategies. *Molecules* 20 (7):13384–13421.
13. Merz Jr. K. M., Ringe D., and Reynolds C. H. 2010. *Drug Design: Structure-and Ligand-Based Approaches*. Cambridge University Press, Cambridge.
14. Bacilieri M., and Moro S. 2006 Ligand-based drug design methodologies in drug discovery process: An overview. *Current Drug Discovery Technologies* 3 (3):155–165.
15. Pavia F., and Curtin W. 2015 Parallel algorithm for multiscale atomistic/continuum simulations using LAMMPS. *Modelling and Simulation in Materials Science and Engineering* 23 (5):055002.
16. Prieto-Martínez F. D., López-López E., Juárez-Mercado K. E., and Medina-Franco J. L. 2019. Computational drug design methods—Current and future perspectives. In K. Roy (ed.) *In Silico Drug Design*, 19–44. Elsevier, Amsterdam.
17. Varma M. V., Kaushal A. M., Garg A., and Garg S. 2004 Factors affecting mechanism and kinetics of drug release from matrix-based oral controlled drug delivery systems. *American Journal of Drug Delivery* 2 (1):43–57.
18. Caraballo I. 2010 Factors affecting drug release from hydroxypropyl methylcellulose matrix systems in the light of classical and percolation theories. *Expert Opinion on Drug Delivery* 7 (11):1291–1301.
19. Song N.-N., Zhang S.-Y., and Liu C.-X. 2004 Overview of factors affecting oral drug absorption. *Asian Journal of Drug Metabolism and Pharmacokinetics* 4 (3):167–176.

20. Jiao J., Yang Y., Wu Z., Li B., Zheng Q., Wei S., Wang Y., and Yang M. 2019 Screening cyclooxygenase-2 inhibitors from Andrographis paniculata to treat inflammation based on bio-affinity ultrafiltration coupled with UPLC-Q-TOF-MS. *Fitoterapia* 137:104259.
21. Guo J., Lin H., Wang J., Lin Y., Zhang T., and Jiang Z. 2019 Recent advances in bio-affinity chromatography for screening bioactive compounds from natural products. *Journal of Pharmaceutical and Biomedical Analysis* 165:182–197.
22. Liu R., Yan H., Jiang J., Li J., Liang X., Yang D., Pan L., Xie T., and Ma Z. 2020 Synthesis, characterization, photoluminescence, molecular docking and bioactivity of Zinc (II) compounds based on different substituents. *Molecules* 25 (15):3459.
23. Cozzini P., Kellogg G. E., Spyrakis F., Abraham D. J., Costantino G., Emerson A., Fanelli F., Gohlke H., Kuhn L. A., and Morris G. M. 2008 Target flexibility: An emerging consideration in drug discovery and design. *Journal of Medicinal Chemistry* 51 (20):6237–6255.
24. Ivetac A., and Andrew McCammon J. 2011 Molecular recognition in the case of flexible targets. *Current Pharmaceutical Design* 17 (17):1663–1671.
25. Schwede T., Kopp J., Guex N., and Peitsch M. C. 2003 SWISS-MODEL: An automated protein homology-modeling server. *Nucleic Acids Research* 31 (13):3381–3385.
26. Krieger E., Nabuurs S. B., and Vriend G. 2003 Homology modeling. *Methods of Biochemical Analysis* 44:509–524.
27. Cavasotto C. N., and Phatak S. S. 2009 Homology modeling in drug discovery: Current trends and applications. *Drug Discovery Today* 14 (13–14):676–683.
28. Janson G., Zhang C., Prado M. G., and Paiardini A. 2017 PyMod 2.0: Improvements in protein sequence-structure analysis and homology modeling within PyMOL. *Bioinformatics* 33 (3):444–446.
29. Janson G., and Paiardini A. 2020 PyMod 3: A complete suite for structural bioinformatics in PyMOL. *Bioinformatics*. doi:10.1093/bioinformatics/btaa849.
30. Webb B., and Sali A. 2016 Comparative protein structure modeling using Modeller. *Current Protocols in Bioinformatics* 54 (1):5.6.1–5.6.37.
31. Chohan K. K., Paine S. W., and Waters N. J. 2006 Quantitative structure activity relationships in drug metabolism. *Current Topics in Medicinal Chemistry* 6 (15):1569–1578.
32. Motoc I., Dammkoehler R. A., Mayer D., and Labanowski J. 1986 Three-dimensional quantitative structure-activity relationships I. General approach to the pharmacophore model validation. *Quantitative Structure-Activity Relationships* 5 (3):99–105.
33. Bleicher K. H., Böhm H.-J., Müller K., and Alanine A. I. 2003 Hit and lead generation: Beyond high-throughput screening. *Nature Reviews Drug Discovery* 2 (5):369–378.
34. Zoete V., Grosdidier A., and Michielin O. 2009 Docking, virtual high throughput screening and in silico fragment-based drug design. *Journal of Cellular and Molecular Medicine* 13 (2):238–248.
35. Bajorath J. 2002 Integration of virtual and high-throughput screening. *Nature Reviews Drug Discovery* 1 (11):882–894.
36. Lengauer T., and Rarey M. 1996 Computational methods for biomolecular docking. *Current Opinion in Structural Biology* 6 (3):402–406.
37. Halperin I., Ma B., Wolfson H., and Nussinov R. 2002 Principles of docking: An overview of search algorithms and a guide to scoring functions. *Proteins: Structure, Function, and Bioinformatics* 47 (4):409–443.
38. Perola E., and Charifson P. S. 2004 Conformational analysis of drug-like molecules bound to proteins: An extensive study of ligand reorganization upon binding. *Journal of Medicinal Chemistry* 47 (10):2499–2510.
39. Pagadala N. S., Syed K., and Tuszynski J. 2017 Software for molecular docking: A review. *Biophysical Reviews* 9 (2):91–102.

40. Li X., Li Y., Cheng T., Liu Z., and Wang R. 2010 Evaluation of the performance of four molecular docking programs on a diverse set of protein-ligand complexes. *Journal of Computational Chemistry* 31 (11):2109–2125.
41. Chaudhary K. K., and Mishra N. 2016 A review on molecular docking: Novel tool for drug discovery databases. *JSM Chemistry* 4 (3):1029.
42. Gaur A. S., Bhardwaj A., Sharma A., John L., Vivek M. R., Tripathi N., Bharatam P. V., Kumar R., Janardhan S., and Mori A. 2017 Assessing therapeutic potential of molecules: Molecular property diagnostic suite for tuberculosis **MPDS^{TB}**. *Journal of Chemical Sciences* 129 (5):515–531.
43. Nagamani S., Gaur A., Tanneeru K., Muneeswaran G., Madugula S., Consortium M., Druzhilovskiy D., Poroikov V., and Sastry G. 2017 Molecular property diagnostic suite (MPDS): Development of disease-specific open source web portals for drug discovery. *SAR and QSAR in Environmental Research* 28 (11):913–926.
44. Gaur A. S., Nagamani S., Tanneeru K., Druzhilovskiy D., Rudik A., Poroikov V., and Sastry G. N. 2018 Molecular property diagnostic suite for diabetes mellitus (MPDSDM): An integrated web portal for drug discovery and drug repurposing. *Journal of Biomedical Informatics* 85:114–125.

10 Diagnosing Chest-Related Abnormalities Using Medical Image Processing through Convolutional Neural Network

Vignessh B. and Reena Raj
Christ (Deemed to Be University)

Balakrishnakumar
Deep Scopy

CONTENTS

10.1 INTRODUCTION

Medical image processing is the technique for conveying clean pics of internal systems of the body. This cycle pursues trouble identification and the board. This cycle goes approximately as a record financial institution of the normal structure of the frame and restricts organs to make it smooth to see the inconsistencies. This cycle fuses with each radiological and natural imaging which used electromagnetic energies (X-beams and gamma), attractive, sonography, extensions, and heat and isotope imaging. There are numerous different imaginative techniques used to report facts, approximately the place and limit of the frame. Those methodologies have diverse obstacles regarded in another way with regard to those balances which produce pics. Every year, billions of photos were accomplished internationally for different exact functions. About a segment of them use ionizing and nonionizing radiation regulates. Clinical imaging produces photographs of the internal structures of the frame without meddling methodologies. The photographs had been made the usage of brisk processors and due to the difference in the energies numerically and fairly to indicators. Those signs and symptoms later are changed over to cutting side pix. The symptoms cope with the special kinds of tissues within the frame. Advanced pix has a critical impact reliably. Scientific imaging planning insinuates looking after snapshots by means of the use of the computer. This plan fuses various types of tactics and errands, as an instance, image picking up, capability, introduction, and correspondence. The picture is a restrict that indicates an extent of traits, as an instance, light or concealing a noticed sight. automatic snapshots have multiple focal factors, faster and humble looking after price, straightforward looking after and correspondence, quick quality assessment, numerous copying with retaining the nice, snappy and unobtrusive age, and adaptable manipulate. The weights of advanced pics are abuse copyright, frailty to resize with securing the exceptional, the want of huge breaking point reminiscence, and the need of quicker processor for control.

An image processing strategy is the usage of computer to manipulate the high-level image. This approach has numerous preferences, as an example, adaptability, flexibility, information taking care of, and correspondence. With the development of different image-resizing strategies, the photos can be saved profitably. The two- dimensional (2D) and three-dimensional (3D) pics may be set up in numerous estimations. The photo processing strategies were set up from the 1960s. Those techniques had been used for distinctive fields, for example, space, scientific purposes, expressions, and TV photograph improvement. During the 1970s with the headway of computer device, the cost of image processing ended up being less and swifter. During the 2000s, the photo processing ended up being swifter, less expensive, and more direct.

10.2 MEDICAL IMAGE PROCESSING

Deep learning with convolutional neural networks (CNNs) has accomplished cutting-edge performance for automated medical image segmentation [1]. Notwithstanding, programmed segmentation strategies have not demonstrated adequately accurate and robust results for clinical use because of the inherent challenges of medical images, for example, helpless image quality, diverse imaging and segmentation conventions, and varieties among patients. On the other hand, intelligent segmentation strategies are generally received, as they incorporate the client's information and consider the application prerequisites for more robust segmentation performance. Thus, interactive segmentation remains the cutting edge for existing business careful arranging and route items. Notwithstanding, there are not many investigations on utilizing CNNs for intuitive segmentation. This is basically because of the prerequisite of a lot of explained images for preparing, the absence of image-explicit variation, and the requesting balance among model unpredictability, surmising time, and memory space effectiveness [5].

Momentous advancement has been made in photograph reputation, mainly due to the accessibility of big scale commented on datasets and deep convolutional neural networks (CNNs). It empowers studying through information-driven, profoundly delegate, and diverse levelled picture highlights from sufficient training statistics. Notwithstanding, acquiring the datasets as thoroughly clarified as ImageNet within the scientific imaging region stays a difficult errand. At present, there are three substantial techniques that efficiently utilize CNNs to medical photo-characterization: training the CNN without any coaching, making use of off-the-rack pre-organized CNN highlights, and conducting solo CNN pre-training with administered calibrating. Another powerful technique is flow getting to know, i.e., calibrating CNN fashions pre-prepared from feature picture dataset to scientific image undertakings. From the past understudied elements of utilizing deep CNN to system supported detection issues. With the aid of assessing and investigating the one-of-a-kind CNN architectures, this model carries 5000 to 160 million limitations and modifications in portions of layers. We at that factor examine the impact of dataset scale and spatial photograph putting on execution. At last, we have a look at when and why circulate gaining from pre-prepared ImageNet (thru tweaking) may be helpful. We take a look at two specific laptop supported detection (CADe) troubles, in particular thoracoabdominal lymph hub (LN) detection and interstitial lung contamination (ILD) association. The reducing part execution on the mediastina LN detection may be completed, and the initial 5-crease go-approval characterization consequences on predicting hub CT cuts with ILD classifications are reported [10]. The CNN model research and vital reviews can be reached out to the plan of elite CAD frameworks for other medical imaging errands.

Second, intelligent division regularly requires image-express sorting out some way to supervise outstanding setting assortments among exceptional pics; anyway present day CNNs are not adaptable to unique take a look at pics, as limits of the model are found from making plan images and a short time later fixed in the testing level, without picture-express exchange. It has been proven that picture-explicit trade of a pre-prepared Gaussian combination version (GMM) enables with improving division precision. Regardless, advancing from clean GMMs to superb but complicated CNNs on this putting has now not but been illustrated.

Third, brisk deduction and reminiscence productivity are referred to clever division. They may be respectably without difficulty finished for 2D images, besides grow to be appreciably more unsafe for 3D pictures [7, 8]. For instance, DeepMedic works on 3D image to decrease the reminiscience necessities besides they bring a slight inference in it. HighRes3DNet goes after 3D complete pics with modestly snappy inferring anyway desires an amazing deal of GPU reminiscence, inciting excessive hardware necessities. To make CNN-based totally instinctive method which is capable to use, permitting CNNs to react speedy to customer collaboration's and to head after a device with confined GPU sources (e.g., a popular work zone computer or a computer) is attractive. DeepIGeoS unites CNNs with purchaser collaboration's and has shown high-quality expertise. Anyway, it has a nonappearance of adaptability to unnoticeable photo settings.

10.3 APPLICATIONS

AI algorithms are built using the state-of-the-art deep learning models, and probabilistic graphic models are trained on millions of medical data and provide qualitative reports for physicians referring to make better diagnosis. With exceptional accuracy, instant triaging and seamless integration, AI algorithms can identify the abnormality within seconds.

10.3.1 Chest X-Ray

Revealing examples on chest X-ray is fundamental for distinguishing and treating sicknesses. AI model aids radiologists by precisely identifying and announcing the ailment present on the X-ray, and empowers insinuating experts to make a superior determination. By utilizing cutting-edge Deep Learning technology which is set up on extraordinary numerous chest X-beams against various illnesses and can precisely arrange the sicknesses close by triaging the polluted zone.

10.3.2 Endoscopy

Endoscopy AI model can be trained for a specific function, for example, to perceive or portray characterized sores, colon polyps, for example. Simulated intelligence model can be prepared by Deep Learning calculations through introduction on various preparing components, for example, an enormous number of predefined polyp-containing video outlines. DL calculations will separate and examine explicit highlights like miniature surface topological example, shading contrasts, miniature vascular example, and pit design, appearance under sifted light, for example, tight band imaging, high amplification, endoscopy appearance, and numerous different highlights from these video-outlines permitting robotized recognition or analysis forecast of sores of premium.

10.3.3 Magnetic Resonance Imaging MRI

Brain MRI (Magnetic Resonance Image) segmentation is vital for the constructive clinical diagnostics of various organ-related ailments. Because of the unpredictable idea of mind MRI (3D), tissue division is a provocative errand. Cerebrum MRI AI model uses the most proficient profound learning strategies to handle these MRI volumes as 3D as opposed to breaking them into 2D pictures, these models are being prepared on immense measures of MRI volumes, AI models can give extraordinary precision in summing up output content and furthermore computationally effective for quick preparing of enormous assortments of information.

10.3.4 Microscope

Malaria parasite AI model detects malaria parasites in thin blood-smeared digital images by using deep learning algorithms which are prepared by training of thousands of blood-smeared microscopic images to predict the infected vs healthy cells and accurately classify them.

10.4 METHOD

Respiratory sicknesses cause a huge number of deaths each year. Determination of these pathologies is a manual, monotonous cycle that has cover and intra-observer changeability, delaying finding and treatment. The progressing COVID-19 pandemic has exhibited the need for making systems to automatize the analysis of pneumonia, while Convolutional Neural Networks (CNNs) have wind up being a splendid option for the modified gathering of clinical pictures. Regardless, given the need of giving a sureness game plan in this setting, it is critical to assess the immovable nature of the model's figures. In this work, we propose an amazing assembly portrayal structure reliant on a Bayesian Deep Learning way to deal with increase execution while assessing the weakness of each request decision. This contraption joins the information isolated from different models by weighting their results according to the weakness of their conjectures. Execution of the Bayesian association is surveyed in a veritable circumstance where at the same time isolating between four novel pathologies: control versus bacterial pneumonia versus viral pneumonia versus COVID-19 pneumonia [11]. In the wake of applying a pre-processing calculation to identify and eliminate stomach areas portraying on pictures, a histogram evening out calculation and a two-sided channel are applied to deal with the first pictures to produce two arrangements of separated pictures. At that point, the first picture and these two separated pictures are utilized as contributions of three channels of the CNN deep learning model, which increment learning data of the model.

To completely take preferences of the pre-improved CNN models, this investigation utilizes an exchange learning strategy to assemble another model to distinguish and group COVID-19 tainted pneumonia. A VGG16-based CNN model was initially prepared utilizing ImageNet and tweaked utilizing chest X-ray pictures in this investigation [6].

10.4.1 Neuron

Neural networks began as an endeavor to replicate the working of the human brain to make things more intelligent. In any event, something like this isn't really consistently complex. Neural network is, typically, a supervised method of learning. This implies there is presence of a training set. In a perfect world, this set contains models with their totally truth esteems (labels, classes and so forth). In the event of sentiment investigation, the training set would be rundown of sentences and their separate right sentiment. Neuron, as shown in Figure 10.1, is the basic building block of artificial neural networks. The entire reason for profound learning is to copy how the human brain functions with the expectation that thusly we will make something stunning. Inside an artificial neural network, a neuron is a numerical capacity that models the working of an organic neuron. Commonly, a neuron figures the weighted normal of its information.

10.4.2 Neural Network Model

An artificial neural network is made up of three components:

- Input layer
- Hidden layer
- Output layer.

The input data information is taken care in the forward direction through the network. Each hidden layer acknowledges the information, measures it according to the actuation capacity, and passes to the progressive layer as shown in Figure 10.2. In request to produce some yield, the information should be taken care in the forward direction as it were. The information ought not to stream in reverse direction during yield age; otherwise, it would frame a cycle, and the yield would never be produced. Such network setups are known as feed-forward network. The feed-forward network helps in forward spread, it acts for one data point at a time, and output is the prediction of input data point. It permits the data to return from the cost backward through the network to register the angle. Along these lines, circle over the hubs beginning at the last hub in reverse topological request to register the subordinate of the last hub yield as for each edge's hub tail. Doing so will assist us in realizing who is answerable for the most blunder and alter the boundaries in that course.

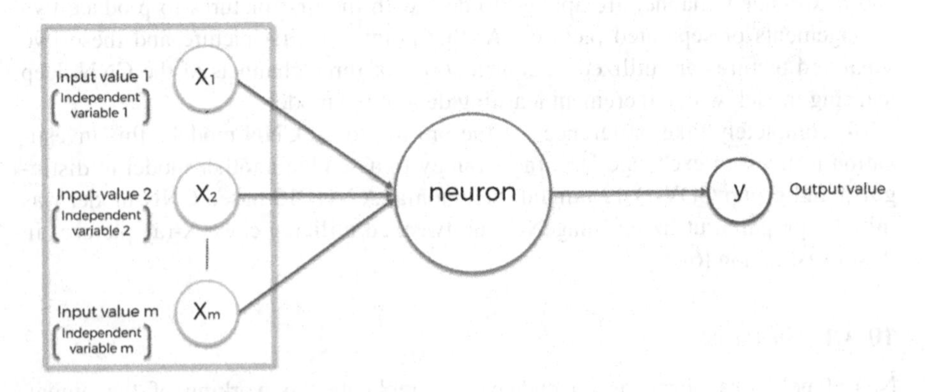

FIGURE 10.1 Neuron activation.

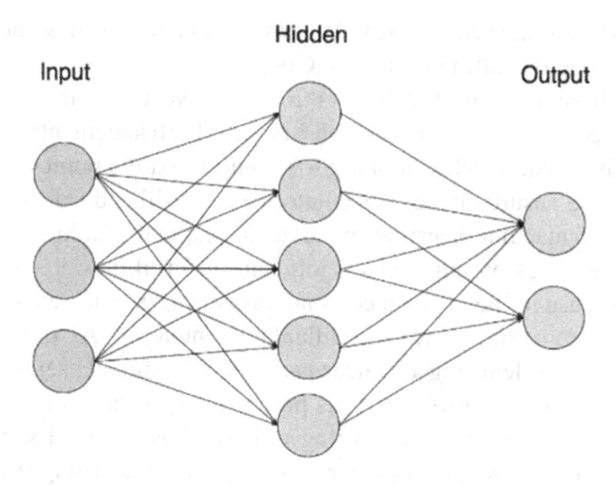

FIGURE 10.2 Neural network model.

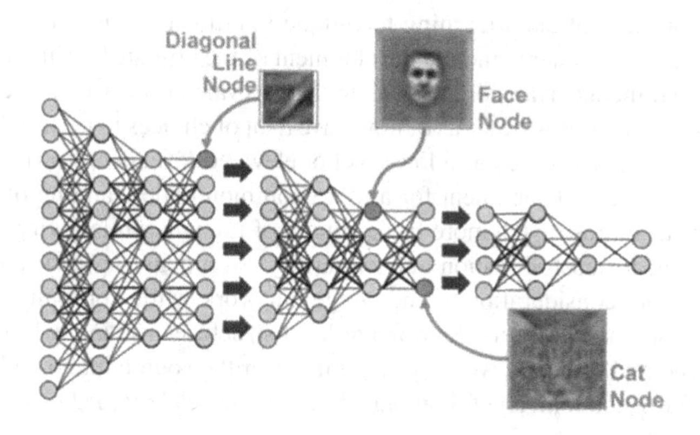

FIGURE 10.3 Deep neural network.

10.4.3 Deep Neural Network

Another significant achievement of the connectionist development was the fruitful utilization of back-engendering to train deep neural networks with interior portrayals and the promotion of the back-proliferation calculation. This calculation has come and gone in ubiquity and it is a predominant way to deal with training deep models.

During the 1990s, significant advancements have been made by scientists in displaying groupings with neural networks as shown in Figure 10.3. Hochreiter et al. recognized some of the major numerical challenges in demonstrating long groupings. The long present moment memory or LSTM network was presented by Hochreiter and Schmidhuber to determine a portion of these challenges [3]. Today, the LSTM is broadly utilized for some arrangement demonstrating undertakings including numerous normal language handling errands at Google.

The next phase of neural networks research went on until the mid-1990s. Adventures based on neural networks and other AI advancements started to make ridiculously driven claims while looking for ventures. At the point when AI research didn't satisfy these absurd desires, speculators were disillusioned. At the same time, different fields of machine learning made advances, and graphical models accomplished great outcomes on numerous significant undertakings. These two elements prompted a decrease in the prevalence of neural networks that went on until 2007.

Right now, deep neural networks outflanked contending AI frameworks dependent on other machine learning advances just as hand-planned usefulness. This third influx of prominence of neural networks proceeds to the hour of this composition; however, the focal point of deep learning research has changed significantly. The third wave started with an emphasis on new unsupervised learning strategies and the capacity of deep models to sum up well from little datasets, yet today there is more revenue in a lot more seasoned supervised learning calculations and the capacity of deep models to use enormous named datasets.

10.4.4 Framework

The appropriation of deep learning technique in clinical envisioning has pushed at an upsetting development, and the development of the climate has likewise moreover demonstrated inconceivable improvement. Due to various enormous tech affiliations and open-source exercises, we as of now have a lot of choices to peruse [2]. The available options can be ordered as a low-level or elevated-level deep learning technique. It may be used as a detachment for a more common understanding of the systems. Low-level structures give a more basic square of thought while giving an enormous heap of room for customization and versatility. Significant level structures are utilized for all out consideration to encourage our work while confining the degree of customization and flexibility. Significant level structures use a low-level framework as a backend and typically work by changing over the source into the ideal low-level structure for execution. The following are a few the celebrated choices of structures for deep learning.

Imperative projects perform calculations as they are experienced along the program flow. "Emblematic projects characterize images and how they should be joined. They bring about what we call a computational chart. Images themselves probably won't have starting qualities" [2]. Images secure qualities after the chart is aggregated and conjured with specific qualities. Light, Chainer and Minerva are instances of basic-style DL frameworks. Emblematic-style DL frameworks incorporate TensorFlow, Theano and CGT. Additionally in emblematic their style are CXXNet and Caffe that characterize the diagram in setup records. Basic frameworks are more adaptable since you're nearer to the language. In representative frameworks, there's less adaptability since you write in a space explicit language. In any case, representative frameworks will in general be more proficient, both as far as memory and speed. On occasion, it may bode well to utilize a blend of both system styles. For instance, boundary refreshes are done significantly, and angle computations are done emblematically. MXNet allows a blend of the two styles. Gluon utilizes a basic style for simpler model turn of events while likewise supporting unique diagrams.

All information is spoken to as tensors (multi-dimensional exhibits). A DL system should along these lines uphold tensors and procedure on them. The capacity to characterize dynamic computational diagrams is wanted by engineers. To be unique implies that chart hubs can be added or taken out at runtime. With PyTorch and Chainer, diagrams can be characterized powerfully. With TensorFlow, you need to characterize the whole calculation chart before you can run it. TensorFlow all the more as of late has TensorFlow Fold for dynamic charts and excited execution for sure fire execution. A basic activity in a DL network during learning is work separation. Programmed differentiation is an element that must be upheld by a DL structure. Deep learning includes preparing and deduction. Preparing is frequently done on cloud groups. Induction can on occasion occur on compelled IoT gadgets, installed frameworks or cell phones. In this manner, prepared models should have the option to run on ARM-based equipment. For instance, Caffe2 is appropriate for cell phones, while TensorFlow is for examination and working alongside for sending. Be that as it may, there's TensorFlow Lite for deduction on compelled gadgets.

TensorFlow is an opensource system created by Google specialists to run AI, deep learning and other factual and prescient investigation remaining burdens. Like comparative stages, it's intended to smooth out the way toward creating and executing progressed investigation applications for clients, for example, information researchers, analysts and prescient modelers. The TensorFlow programming handles informational indexes that are displayed as computational hubs in chart structure. The edges that interface the hubs in a chart can speak to multidimensional vectors or lattices, making what are known as tensors. Since TensorFlow projects utilize an information flow design that works with summed up moderate aftereffects of the calculations, they are particularly open to exceptionally enormous scope equal handling applications, with neural organizations being a typical model. The structure incorporates sets of both high-level and low-level APIs. Google suggests utilizing the high-level ones when conceivable to rearrange information pipeline advancement and application programming. Notwithstanding, realizing how to utilize the low-level APIs – called TensorFlow Core – can be important for experimentation and investigating of uses, the organization says; it likewise gives clients a "psychological model" of the AI innovation's internal functions, in Google's words. TensorFlow applications can run on either ordinary CPUs or higher-execution illustrations handling units (GPUs), just as Google's own tensor preparing units (TPUs), which are custom gadgets explicitly intended to accelerate TensorFlow positions. Google's first TPUs, itemized freely in 2016, and were utilized inside related to TensorFlow to control a portion of the organization's applications and online administrations, including its RankBrain search calculation and Street View planning innovation.

In mid-2018, Google advanced its outside TensorFlow endeavors by making the second era of TPUs accessible to Google Cloud Platform clients for preparing and running their own AI models. TensorFlow put together remaining burdens is charged with respect to every subsequent premise; the Cloud TPU administration at first was dispatched as a beta program with just "restricted amounts" of the gadgets accessible for use, as indicated by Google.

Generally, TensorFlow applications are progressed and has huge scope in the domains of AI and deep learning. In fueling Google's RankBrain AI framework, TensorFlow has been utilized to improve the data recovery abilities of the organization's lead internet searcher. Google has likewise utilized the structure for applications that incorporate programmed email reaction age, picture grouping and optical character acknowledgment, just as a medication revelation application that the organization chipped away at with scientists from Stanford University. Different organizations recorded on the TensorFlow site as clients of the system incorporate Airbnb, Coca-Cola, eBay, Intel, Qualcomm, SAP, Twitter, Uber and Snapchat designer Snap, Inc. Another client is STATS LLC, a games counseling organization that runs TensorFlow-based deep learning models to break down things, for example, the developments of players during elite athletics games. TensorFlow-based deep learning has likewise been a piece of trials and tests including one of the bigger-scaled proposed developments today that is self-driving vehicles.

Training large models consumes a great deal of time, and it is a smart thought to spare the prepared models to records to try not to prepare them over and over. There are various motivations to do this. For instance, you should do surmising on a machine that is not the same as the one where the model was prepared. Sometimes model's presentation on validation set decreases toward the finish of the training on account of over fitting. On the off chance that you spared your model boundaries after each age, toward the end you can choose to utilize the model that performs best on the validation set. Another explanation is train your model utilizing one language (like Python that has a ton of instruments for training) and run surmising utilizing an alternate language (like Scala presumably on the grounds that your application is based on Scala). When compared with TensorFlow, PyTorch is more natural. One snappy undertaking with both these structures will make that bounteously understood. Regardless of whether you don't have a strong mathematics or an unadulterated machine learning foundation, you will have the option to comprehend PyTorch models. You can characterize or control the chart as the model continues which makes PyTorch more instinctive. PyTorch doesn't have any representation apparatus like TensorBoard; however, you can generally utilize a library like matplotlib. I wouldn't state PyTorch is superior to TensorFlow; however, both these profound learning systems are inconceivably helpful.

While deep neural networks are extremely popular, the intricacy of the significant frameworks has been a boundary to their utilization for engineers new to AI. There have been a few recommendations for improved and disentangled elevated-level APIs for building neural network models, all of which will in general seem to be comparable from a good way yet show contrasts on nearer assessment. Keras is one of the main significant level neural networks of APIs. It is written in Python and supports various back-end neural network calculation motors. Keras was made to be easy to use, particular, simple to expand, and to work with Python. The API was "intended for individuals, not machines," and "follows best practices for lessening psychological load." Neural layers, cost capacities, enhancers, instatement plans, enactment capacities, and regularization plans are all independent modules that you can join to make new models. New modules are easy to add, as new classes and capacities. Models are characterized in Python code, not independent model design records.

The main motivations to utilize Keras come from its core values, essentially the one about being easy to understand. Past simplicity of learning and simplicity of model structure, Keras offers the benefits of expansive reception, uphold for a wide scope of creation organization alternatives, reconciliation within any event five back-end motors (TensorFlow, CNTK, Theano, MXNet, and PlaidML), and solid help for different GPUs and appropriated preparing. Additionally, Keras is sponsored by Google, Microsoft, Amazon, Apple, Nvidia, Uber, and others. Keras appropriately doesn't do its own low-level tasks, for example, tensor items and convolutions; it depends on a back-end motor for that. Despite the fact that Keras bolsters various back-end motors, its essential (and default) back end is TensorFlow, and its essential ally is Google. The Keras API comes bundled in TensorFlow as tf.keras, which as referenced prior will turn into the essential TensorFlow API as of TensorFlow 2.0. Figure 10.4 shows the framework of the algorithm.

10.4.5 Supervised Learning

Supervised learning is the most widely recognized sub-branch of AI today. Commonly, new AI professionals will start their excursion with supervised learning algorithms. Along these lines, the first of this three-post arrangement will be about supervised learning. Supervised AI algorithms are intended to learn as a visual cue. The name "supervised" taking in begins from the possibility that training this kind of algorithm resembles having an educator direct the entire cycle. When training a supervised learning algorithm, the training information will comprise of inputs matched with the right outputs. During training, the algorithm will look for designs in the information that relate with the ideal outputs. Subsequent to training, a supervised learning algorithm will take in new concealed inputs and will figure out which

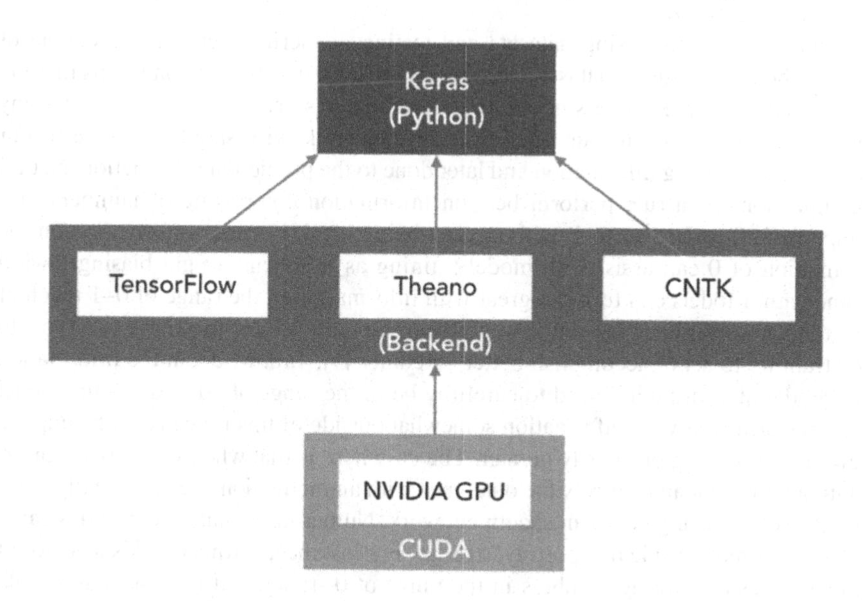

FIGURE 10.4 Framework.

name the new inputs will be named dependent on earlier training information. The target of a supervised learning model is to anticipate the right name for recently introduced input information.

During training, the classification technique that will be talked about in this part are those centered on foreseeing a subjective reaction by examining information and perceiving designs. For instance, this kind of method is utilized to arrange whether a Visa exchange is deceitful.

A classification algorithm will be given information focuses with an allotted classification. The occupation of a classification algorithm is to then take an info esteem and relegate it to a class, or it finds a way into dependent on the training information gave. The most well-known illustration of classification is deciding whether an email is spam or not. With two classes to browse (spam, or not spam), this issue is known as a paired classification issue. The algorithm will be given training information with messages that are both spam and not spam. The model will discover the highlights inside the information that connect to one or the other class and make the planning capacity referenced before: $Y=f(x)$. At that point, when given a concealed email, the model will utilize this capacity to decide if the email is spam.

Regression is a predictive statistical cycle where the model endeavors to locate the significant relationship among dependent and independent variables. The objective of a regression calculation is to foresee a persistent number, for example, deals, pay, and grades. Direct regression is a regulated learning procedure regularly utilized in foreseeing, gauging, and discovering relationships between quantitative information. It is one of the fastest learning procedures, which is still generally utilized. For instance, this procedure can be applied to inspect if there was a relationship between an organizations' promoting financial plan and its deals. You could likewise utilize it to decide whether there is a straight relationship between a specific radiation treatment and tumor sizes.

Since we are discussing datasets and testing, it merits referencing a couple of things about the training dataset and activities that we can perform on it; this method is alluded to as pre-processing. Notwithstanding, it's critical to recollect that any pre-processing we do to our training information likewise should be done to our approval and testing information and later done to the prediction information. Neural organizations as a rule perform best on information comprising of numbers in a range from 0 to 1 or –1 to 1, with the last being ideal. Fixating information on the estimation of 0 can assist with model training as it lessens weight biasing toward some path. Models can turn out great with information in the range of 0–1 much of the time, however once in a while we will have to rescale them to a range of –1 to 1 to get training to act or accomplish better outcomes [9]. Talking about the information range, the qualities don't need to carefully be in the range of –1 and 1 – the model will perform well with information somewhat outside of this range or with simply a few qualities being ordinarily greater. The case here is that when we increase information by weight and entirety the outcomes with an inclination, we're typically passing the subsequent yield to an enactment work. Numerous actuation capacities carry on appropriately inside this portrayed range. For instance, softmax yields a vector of probabilities containing numbers in the range of 0–1; sigmoid likewise has a yield range of 0–1 yet tanh yields a range from –1 to 1.

Another motivation behind why this scaling is ideal is a neural organization's dependence on numerous duplication tasks. On the off chance that we increase by numbers over 1 or underneath –1, the subsequent worth is bigger in scale than the first one. Inside the –1 to 1 range, the outcome turns into a small amount, a more modest worth. Increasing enormous numbers from our training information with loads may cause coasting point flood or precariousness – loads becoming excessively quick. It's simpler to control the training cycle with more modest numbers. There are numerous terms identified with information pre-processing: normalization, scaling, change scaling, mean evacuation (as referenced above), nonstraight changes, scaling to exceptions, and so on, yet they are out of the extent of this book. We're simply going to scale information to a range by essentially separating the entirety of the numbers by the limit of their supreme qualities. For the case of a picture that comprises of numbers in the range somewhere in the range between 0 and 255, we partition the entire dataset by 255 and return information in the range from 0 to 1. We can likewise deduct 127.5 (to get a range from –127.5 to 127.5) and partition by 127.5, returning information in the range from –1 to 1.

10.4.6 Convolutional Neural Network

Convolutional neural networks (CNNs) rose up out of the investigation of the mind's visual cortex, and they have been utilized in picture acknowledgment since the 1980s. Over the most recent couple of years, because of the expansion in computational power, the measure of accessible preparing information, CNNs have figured out how to accomplish superhuman execution on some complex visual errands. The force picture search administrations, self-driving vehicles, programmed video classification frameworks, and that's just the beginning. In addition, CNNs are not limited to visual discernment: they are additionally fruitful at numerous different errands, for example, voice acknowledgment and common language handling [5]. The biggest drawback of A-NN is that the efficiency goes low as the input size increases, In A-NN, the images needs to be centered all the time, if not the model will not learn properly. Therefore we need to spot the features in a photograph if the picture is not centered and the need arises for convolution NN.

Convolutional Neural Network is a concept of feed forward neural nets in artificial intelligence. CNNs are used in high level applications like image or speech recognition, NLP, analyzing in organs, and recommendation systems. This network was proposed by Yun Zhou in the 1980s [4]. CNNs have multiple layers of neurons connected to each other, like human brain. Basically, these neurons are a math function, calculating the sum of weighted input tensors and passing it through an activation function which tries to learn the nonlinearity in the data. CNNs are able to detect the spatial features and thermal features. When an image is fed to ConvNets, the first layer identifies the edges, horizontal, and vertical lines. If the image goes deeper into the ConvNets, they can identify complex structures of the objects.

In each neuron, there are two operations used. First, the input image is multiplied by the random weights generated using Gaussian distribution and adding all the weighted pixels. Second, the weighted pixels are passed to an activation function which helps the system to decide the output corresponding to the given input tensor.

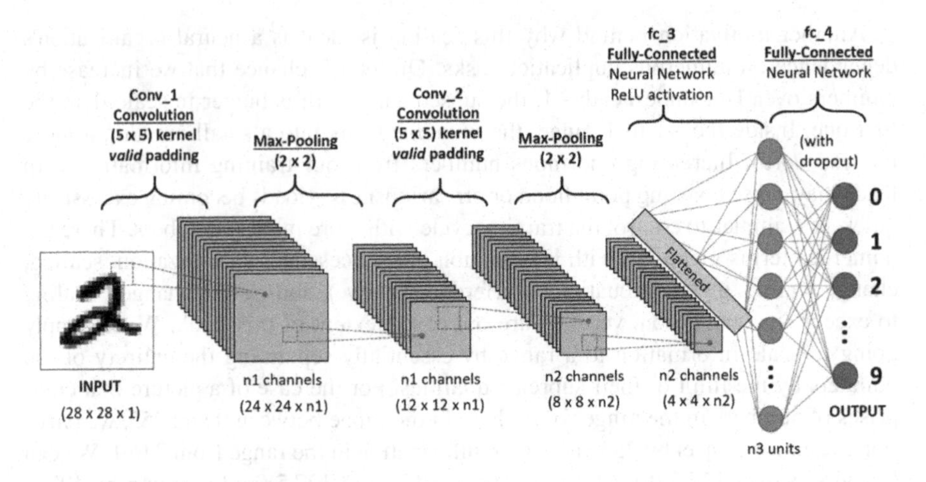

FIGURE 10.5 Convolutional neural network.

ConvNets are used to encode the data in smaller values and are easier to process without losing the features of the input tensors.

CNN is composed of two parts

When training the ConvNets, there are some hyper parameters that are needed to consider which are learn able parameters. These are basically the building blocks of CNN as shown in Figure 10.5. All images are in the same shape when training in CNNs. Different shapes of Kernels or filters are used in the convolutional operation. These kernels can cause down sampling of the image with respect to its shape. Each kernel can help to identify different patterns in the image.

Strides are used to define how many steps to move the kernel on the image. Padding is used to prevent down sampling by maintaining the same shape of the input image. This can be done by adding zeros as the border for the image. Pooling layers are used for converting the input image in small size; this helps reduce the computational cost without losing the features of the patterns. There are two types of pooling layers, namely, Max Pooling and Average Pooling. Max Pooling gives the maximum value of the group of pixels. Average Pooling calculates the average of the group of pixels [11]. Thus, it reduces the size and shape of the input tensors which helps in reducing the computational cost. Max Pooling reduces the noise in the image. Thus, it performs better than Average Pooling.

Activation Functions help to determine the output of the image by adding nonlinearity in the tensors. From this, the network can learn the very complex or difficult patterns in the image. Many types of activation functions are used to learn the patterns. They are Sigmoid, Hyperbolic, Rectified Linear Unit, Leaky Rectified Linear Unit, etc. The Rectified Linear Unit activation function is widely used because it rectified the negative values. If the value is less than zero, then it returns zero. Otherwise, it returns the same value.

VGG-19 Architecture was proposed by Karen Simonyan and Andrew Zisserman from the University of Oxford in 2015. In this project, we are using the VGG-19 architecture to identify the patterns of different disorders in the chest X-Ray images.

This architecture contains 16 ConvNets, five max pooling layers. The input shape is 224×224×3, kernel shape is 3×3, 1 pixel stride, and 2×2 of max pooling with stride of 2 pixels are used to build this architecture. ReLU activation function is used to perform better to learn the disorder patterns. There are 143,667,240 parameters used to train the dataset by ConvNets. And the depth is 26. From this architecture, we achieved high accuracy in determining the patterns of different types of lung disease.

10.5 METHODOLOGY

10.5.1 Dataset Description

To overcome this issue, datasets of 1, 12, 121 images from the National Institute of Health are used, and the dataset consists of 16 columns indicating image index, train or test dataset type and 14 different abnormalities that affect chest. Figure 10.1 shows the sample of the dataset.

In binary classification, it consists of image index and label of one abnormality that affects the chest as shown in Table 10.1; label 0 indicates the absence, and label 1 indicates the presence of abnormalities.

From Table 10.2, the multiple classification consists of image index and multiple abnormalities that affect the chest: label 0 indicates the absence, and label 1 indicates the presence of abnormalities (Figure 10.6).

10.5.2 Abnormalities

Chest X-ray algorithm is built using the state-of-the-art Deep Learning models and probabilistic Graphical Models which are trained on millions of medical data and thus provide physicians qualitative reports for referring to make a better diagnosis. This algorithm can be used to detect up to 14 abnormalities that are found in CXR such as cardiomegaly, effusion, hernia, and infiltration along with triaging the infected area. The primary objective is to create this algorithm with accuracy metrics on par with practicing radiologists.

TABLE 10.1
Binary Classification

Image Index	Labels
X-Ray_Image_1.dcm	1
X-Ray_Image_2.dcm	0
X-Ray_Image_3.dcm	1
X-Ray_Image_4.dcm	1
X-Ray_Image_5.dcm	1
X-Ray_Image_6.dcm	1
X-Ray_Image_7.dcm	0
X-Ray_Image_8.dcm	0
X-Ray_Image_9.dcm	1
X-Ray_Image_10.dcm	0

TABLE 10.2
Multiple Classification

	Labels			
Image Index	**Pneumonia**	**Tuberculosis**	**Nodule**	**Hernia**
Chest_X-Ray_Image_1.dcm	1	0	0	0
Chest_X-Ray_Image_2.dcm	1	0	0	0
Chest_X-Ray_Image_3.dcm	0	1	0	1
Chest_X-Ray_Image_4.dcm	0	0	1	0
Chest_X-Ray_Image_5.dcm	0	0	0	1
Chest_X-Ray_Image_6.dcm	0	0	0	1
Chest_X-Ray_Image_7.dcm	0	0	1	0
Chest_X-Ray_Image_8.dcm	0	1	0	0
Chest_X-Ray_Image_9.dcm	0	0	1	0
Chest_X-Ray_Image_10.dcm	1	0	1	0

Image Index	fold	Cardiomeg	Emphysem	Effusion	Hernia	Infiltration	Mass	Nodule	Atelectasis	Pneumotho	Pleural_Thi	Pneumonia	Fibrosis	Edema	Consolidation
00000001_000.png	train	1	0	0	0	0	0	0	0	0	0	0	0	0	0
00000001_001.png	train	1	1	0	0	0	0	0	0	0	0	0	0	0	0
00000001_002.png	train	1	0	1	0	0	0	0	0	0	0	0	0	0	0
00000002_000.png	train	0	0	0	0	0	0	0	0	0	0	0	0	0	0
00000003_000.png	train	0	0	0	1	0	0	0	0	0	0	0	0	0	0
00000003_001.png	train	0	0	0	1	0	0	0	0	0	0	0	0	0	0
00000003_002.png	train	0	0	0	1	0	0	0	0	0	0	0	0	0	0
00000003_003.png	train	0	0	0	1	1	0	0	0	0	0	0	0	0	0
00000003_004.png	train	0	0	0	1	0	0	0	0	0	0	0	0	0	0
00000003_005.png	train	0	0	0	1	0	0	0	0	0	0	0	0	0	0

FIGURE 10.6 NIH opensource dataset.

Cardiomegaly implies enlargement of the heart. The definition is the point at which the cross over diameter of the heart outline is more prominent than or equivalent to half of the cross over diameter of the chest (expanded cardiothoracic proportion) on a back foremost projection of a chest radiograph or a figured tomography. It ought not to be mistaken for an enlargement of the cardiomediastinal diagram. Cardiomegaly is normally a sign of another pathologic cycle and presents with a few types of essential or procured cardiomyopathies. It might include enlargement of the right, left, or the two ventricles or the atria.

Pneumonia is an infection that influences one or two lungs. It causes the air sacs, or alveoli, of the lungs to top off with liquid or discharge. Bacteria, viruses, or fungi may cause pneumonia. Side effects can go from mellow to genuine and may incorporate a hack with or without bodily fluid (a disgusting substance), fever, chills, and inconvenience relaxing. How genuine your pneumonia is relies upon your age, your general wellbeing, and what is causing your infection. To analyze pneumonia, your PCP will survey your clinical history, play out an actual test, and request analytic tests, for example, a chest X-beam. This data can assist your primary care physician with figuring out what sort of pneumonia you have. Treatment for pneumonia may incorporate anti-infection agents or viral or parasitic medicines. It might take half a month to recuperate from pneumonia. On the off chance that your side effects deteriorate, you should see a specialist immediately. On the off chance that you have serious pneumonia, you may have to go to the clinic for anti-microbial given through an intravenous (IV) line and oxygen treatment.

A pleural effusion is an unordinary measure of fluid around the lung. Numerous ailments can prompt it, so despite the fact that your pleural effusion may must be depleted, your primary care physician probably will focus on the treatment at whatever caused it. The pleura is a flimsy layer that lines the outside of your lungs and within your chest divider. At the point when you have a pleural effusion, fluid develops in the space between the layers of your pleura. Regularly, just teaspoons of watery fluid are in the pleural space, which permits your lungs to move easily in your chest hole when you relax.

About 96% of hernias are serious, and mostly happen in men because of the characteristic weakness of this area in their body. In an incisional hernia, the digestive system pushes through the stomach at the site of past stomach a medical procedure. This sort is generally normal in old or overweight in individuals who are latent after stomach surgery. A femoral hernia happens when the digestive system enters the trench conveying the femoral vein into the upper thigh. Femoral hernias are generally basic in ladies, particularly the individuals who are pregnant or obese. In an umbilical hernia, some portion of the small digestive tract goes through the stomach divider close to the navel. Normal in babies, and it likewise regularly besets stout ladies or the individuals who have had numerous children. A hiatal hernia happens when the upper stomach squeezes through the rest, an opening in the stomach through which the throat passes.

Lung nodules is the formation of little masses of tissue in the lung which are extremely typical. They appear as round, white shadows on a chest X-beam or modernized tomography (CT) examine. Lung nodules are commonly about 0.2 inch (5 mm) to 1.2 inches (30 mm) in size. A greater lung handle, for instance, one that is 30 mm or greater, will undoubtedly be perilous than is a more unobtrusive lung handle. Essentially the doctor perceives a lung handle on an imaging test, it's helpful to differentiate your current imaging analyze and a previous one. In case the handle on earlier pictures hasn't changed in size, shape or appearance in 2 years, it's most probably noncancerous. Noncancerous lung nodules are routinely achieved by past defilements. Noncancerous lung nodules generally speaking require no treatment. Once in a while considering the doctor may endorse yearly chest imaging to check whether a lung handle creates or changes after some time. In case a lung handle is new or has changed in size, shape or appearance, your PCP may recommend further testing – for instance, a CT check, positron outpouring tomography (PET) analyze, bronchoscopy or tissue biopsy – to conclude whether it's threatening.

A pneumothorax is an imploded lung. A pneumothorax happens when there is air spill space between your lung and chest divider. This air pushes apparently of your lung and makes it breakdown. Pneumothorax can be a completed lung breakdown or a breakdown of a tad of the lung. It can be achieved by an unpolished or entering chest injury, certain activities, or harm from essential lung infection. Or then again it may occur for no verifiable clarification. Signs typically fuse unexpected chest torture and shortness of breath. On specific occasions, a cell lung can be a perilous event. Treatment for a pneumothorax by and large incorporates implanting's a needle or chest tube between the ribs to dispose of the plenitude air. In any case, a little pneumothorax may patch in isolation.

Pulmonary edema is a condition brought about by overabundance fluid in the lungs. This fluid gathers in the various air sacs in the lungs, making it hard to breathe. In most cases, heart issues cause pulmonary edema. In any case, fluid can gather in the lungs for different reasons, including pneumonia, introduction to specific poisons and drugs, injury to the chest divider, and heading out to or practicing at high elevations. Pulmonary edema that grows abruptly (intense pulmonary edema) is a health-related crisis requiring prompt consideration. Pulmonary edema can some of the time cause demise. The standpoint improves in the event that you get treated rapidly.

Emphysema causes shortness of breath. In individuals with emphysema, the air sacs in the lungs (alveoli) are harmed. Over the long run, the internal dividers of the air sacs debilitate and crack-making bigger air spaces rather than numerous little ones. This lessens the surface territory of the lungs and, thusly, the measure of oxygen that arrives at your bloodstream. When you breathe out, the harmed alveoli don't work appropriately and old air gets caught, ruling out new, oxygen-rich air to enter. Most individuals with emphysema likewise have chronic bronchitis. Chronic bronchitis is irritation of the cylinders that convey air to your lungs (bronchial cylinders), which prompts a diligent hack. Emphysema causes chronic obstructive pulmonary disease (COPD). Smoking is the main source of COPD. Treatment may slow the movement of COPD, yet it can't switch the harm.

Atelectasis is a finished or fractional collapse of the entire lung or territory (projection) of the lung. It happens when the small air sacs (alveoli) inside the lung become emptied or perhaps loaded up with alveolar liquid. Atelectasis is one of the most well-known breathing (respiratory) inconveniences after a medical procedure. It's additionally a potential entanglement of other respiratory issues, including cystic fibrosis, lung tumors, chest wounds, liquid in the lung and respiratory shortcoming. You may create atelectasis in the event that you take in an unfamiliar item. Atelectasis can make breathing troublesome, especially on the off chance that you as of now have lung illness. Treatment relies upon the reason and seriousness of the collapse.

When imaging the chest divider, pleura, and stomach, chest radiography is useful in critical thinking, though in the mediastinum, CT is considerably more helpful. With extra pulmonary sores emerging in the unrivaled sulcus (apical) district, or chest divider masses, attractive reverberation imaging (MRI) is great as a result of its tissue portrayal capacities.

By and large, typical variations, in contrast to illness, are sensibly symmetric and frequently respective, and accordingly a one next to the other correlation can be made. The delicate tissues, fat, and musculature should be fairly symmetric. While surveying for skeletal anomalies, which are oftentimes testing to see, it is basic to analyze the individual bones cautiously, individually. To help separate an extrapulmonary (chest divider, pleural, or diaphragmatic) sore from an aspiratory parenchymal sore, evaluating the point the mass makes with the lung edge (uncaring plot for extra-parenchymal masses and intense plots for pneumonic masses) might be useful. With extrapulmonary masses, it tends to be hard to decide whether it is emerging from the chest divider or pleura, as their shapes might be comparable, yet the presence of bone annihilation recommends an extrapleural root.

Cystic fibrosis (CF) is a procured issue that makes outrageous damage to the lungs, digestive structure and various organs in the body. It impacts the cells that produce natural liquid, sweat and digestive juices. These released fluids are customarily modest and tricky. However, in people with CF, a blemished quality makes the releases become shabby and thick. Instead of going about as oils, the releases plug up chambers, channels and ways, especially in the lungs and pancreas. Though cystic fibrosis is reformist and requires each day care, people with CF are commonly all set to class and work. They consistently have a predominant individual fulfillment than people with CF had in before numerous years. Redesigns in screening and prescriptions infer that people with CF presently may live into their mid- to late 30s or 40s, and some are living into their 50s.

Pulmonary edema is a condition brought about by excess fluid in the lungs. This fluid gathers in the various air sacs in the lungs, making it hard to breathe. As a rule, heart issues cause pulmonary edema. In any case, fluid can gather in the lungs for different reasons, including pneumonia, introduction to specific poisons and meds, injury to the chest divider, and venturing out to or practicing at high rises. Pulmonary edema that grows unexpectedly (intense pulmonary edema) is a health-related crisis requiring prompt consideration. Pulmonary edema can here and there cause passing. The viewpoint improves in the event that you get treated rapidly. Treatment for pulmonary edema differs relying upon the reason however by and large incorporates supplemental oxygen and prescriptions.

Lung consolidation happens when the air that generally fills the little aviation routes in your lungs is supplanted with something different. Contingent upon the reason, the air might be supplanted with a liquid, for example, discharge, blood, or water, a strong, for example, stomach substance or cells the presence of your lungs on a chest X-ray, and your indications, are comparative for every one of these substances. Along these lines, you'll commonly require more tests to discover why your lungs are merged. With proper treatment, the consolidation as a rule disappears, and air returns. Consolidation quite often makes it hard for you to relax. Air can't overcome the consolidation, so your lung can't take care of its responsibility of acquiring the outside air and eliminating the air your body has utilized. This may cause you to feel winded. It might likewise make your skin look pale or pale blue because of an absence of oxygen. At the point when you have a disease in your lung, your body sends white platelets to battle it. Dead cells and flotsam and jetsam develop making discharge, which fills the little aviation routes. Pneumonia is normally because of microbes or an infection, yet it can likewise be brought about by a parasite or other abnormal creatures.

10.5.3 Pre-processing

Every X-ray image is in the form of greyscale values ranging from 0 to 256, where 0 denotes high black intensity and 256 indicates high white intensity. A single X-ray image is a matrix of 2 dimensions, stacked one after another. The images are to be normalized by following Gaussian distribution (values ranges between 0 and 1), standardized (i.e., mean = 0 and standard deviation = 1) and also resized to (256px, 256px) (height, width).

Images are computationally intensive. Image recognition systems tend to use small image sizes. They are scaled down to that smaller size before being fed into a neural network.

Gaussian or Normal Distribution is exceptionally regular term in statistics. These are commonly used to speak to random variables which coming into Machine Learning we can say which is something like the blunder when we don't know the weight vector for our Linear Regression Model. In a Gaussian distribution the more the data close to the mean it resembles a ringer bend all in all we have two fundamental parameters to clarify or educate with respect to our Gaussian distribution model they are mean and difference. Mean is typically spoken to by μ and change with σ^2 (σ is the standard deviation). The diagram is symmetric about mean for a Gaussian distribution.

The mean, median and mode are equivalent. Usually more data is nearer to the mean value and the not many or less continuous data is seen toward the boundaries, which is only a Gaussian distribution that resembles this ($\mu = 0$ and $\sigma = 1$) as shown in Figure 10.7. The central limit theorem (CLT) builds up that, in certain circumstances, when autonomous random variables are added, they are appropriately normalized which inclines toward a normal distribution (casually a "ringer bend") regardless of whether the first variables are not normally circulated or not. So due to these properties and Central Limit Theorem (CLT), Gaussian distribution is regularly utilized in Machine Learning Algorithms.

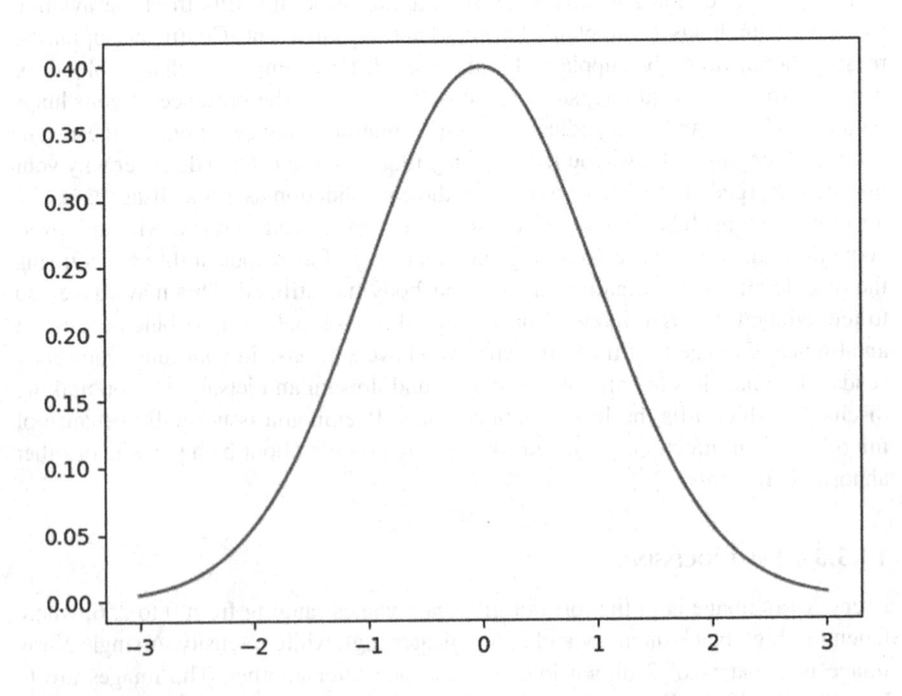

FIGURE 10.7 Bell curve.

10.5.4 Modeling

The chest X-ray deep learning algorithm is created using Python Deep Learning Framework (Keras, Tensorflow) and Convolutional Neural Network (CNN). In A-NN, the images need to be centered all the time, if not the model will not learn properly. Therefore, we need to spot the features in a photograph if the picture is not centered and the need arises for convolution NN. The various steps involved in CNN are convolutional layer, pooling layer and dense layer. In the wording of CNN, we call the examples 'kernel', 'filter', or 'feature detector'. The plan of kernels depends on significant levels of mathematics. So what CNN does is recognizing the needed features from the image data utilizing relating filters and extricating the critical features for expectation.

Padding: You may as of now notice that the pixels of the image aren't prepared with a similar number. The pixels at the corner are less included than those in the center. This implies that the pixels don't get similar measure of loads. Moreover, if we simply continue applying the convolution, we may lose the data excessively quick. Padding is the stunt we can use here to fix this issue. As its name, padding implies giving extra pixels at the limit of the data.

Stride: By the way, does a filter consistently need to move each pixel in turn, i.e., the moving pace of the filters over the image is stride rate. Obviously not. We can likewise make it move two stages or three stages all at once both in the flat and vertical manners. This is called 'stride.'

The size of the information sources can be decreased using pooling layers and consequently accelerate the calculation as shown in Figure 10.8. So it's essential to decrease the size of the data. Sliding a window, we just take the greatest incentive inside the crate on the left case. This is 'max pooling.' We can likewise take the normal qualities like the image on the right. This is 'normal pooling.' It may appear to be that we are losing data, yet the opposite is valid. We are just eliminating commotion and keeping the important data in our photos.

Grad-CAM technique is used to demystify the CNN, and Grad-CAM utilizes the gradients of any objective idea (state logits for "dog" or even an inscription), streaming into the last convolutional layer to deliver a coarse localization map featuring

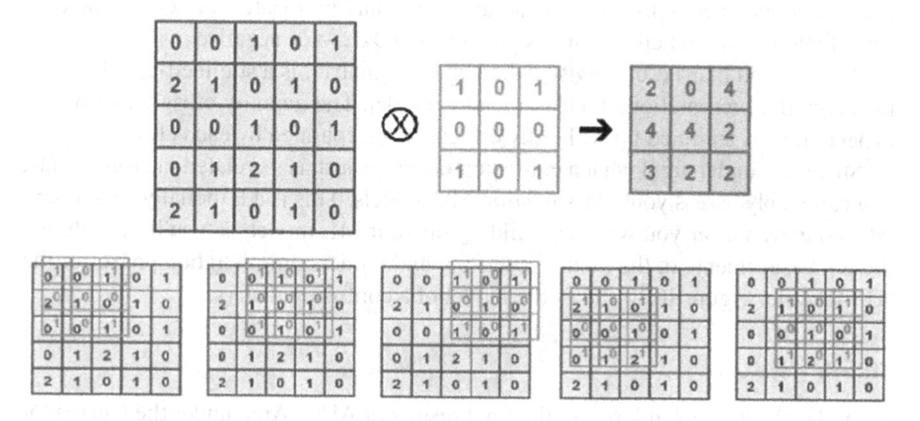

FIGURE 10.8 Stride.

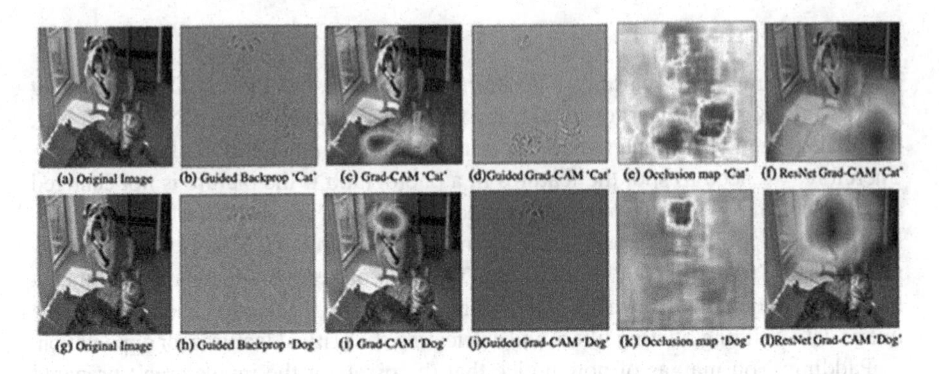

FIGURE 10.9 Grad-CAM model.

the significant districts in the picture for foreseeing the idea as shown in Figure 10.9. Utilizing Grad-CAM, we can outwardly approve where our organization is looking, verifying that it is surely taking a gander at the right patterns in the picture and activating around those patterns. In the event that the organization isn't activating around the proper patterns/objects in the picture, we realize that the organization hasn't properly taken in the hidden patterns in our dataset, the preparation strategy should be returned to, and above all, our model isn't prepared for arrangement. Grad-CAM is an instrument that should be in any profound learning specialist's tool stash. Grad-CAM, in contrast to CAM, utilizes the gradient data streaming into the last convolutional layer of the CNN to see every neuron for a choice of interest. To get the class discriminative localization guide of width u and stature v for any class c, we initially figure the gradient of the score for the class c, yc (before the softmax) regarding highlight maps ak of a convolutional layer. These gradients streaming back are worldwide normal pooled to acquire the neuron significance loads ak for the objective class.

10.5.5 Evaluation

The accuracy of the algorithm is calculated with the help of confusion matrix which is also known as error matrix, The actual values and predicated values will be converted into 0 and 1 where 1 denotes positive and 0 denotes negative.

A confusion matrix, otherwise called an error matrix, is a summed-up table used to survey the presentation of a classification model. The quantity of right and wrong expectations is summed up with tally esteems and separated by each class.

Since you understand what a confusion matrix is just as its related measurements, you can viably assess your classification ML models. This is additionally fundamental to see even after you wrap up building up your ML model, as you'll be utilizing these measurements in the model observing and model administration phases of the AI life cycle. Figure 10.10 shows the model of a confusion matrix.

10.5.6 Results

From the chest X-ray algorithm, the final results of AUC (Area under the Curve) for each abnormality are mentioned.

AUC-ROC bend is a presentation estimation for the arrangement issues at different edge settings. ROC is a probability bend and AUC speaks about degree or proportion of distinctness. It tells how much the model is equipped for recognizing classes as shown in Figure 10.11. Higher the AUC, the better the model is at predicting 0s as 0s and 1s as 1s. By similarity, the Higher the AUC, the better the model is at recognizing patients with the illness and no sickness.

From the above results, conclusions can be drawn that emphysema has the highest AUC value of 0.92 and infiltration has the least AUC value of 0.713 as shown in Figure 10.12.

In order to check the accuracy of X-ray algorithm, it is deployed and tested with real-time data from the lab where the chest X-ray image of the patient model is Fed into the tested X-ray deep learning algorithm.

Figure 10.13 shows that the diagnosed image feed into the algorithm based on the algorithm, we can predict whether the patient is diagnosed or not.

	Predicted 0	Predicted 1
Actual 0	TN	FP
Actual 1	FN	TP

FIGURE 10.10 Confusion matrix.

	TP	TN	FP	FN	Accuracy	Prevalence	Sensitivity	Specificity	PPV	NPV	AUC	F1	Threshold
Cardiomegaly	127	21703	148	455	0.973	0.026	0.218	0.993	0.462	0.979	0.909	0.296	0.5
Emphysema	146	21789	135	363	0.978	0.023	0.287	0.994	0.52	0.984	0.921	0.37	0.5
Effusion	1071	18945	734	1683	0.892	0.123	0.389	0.963	0.593	0.918	0.883	0.47	0.5
Hernia	0	22391	0	42	0.998	0.002	0	1	NaN	0.998	0.884	0	0.5
Infiltration	311	18190	305	3627	0.825	0.176	0.079	0.984	0.505	0.834	0.713	0.137	0.5
Mass	187	21140	160	946	0.951	0.051	0.165	0.992	0.539	0.957	0.833	0.253	0.5
Nodule	122	20965	133	1213	0.94	0.06	0.091	0.994	0.478	0.945	0.767	0.153	0.5
Atelectasis	374	19648	365	2046	0.893	0.108	0.155	0.982	0.506	0.906	0.816	0.237	0.5
Pneumothorax	202	21140	204	887	0.951	0.049	0.185	0.99	0.498	0.96	0.876	0.27	0.5
Pleural_Thickening	1	21697	2	733	0.967	0.033	0.001	1	0.333	0.967	0.786	0.003	0.5
Pneumonia	0	22191	0	242	0.989	0.011	0	1	NaN	0.989	0.764	0	0.5
Fibrosis	1	22069	2	361	0.984	0.016	0.003	1	0.333	0.984	0.82	0.005	0.5
Edema	14	21993	27	399	0.981	0.018	0.034	0.999	0.341	0.982	0.893	0.062	0.5
Consolidation	1	21475	1	956	0.957	0.043	0.001	1	0.5	0.957	0.803	0.002	0.5

FIGURE 10.11 AUC value of the model.

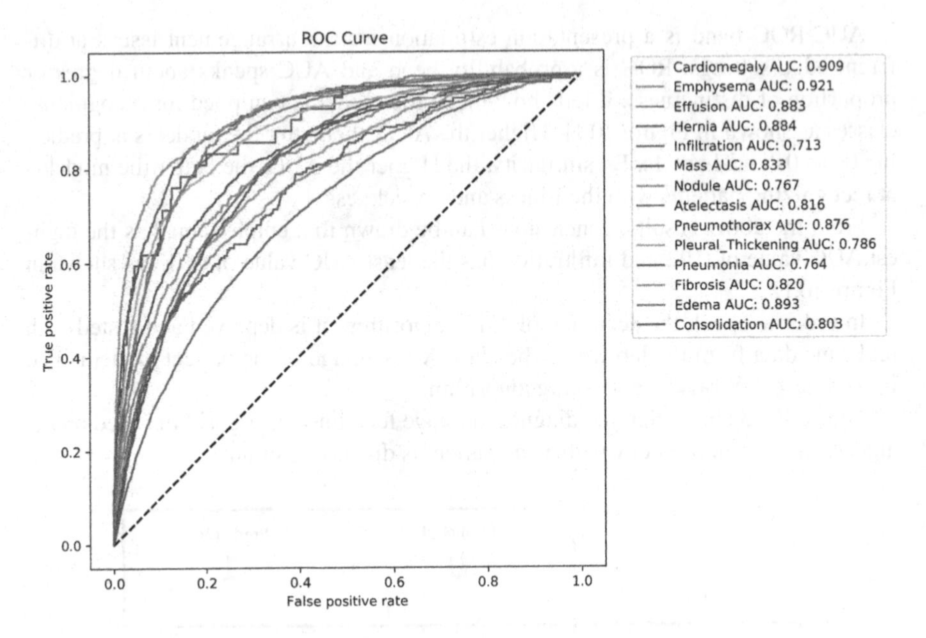

FIGURE 10.12 ROC curve.

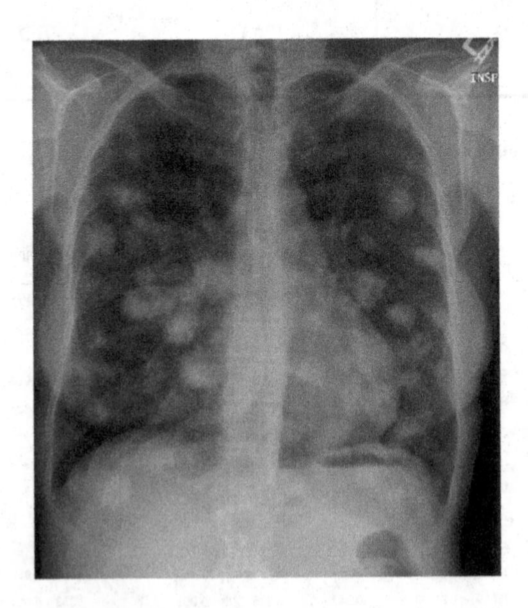

FIGURE 10.13 Input IMAGE.

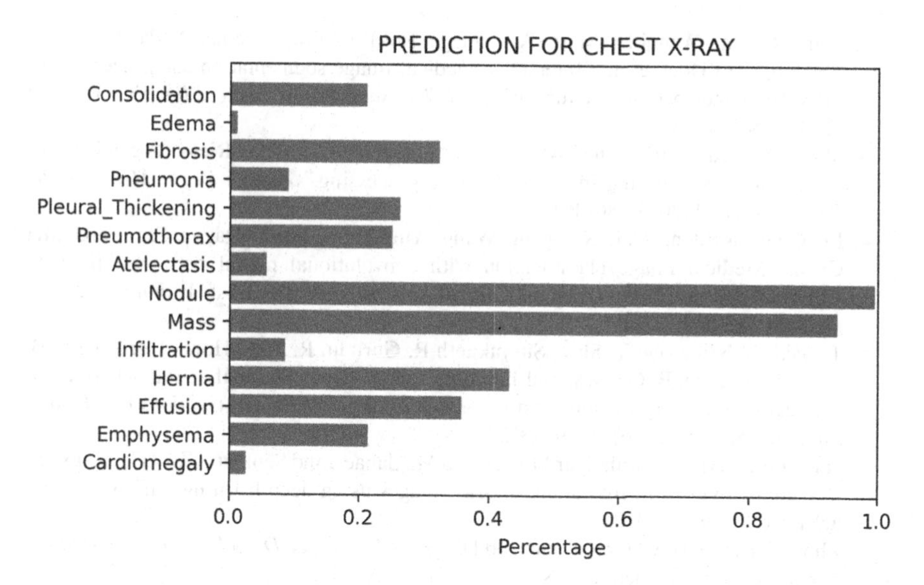

FIGURE 10.14 Output image.

Figure 10.14 indicates that the patient is diagnosed by nodule, nodules can be cancerous they are caused by scar tissue or infections. From the algorithm results we can conclude that the patient is diagnosed by nodules that shows more than 97% accuracy, followed by indication of mass.

10.6 CONCLUSION

With a large number of diagnostic examinations performed every year, chest X-rays are a significant and available clinical imaging instrument for the location of numerous diseases. Out of 1 billion X-rays taken every year, around 40 million X-rays are misdiagnosed leading to high fatality. Notwithstanding, their helpfulness can be restricted by difficulties in translation, which requires fast and intensive assessment of a 2D picture portraying complex, 3D organs and disease measures; so with the help of this chest X-ray algorithm, the beginning phase lung cancers or pneumothoraxes (collapsed lungs) can be diagnosed. Thus, this algorithm can be used as sophisticated algorithms for custom medical requirements and improve technicians' productivity, and it also acts as an assistance to the doctors; this algorithm can be replicated by both private and public healthcare organizations with less cost compared to current practicing methods, and it also reduces misinterpretations significantly.

REFERENCES

1. Nithyashri, J., et al. "Intelligent classification of liver images using back propagation neural network." *International Journal of Engineering Science* 9 (2019): 20208.

2. Wang, Guotai, Wenqi Li, Maria A. Zuluaga, Rosalind Pratt, Premal A. Patel, Michael Aertsen, Tom Doel, et al. "Interactive medical image segmentation using deep learning with image-specific fine tuning." *IEEE Transactions on Medical Imaging* 37, no. 7 (2018): 1562–1573.
3. Maier, Andreas, Christopher Syben, Tobias Lasser, and Christian Riess. "A gentle introduction to deep learning in medical image processing." *Zeitschrift für Medizinische Physik* 29, no. 2 (2019): 86–101.
4. Li, Qing, Weidong Cai, Xiaogang Wang, Yun Zhou, David Dagan Feng, and Mei Chen. "Medical image classification with convolutional neural network." In *2014 13th International Conference on Control Automation Robotics & Vision (ICARCV)*, pp. 844–848. IEEE, 2014.
5. Tajbakhsh, Nima, Jae Y. Shin, Suryakanth R. Gurudu, R. Todd Hurst, Christopher B. Kendall, Michael B. Gotway, and Jianming Liang. "Convolutional neural networks for medical image analysis: Full training or fine tuning?" *IEEE Transactions on Medical Imaging* 35, no. 5 (2016): 1299–1312.
6. Haghanifar, Arman, Mahdiyar Molahasani Majdabadi, and Seokbum Ko. "Covid-cxnet: Detecting covid-19 in frontal chest x-ray images using deep learning." arXiv preprint arXiv:2006.13807, 2020.
7. Zhou, S. Kevin, Hayit Greenspan, and Dinggang Shen, eds. *Deep Learning for Medical Image Analysis*. Academic Press, Cambridge, MA, 2017.
8. Gang, Peng, Wang Zhen, Wei Zeng, Yuri Gordienko, Yuriy Kochura, Oleg Alienin, Oleksandr Rokovyi, and Sergii Stirenko. "Dimensionality reduction in deep learning for chest X-ray analysis of lung cancer." In *2018 Tenth International Conference on Advanced Computational Intelligence (ICACI)*, pp. 878–883. IEEE, 2018.
9. Lo, Shih-Chung B., Heang-Ping Chan, Jyh-Shyan Lin, Huai Li, Matthew T. Freedman, and Seong K. Mun. "Artificial convolution neural network for medical image pattern recognition." *Neural Networks* 8, no. 7–8 (1995): 1201–1214.
10. Shin, Hoo-Chang, Holger R. Roth, Mingchen Gao, Le Lu, Ziyue Xu, Isabella Nogues, Jianhua Yao, Daniel Mollura, and Ronald M. Summers. "Deep convolutional neural networks for computer-aided detection: CNN architectures, dataset characteristics and transfer learning." *IEEE Transactions on Medical Imaging* 35, no. 5 (2016): 1285–1298.
11. Heidari, Morteza, Seyedehnafiseh Mirniaharikandehei, Abolfazl Zargari Khuzani, Gopichandh Danala, Yuchen Qiu, and Bin Zheng. "Improving the performance of CNN to predict the likelihood of COVID-19 using chest X-ray images with preprocessing algorithms." *International Journal of Medical Informatics* 144 (2020): 104284.

11 Recent Trends in Healthcare System for Diagnosis of Three Diseases Using Health Informatics

Shawni Dutta and Samir Kumar Bandyopadhyay
The Bhawanipur Education Society College

CONTENTS

11.1 INTRODUCTION

Data mining techniques are considered to be Artificial Intelligence (AI)-empowered tools that are capable of uncovering useful information from a database. These techniques ensure the construction of knowledge base to improve actions for the specified problem domain. In recent days, the uses of data mining or knowledge discovery processes are rapidly increasing in the healthcare industry. These techniques utilize health records systematically for revealing the unseen patterns from a massive amount of information database [1]. These techniques will benefit the healthcare industries for acquiring proficient treatment, reducing risks from patients' life, and sustaining a low amount of medical expense. Data mining techniques are useful in healthcare systems because they can detect diseases in advance as well as assist the physicians to yield safeguards for the diagnostic process.

Disease classification task is the process of analyzing enormous amount of patients' data and making ideas related to decision-making process. This gathered knowledge will predict the patients' tendency of being affected by a particular disease [2]. This study demonstrates the modeling of disease classification tool for three diseases, namely, Chronic Kidney disease (CKD), cardiovascular disease (CVD), and Liver disease. All these diseases are important to be considered in case of the healthcare industry.

The prevalence of public health due to CKD has dramatically increased with the aging population and their chronic diseases. CKD is often accelerated by the influence of several parameters such as age, diabetes, hypertension, obesity, and primary renal disorders [3].

CKD may be one of the accelerating causes of CVD. About 28.1% of total deaths and 14.1% of total deaths are due to CVD in India in 2016 as compared with 15.2% and 6.9%, respectively, in 1990 [4]. Acute kidney injury (AKI) is not an isolated event, but it affects other vital organs, such as heart, liver, and many more [5]. Liver diseases become one of the principal reasons of worldwide death and illness. In 2010, the major liver diseases such as acute hepatitis, cirrhosis, and liver cancer resulted in more than 2 million deaths, which accounted for around 4% of all deaths worldwide [6]. Due to the mortality rate caused by the aforementioned three diseases, it is necessary to concentrate on these considered diseases. Early-stage detection can reach higher efficiency in terms of securing patients' life.

11.1.1 Machine Learning and Healthcare

Machine learning (ML), a specialized field of AI, can be used in healthcare that analyzes numerous different data points, recommends outcomes, provides the well-timed risk scores, defines the resource allocation, and delivers many other applications. It enables opportunities for improving the clinical decision support. ML helps for developing, validating, and implementing ML models to increase the chances of eventually improving patient care [7]. The application of ML in the healthcare industry provides an insight in the future where the analysis and prediction of data can help healthcare workers to save countless patients' life. ML techniques are often related to data mining procedure. From the data mining point of view, ML techniques can simulate the target of data mining techniques by teaching the computer how to learn and comprehend. In brief, it can be said that data mining examines an enormous amount of data and sets a particular outcome based on those examined data. ML focuses on achieving that goal by using harvested data for modeling smart intelligent automated tool [8].

The modeling of all these mentioned diseases is perceived using various ML algorithms such as support vector machine (SVM) [9], decision tree (DT) [10], k-nearest neighbor (k-NN) [11], Naïve Bayes (NB) [12], multilayer perceptron (MLP) [13], Random Forest (RF) [14], gradient boosting (GB) [15], and AdaBoost [16] classifiers. A comparative analysis is done among all the aforementioned ML models in terms of their efficiency in the disease classification task. Different datasets are utilized for each of the considered diseases. A clean dataset is required for each case after applying preprocessing techniques. Apart from this step, it is also necessary to fine-tune the parameters of the classifier models so that the highest efficiency is obtained.

11.1.2 Objective of This Study

In brief, the outline of this study can be summarized as follows:

- Implement the disease classification model for three diseases, namely, CKD, heart disease, and liver disease.
- For each disease, datasets are collected, and preprocessing techniques are applied to acquire the transformed and cleaned dataset.
- Apply several ML algorithms such as SVM, DT, k-NN, NB, MLP, RF, GB, and AdaBoost classification techniques. All these models are implemented using the necessary adjustment of input parameters.
- Performances of these models are analyzed for each disease. The prediction efficiencies of these models are compared, and the best model for each disease classification task is identified.

11.2 LITERATURE SURVEY

This section provides a brief discussion on the existing researches carried out for CKD, CVD, and liver diseases. Researches have been conducted for the prediction of CKD at an early stage. Four ML methods, namely, RPART, LogR, SVM, and MLP, have been implemented and applied to CKD dataset. As a result, an AUC score of 0.995 was observed as the highest [17]. Another study implemented MLP, probabilistic neural networks (PNNs), SVM, and radial basis function (RBF) algorithms for determining the severity stage in CKD. The comparative analysis indicated the superiority of PNN algorithm in terms of better classification and prediction performance [18]. Another research employed and compared SVM and artificial neural networks

(ANNs) in order to predict the kidney disease. After comparing the performance of these two predictive models, it has been concluded that ANN outperforms SVM with an accuracy of 87% [19]. Researchers exemplified the use of ANN by implementing learning vector quantization (LVQ), two-layer feed-forward perceptron trained with backpropagation training algorithm, and RBF networks for the diagnosis of kidney stone disease [20]. Their experimental results concluded the superiority of MLP in the diagnostic process.

Liver disease classification task has been carried out by several studies. For implementing the automatic rule extraction from medical databases, differential evolution technique is presented in Ref. [21]. The automatic classification of items in medical databases is the basic objective of this study. The presented method has been applied the liver disorder dataset that reached an accuracy of 64.74%, a specificity of 45.08%, a sensitivity of 79.84%, and an ROC curve area of 62.46 [21]. Another research ensured that the application of fuzzy techniques such as fuzzy beans, Bocklisch membership function, and differential evolution algorithm was found in Ref. [22]. This research diagnosed liver disorders with an accuracy of 73.9% [22]. Elizondo et al. in Ref. [23] measured the complexity level of the classification datasets. By analyzing the blood tests on liver functionality, Bayesian classifier was implemented for the automatic diagnosis of liver diseases [24]. Liver disease severity is assessed by implementing SVM, Boosted C5.0, and NB classification algorithms [25]. Binish Khan et al. in Ref. [26] have analyzed the performance of classification algorithms such as RF, logistic regression, and separation algorithm to identify the best classifier for determining the liver diseases. The accuracy of RF method outperformed than those of other algorithms in case of the prediction of liver disease. Hoon Jin et al. in Ref. [27] implemented numerous classification techniques that assist the doctors to conclude the disease quickly and efficiently. For this purpose, different classification methods are applied. The experimental results showed that in terms of precision, NB provided the superior classification outcome, whereas logistic regression and RF provided the better results in terms of recall and sensitivity.

This section summarizes the research implications for the heart disease identification as carried out by Ref. [16,17]. By implementing data mining rules, data related to coronary illness is extracted from a large database. For this purpose, weighted association is implemented in Ref [28]. Heart disease is predicted using the rule mining algorithms on patients' dataset. The results achieved 61% training accuracy and 53% testing accuracy. In Ref. [29], historical medical data is utilized in order to predict CHD using the three supervised ML algorithms, namely, NB, SVM, and DT. Four hundred and sixty-two instances of South African Heart Disease dataset are used for the prediction purpose. All these algorithms were performed using ten-fold cross-validation method. It is concluded in Ref. [29] that the probabilistic NB classifier achieves better performance over other classifiers. In Ref. [30], patients with heart failure (HF) are classified into the categories, namely, HF with preserved ejection fraction (HFPEF) and HF with reduced ejection fraction (HFREF). Several classification methods such as classification trees, bagged classification trees, RFs, boosted classification trees, SVMs for prediction, logistic regression, regression trees, bagged regression trees, and boosted regression trees are utilized for detecting patients with the aforementioned three categories of heart failure. Conventional classification and regression trees for predicting and classifying HF subtypes have shown lesser performance than the tree-based methods. K. Gomathi et al. in Ref. [31] predicted the heart disease using NB classifier and J48 classifier. J48 classifier reaches an accuracy of 77%, whereas NB classifier reaches an accuracy of 79%. P. Sai Chandrasekhar Reddy et al. in Ref. [32] used ANN while predicting heart disease. The method is used to predict the condition of the patient by considering various parameters like heartbeat rate, blood pressure, cholesterol etc. J48, DT, k-NN, SMO, and NB were implemented by Boshra Brahmi et al. in Ref. [33] while evaluating the prediction and diagnosis of heart disease. J48 classifier and DT have shown the best result for the prediction of heart disease after comparing these classifiers with respect to the evaluation metrics. J48 classifier reached the best accuracy of 83.732%. A hybrid RF with linear model (HRFLM) is proposed in Ref. [34] for detecting patients with cardiac disease. This model uses all features without any restrictions of feature selection.

11.3 MATERIALS AND METHODS

Recently, AI has been immensely studied in the field of healthcare. In the field of AI, intelligent systems can be modeled so that they perceive the inputs from the underlying environments and take necessary actions for maximizing the success probability. The intelligent model gathers knowledge and utilizes that knowledge for supporting the decision-making process.

ML is considered to be the subfield of AI. Classification technique or predictive analysis can be achieved by ML algorithms. ML algorithms can be categorized into broad sections such as supervised ML, unsupervised ML, semi-supervised ML, and reinforcement learning.

Supervised ML algorithms receive the input examples and produce the output labels (also known as prediction value). The model involved to acquire such output value prediction is considered to be as a classifier. Based on the obtained knowledge during the training procedure, the classifier model can investigate unknown data samples for predictive analysis. In other words, classification is a supervised ML technique that analyzes a specified set of features and identifies data as belonging to a particular class.

Unsupervised ML algorithms follow the concept of "learning from observations." These techniques are well suited when the prediction label is absent. In such situations, the underlying model attempts to identify the hidden structures within the unlabeled data.

Semi-supervised ML algorithms can model both labeled and unlabeled data. A considerable improvement in terms of learning efficiency is observed when unmarked data is used in conjunction with the marked data. The process of creating the marked data requires the involvement of human expert with higher degree of difficulties and increased cost. Relatively, the cost decreases when it comes to the question of untagged data.

Reinforcement learning is one of the most exciting fields in ML. The main objective of this learning is to maximize the specified goal by considering the current state of the model and the external environment conditions. This technique has gained its popularity when the underlying situation is constantly evolving and/or there is an enormous amount of state space to be considered [35].

In recent days, AI is gaining a popularity in the healthcare field due to its power of automation. ML algorithms can eventually be employed in the healthcare industry in order to improve the diagnosis and prediction of diseases. Accurate predictions for patients' diseases are required by the doctors. However, along with the accurate prediction, timeliness is considered to be another important factor that influences the treatment decisions. With these provided conditions/factors, this study focuses on implementing the classifier models based on supervised ML techniques. All implemented models receive the training set to learn from the given database. Later, the learning outcome is utilized for the upcoming new data.

11.3.1 ML Algorithms Description

Intelligent automation systems can be developed by the ML algorithms. There are many existing ML techniques based on several logical entities for constructing the intelligent predictive systems. This study demonstrates the utility of ML algorithms for disease classification tool modeling. The current section elaborates various ML algorithms.

11.3.1.1 Support Vector Machine (SVM)

SVM has been successful in modeling the real-world applications. It can tackle the classification tasks by exhibiting the superior generalization performance. This method can also handle sparse data. It reduces the upper limit of the generalization error established on the structural risk minimization principle. SVM constructs a maximal separating hyperplane for mapping the input vector to a higher dimensional space. A kernel function is used to map the input data into the higher dimensional space. The kernel function should be chosen wisely based on the characteristics of the dataset. RBF, polynomial, and sigmoid are the most popularly used kernel functions. On each side of the hyperplane, two parallel hyperplanes are built that split up the data. This method maximizes the distance between the two parallel hyperplanes that are used to separate the hyperplane. In order to exhibit the reduced generalization error, the maximum distance between these parallel hyperplanes is taken into consideration.

It is to be noted that SVM acts as a generalization technique in order to distinguish between linearly separable data points and nonlinearly separable data points. For implementing the classification process, this classifier makes $N-1$ number of hyperplanes for N-dimensional data. SVM can learn with a small amount of data for creating a decision boundary [9].

11.3.1.2 K-Nearest Neighbor (k-NN)

k-NN, also known as lazy learners, follows a supervised learning approach. When a new sample appears, this technique picks the nearest k sample from the existing training data. The new sample point is classified according to the most similar class. In order to find out the closeness between two data points, several popular distance measurements such as Euclidean distance, Manhattan distance, and Minkowski distance may be used. Picking up the appropriate value of k is the foremost challenge of this technique. This algorithm goes through a trial process for identifying the value of k [11].

11.3.1.3 Multilayer Perceptron (MLP)

Neural networks are designed to model the function of human brain in order to perceive a complicated task. MLP classifier relies on the neural network architecture for performing the task of classification. It follows a feed-forward neural network that accepts input features and maps them into appropriate output sets. Any MLP classifier comprises the three layers, namely, the input layer, the hidden layer, and the output layer. The hidden layer exists between the input layer and the output layer. The number of hidden layers depends on the problem-specific domain. When only one hidden layer exists in the architecture, it is often referred as Vanilla neural network. Introduction of several layers is determined by the requirement to increase the complexity of decision regions. The connections between perceptron in an MLP are forward, and every perceptron is connected to all the perceptrons in the next layer except the output layer that directly gives the result. MLP is advantageous since it can distinguish data that are linearly nonseparable [13]. Linear as well as nonlinear activation functions can be used by MLP. Activation function is used as a step to transform the input into the output signal within a definite range [36]. Except the input layer neurons, nonlinear activation functions are applied. The use of multiple layers along with nonlinear activation functions makes MLP superior to the linear perceptron. MLP follows the supervised learning method that utilizes the backpropagation algorithm for training purposes.

11.3.1.4 Naïve Bayes (NB)

The NB classifier is a statistical model that follows Bayes theorem for carrying out the classification. This classifier is the simplest form of Bayesian network. By exemplifying the use of statistical method along with the supervised technique, this method acquires the classification result. By influencing the probabilities of the results, the prediction results are provided by this method. NB classifier performs significantly well in practice even if the inaccurate estimates are assumed. The accuracy of this classifier does not dependent on the feature relationships. Instead, it is dependent on the quantity of information loss of the class due to the independence assumption [12].

11.3.1.5 Decision Tree (DT)

DT analysis follows the divide-and-conquer approach for discovering features or patterns from large database. These features or patterns are important for discrimination and predictive modeling. A recursive partitioning method is applied on the feature space of training dataset. A set of decision rules are induced from this partitioning strategy that will obtain natural partitioning of dataset for providing the informative and hierarchical structure of the data. A scoring criterion is imposed for evaluating this partitioning strategy. The evaluation process depends on the two popular scoring methods, namely, information gain and Gini index. Information gain identifies the possible partition value that maximizes the information change. On the other hand, Gini index measures the class impurity from the feature space partitions.

For constructing DT model, a tree-like structure is exemplified. The leaf nodes present in the tree-like structure represent the outcome of the prediction, whereas the nonleaf nodes indicate the certain tests, and the test results are identified by branches of the test nodes. Starting from the top of this tree and traversing through it until a leaf node is touched is the procedure to retrieve the classification outcome [10].

11.3.1.6 Ensemble Techniques

These techniques ensure to assemble the prediction results of individually trained set of classifiers within a single classifier. This allows obtaining more accurate prediction results than the individual classification outcome. Bagging and boosting are the well-established ensemble techniques.

- Bagging techniques follow the bootstrap sampling methodology. In each of the iterations, different set of bootstrap samples are obtained from the original dataset randomly with replacement. In order words, during sampling, some instances can be repeated or missed out from the actual dataset. Individual classifiers are trained on these samples, and these classification results are combined by a means of voting. However, bagging technique can lead to the unstable learning method since a small change in the training data can affect the prediction outcome in a large amount.
- Boosting techniques follow the sequential ensemble strategy, which is capable of converting weak learners into strong learners. Boosting constructs new classifiers that are able to predict instances with superior efficiency for which the current ensemble's performance is poor [37].

11.3.1.6.1 AdaBoost Classifier

AdaBoost is known to be the first boosting technique presented by Freund and Schapire [16]. This method uses the distribution of one set of probabilities for training samples and adjusts this probability distribution for each sample during each of the iterations. Member classifiers are generated, and the error rate is calculated on the training sample by implementing a particular learning strategy. The role of changing weights is to set a greater weight for the incorrectly classified sample and reduce its weight if the sample is classified correctly. A strong classifier will be established finally by the way of the weighted voting of single classifiers.

It belongs to the category of interpolating classifiers. It fits the training data completely without an error. It also shows the property of self-averaging property. It obtains the low generalization error. This classifier is also regarded as a meta-estimator that fits a classifier on the original dataset, and then, supplementary copies of the classifiers are fitted after re-weighting the incorrectly classified instances in such a manner that the classifier is superior in tackling more challenging cases [16].

11.3.1.6.2 Gradient Boosting Classifier

GB [15] algorithm successively fits the new models for attaining the promising accuracy for response variable approximation. This ensures new base learners to be maximally correlated with the negative gradient of the loss function, accompanying with the whole ensemble. The high flexibility of this algorithm allows different loss functions to be applied on the related problem domains while involving data-specific base learners.

Depending on the type of the response variable, the loss function should be picked up. Gaussian L2 loss function, Laplace L1 loss function, Huber loss function (δ specified), and quantile loss function (α specified) are used for the continuous response variable. For categorical response variable, loss functions to be used are binomial loss function and AdaBoost loss function. Loss functions for survival models, loss functions counts data, and custom loss functions are used for other categories of response variables. Choosing the appropriate loss function highly depends on the type of problem, and it is of course a matter of trial and error. This makes GB to be highly flexible and customizable to be applied to any particular data-driven task [15].

11.3.1.6.3 Random Forest Classifier

RF classifier is another supervised ensemble ML technique. In 2001, Breiman presented RF to be built on DT base learners. It creates DTs on randomly selected data samples and then gets the prediction from each tree. It selects then the best solution by means of voting. These features are randomly selected in each decision split. The correlation between trees is reduced by randomly selecting the features, which improves the prediction power and results in higher efficiency [14].

11.3.2 Evaluating ML Model's Efficiency

It is necessary to justify the quality of the predictive results. Justifying the performance of model requires some evaluating metrics.

The ratio of true predictions to the sum of all the considered instances is measured by accuracy. It does not consider the wrongly predicted cases. So precision and recall are necessary for finding the performance of the method.

The proportion of correct positive results over the number of positive results predicted by the classifier model is defined as precision. The quantity of correct positive results divided by the quantity of total relevant instances is denoted as recall. F1-score or F-measure is calculated as the harmonic mean of precision and recall.

The absolute difference between the prediction and the actual observation of the test samples is assessed by mean-squared error (MSE).

Based on true positive (TP), true negative (TN), false positive (FP), and false negative (FN), the following calculations are made:

$$\text{Accuracy} = (\text{TP} + \text{TN})/(\text{TP} + \text{FP} + \text{TN} + \text{TP}) \quad (11.1)$$

$$\text{Recall} = \text{TP}/(\text{TP} + \text{FN}) \quad (11.2)$$

$$\text{Precision} = \text{TP}/(\text{TP} + \text{FP}) \quad (11.3)$$

$$\text{F1} - \text{Measure} \quad \text{or} \quad \text{F1} - \text{Score} = (2 * \text{Recall} * \text{Precision})/(\text{Recall} + \text{Precision}) \quad (11.4)$$

$$\text{MSE} = \left(\sum_{i=1}^{N} (X_i - X_i')^2 \Big/ \text{N} \right) \text{where } X_i \text{ is the actual value and} \quad (11.5)$$

$$X_i' \text{ is the predicted value}$$

Any classifier model should exhibit lower MSE value and higher values of accuracy, and its F1-score is regarded as the best one [38].

11.4 PROPOSED SYSTEM FOR DISEASE CLASSIFICATION TASK

For implementing the automated tool for CKD, CVD, and liver disease classification, several well-known ML models are employed. For each of the cases, all the models are tuned for attaining the highest efficiency and low error prediction results. This section provides a detailed description for each disease classification process. The understanding of dataset for each disease is specified in the following sections. The necessary parameters are also specified in these upcoming sections.

11.4.1 Disease Classification for Chronic Kidney Disease Prediction

CKD prerequisites are to be assessed at an early stage so that expensive end-stage treatments like dialysis and kidney transplantations can be avoided. In India, at least 70% people in rural areas experience CKD, which is often detected at later stages. Throughout the last stage, less than 10% of renal disease patients can pay for any kind of renal replacement therapy due to quiet significantly high cost of treatment [39]. CKD can be predicted at an early stage by ML methods. This research targets to recognize patients with CKD by analyzing interfering factors such as diabetic tendency, blood reports, and many more.

11.4.1.1 Dataset Used and Preprocessing

This research accumulates Chronic Kidney Disease Data Set from UCI machine learning repository [40]. This dataset contains 400 numbers of records, and each record size consists of 26 variables. These attributes are provided in Table 11.1. Whether the patient has CKD or not depends on attribute "classification". During classification process, this variable is designated as dependent or target variable. The rest of the variables are fed as an input to identify the target class. The scattering of the target variable in the dataset is portrayed in Figure 11.1.

The presence of missing values will modify the prediction efficiency. However, the occurrence of missing values can be overlooked or deleted when the quantity of missing values is not as much of in percentage. Unknown or missing values in the dataset in some cases may contribute to the disease. In our implementation, the missing values are replaced by substituting the mean or average value of considered attributes. The nominal variables are altered to numerical values of range 0–1. These steps will support to acquire the preprocessed dataset. This preprocessed dataset can be now fitted to any classifier model. It is distributed then with the ratio of 67:33 for

TABLE 11.1
Description of Chronic Kidney Disease Dataset

Attribute	Explanation	Type of Attribute	Values Present	Count of Missing Values
Age	Patients' age	Numerical	2–90	9
Bp	Blood pressure in mm/Hg	Numerical	50–100	12
Sg	Specific gravity	Nominal	1.005–1.025	47
Al	Albumin	Nominal	0–5	46
Su	Sugar	Nominal	0–5	49
Rbc	Red blood cells	Nominal	Normal, abnormal	152
Pc	Pus cell	Nominal	Normal, abnormal	65
Pcc	Pus cell clumps	Nominal	Present, not present	4
Ba	Bacteria	Nominal	Present, not present	4
Bgr	Blood glucose random in mgs/dl	Numerical	22.0–490.0	44
Bu	Blood urea in mgs/dl	Numerical	1.5–391.0	19
Sc	Serum creatinine in mgs/dl	Numerical	0.4–76.0	17
Sod	Sodium in mEq/L	Numerical	4.5–163.0	87
Pot	Potassium in mEq/L	Numerical	2.5–47.0	88
Hemo	Hemoglobin in gms	Numerical	3.1–17.8	52
Pcv	Packed cell volume	Numerical	9–54	70
Wc	White blood cell count	Numerical	3800–21,600	105
Rc	Red blood cell count	Numerical	2.3–8.0	130
Htn	Hypertension	Nominal	Yes, no	2
Dm	Diabetes mellitus	Nominal	Yes, no	2
Cad	Coronary artery disease	Nominal	Yes, no	2
Appet	Appetite	Nominal	Good, poor	1
Pe	Pedal edema	Nominal	Yes, no	1
Ane	Anemia	Nominal	Yes, no	1
Classification	Patients having CKD or not	Nominal	CKD, non-CKD	0

locating training and testing datasets, respectively. These datasets are used for the classification and prediction of the disease.

11.4.1.2 Detailed Description of Classifiers

This section clarifies the execution of employed classifier models. After certain trial-and-error process, the most appropriate hyperparameters are identified for each model. This section provides the detailed specification of these hyperparameters. Table 11.2 shows the classification details.

11.4.2 Disease Classification for Heart Disease

Heart, the important organ of human body, pumps signals throughout the body for functioning different parts of the body. The signal is created by a node, called sinus node. Heart is divided into two halves. One half is atria, and another part is ventricle.

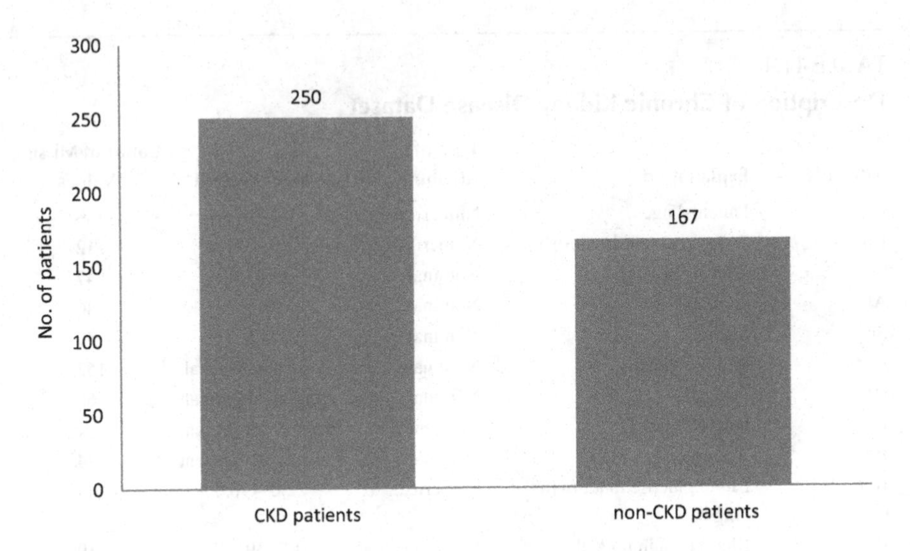

FIGURE 11.1 Patients' distribution based on the target variable on the dataset.

TABLE 11.2
Classifier Implementation Details for CKD Detection

Classifier Models	Parameters Used	Values
NB	Type of classifier	Gaussian NB
	Smoothing variable	1e−09
MLP	Activation function	ReLu
	Optimizer	Adam
	Number of hidden layers	4
	Size of hidden layers	64,32,16,8
	Learning rate	0.001
K-NN	K	10
	Distance metric	Minkowski
	Leaf size	7
SVM	Regularization parameter (C)	$C = 100$
	Kernel used	RBF
DT	Criterion	Gini
	Splitter	Best
	Number of leaves	169
	Depth of the tree	21
RF	Criterion	Gini
	Base estimator	DT

(Continued)

TABLE 11.2 (*Continued*)
Classifier Implementation Details for CKD Detection

Classifier Models	Parameters Used	Values
	Number of base estimators	500
GB	Criterion	Friedman MSE
	Loss	Deviance
	Learning rate	0.5
	Number of estimators	500
AdaBoost	Algorithm	SAMME.R
	Base estimator	DT
	Number of base estimators	500
	Learning rate	0.5

There are two atria (left and right) and two ventricles (left and right). The atria accumulate blood, and the ventricles push blood out of the heart. The right half of the heart blood sends oxygen to the lungs so that blood cells can get hold of more oxygen. Then, oxygen travels from the lungs into the left atrium and the left ventricle. It then pumps it into the organs and tissues of the body. This oxygen provides body with energy and is essential to keep body healthy [41]. Hence, detecting troubles in this important organ of human body is necessary in the medical field. Timely detection and screening play a leading role in the prevention of heart attacks.

11.4.2.1 Dataset Used

In this framework, heart disease dataset from UCI machine learning repository [42] is utilized for predicting cardiac trouble tendency of a patient. The dataset consists of numerous attributes or variables that include different conditions for detecting heart disease tendency. The understanding of the dataset is provided in Table 11.3. The dataset consists of an attribute "target" that identifies whether a patient suffers from CVD or not. However, the variable "target" is exploited as the output class of the prediction. The distribution of the output variable for the dataset is shown in Figure 11.2.

Preprocessing techniques such as missing value handling and scaling some attributes are performed for obtaining a balanced dataset. Performing these techniques will yield a transformed dataset that can be fitted to the classifier. This transformed dataset is separated into training dataset and testing dataset. The training dataset and the testing dataset are obtained by partitioning the transformed dataset with the ratio of 7:3. Next, all the classifier models are implemented using the necessary parameter tuning. Implementation details of the models are summarized in Table 11.4.

11.4.3 Disease Classification System for Liver Disease

Liver diseases are caused by factors like genetic predisposition, infections, and the environment. These diseases require diverse and targeted treatment options. The

TABLE 11.3
Understanding of Heart Disease Dataset

Attribute (Explanation)	Attribute Type	Values
Age	Numeric	29–77
Sex	Categorical	1—male, 0—female
Cp (chest pain)	Categorical	0: asymptomatic, 1: atypical angina, 2: nonanginal pain, 3: typical angina
(The patients' resting blood pressure in mm Hg on admission to the hospital): trestbps	Numeric	94–200
chol: The patients' cholesterol measurement in mg/dl	Numeric	126–564
fbs: The patients' fasting blood sugar	Binary	(> 120 mg/dl, 1 = true; 0 = false)
restecg: resting electrocardiographic results	Categorical	Zero value shows probable or definite left ventricular hypertrophy by Estes' criteria 1: normal Two having ST-T wave abnormality (T wave inversions and/or ST elevation or depression of > 0.05 mV)
thalach: The person's maximum heart rate achieved	Numeric	71–202
exang: Exercise-induced angina	Categorical	1 = yes; 0 = no
ST depression induced by exercise relative to rest: oldpeak	Numeric	0.0–6.2
The slope of the peak exercise ST segment	Categorical	0: down-sloping; 1: flat; 2: up-sloping
ca: The number of major vessels	Categorical	0–3
thal: thalassemia	Categorical	Zero: NULL One: fixed defect (no blood is flowing in some portions of the heart) Two: normal blood flow Three: reversible defect (an abnormal blood flow is observed)
target: Presence of heart disease	Binary	1 = no, 0= yes

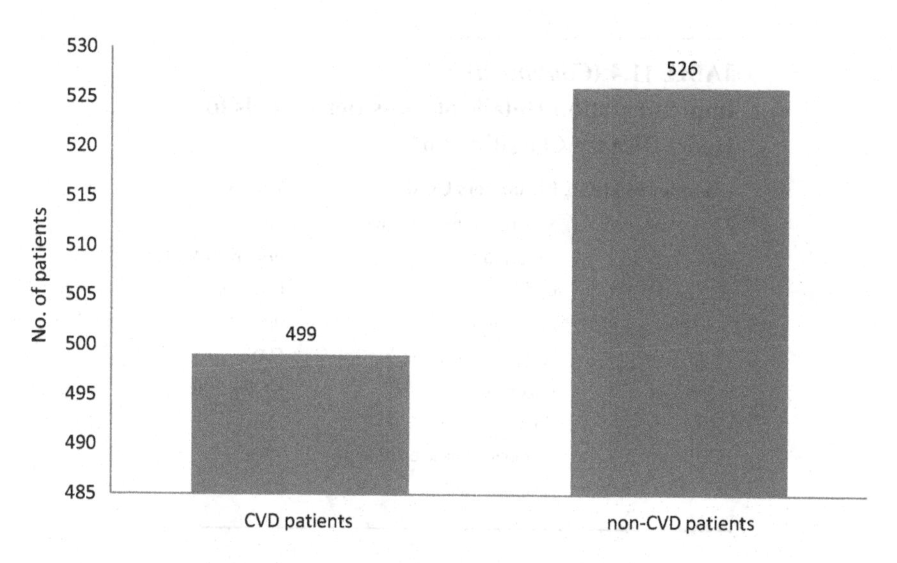

FIGURE 11.2 Distribution of heart disease patients.

TABLE 11.4
Implementation Details of Classifier Models for Heart Disease Classification

Classifier Models	Parameters Used	Values
NB	Type of classifier	Gaussian NB
	Smoothing variable	1e−09
MLP	Activation function	ReLu
	Optimizer	Adam
	Number of hidden layers	4
	Size of hidden layers	64,32,16,8
	Learning rate	0.001
K-NN	K	9
	Distance metric	Minkowski
	Leaf size	7
SVM	Regularization parameter (C)	$C=100$
	Kernel used	RBF
DT	Criterion	Gini
	Splitter	Best
	Number of leaves	49
	Depth of the tree	9
RF	Criterion	Gini
	Base estimator	DT

(Continued)

TABLE 11.4 (*Continued*)
Implementation Details of Classifier Models for Heart Disease Classification

Classifier Models	Parameters Used	Values
	Number of base estimators	500
GB	Criterion	Friedman MSE
	Loss	Deviance
	Learning rate	0.5
	Number of estimators	500
AdaBoost	Algorithm	SAMME.R
	Base estimator	DT
	Number of base estimators	500
	Learning rate	0.5

TABLE 11.5
Liver Disease Dataset Descriptions

Attribute Name	Values Present	Number of Missing Values
Age	4–90	0
Gender	"Female," "Male"	0
Total bilirubin	0.4–75.0	0
Direct bilirubin	0.1–19.7	0
Alkaline phosphatase	63–2110	0
Alanine aminotransferase	10–2000	0
Aspartate aminotransferase	10–4929	0
Total proteins	2.7–9.6	0
Albumin	0.9–5.5	0
Albumin/globulin ratio	0.3–2.8	4
Selector	1—liver disease, 2—nonliver patients	0

lifestyle factors such as alcohol consumptions and unnecessary use of drugs increase hepatic conditions worldwide [43]. These factors control decisions of therapy selection and timing of treatment, and guide the decision to be taken by doctor.

11.4.3.1 Dataset Used and Preprocessing

The dataset used for this purpose was acquired from the Machine Learning Repository University of California, Irvine [44]. The detailed description of the attributes of dataset along with the value range and missing values interpretation is given in Table 11.5. The distribution of patients having liver disease and without having liver disease is shown in Figure 11.3.

Operations like missing values replacement, irrelevant attribute elimination etc. are carried out as the cleaning steps after the collection of datasets. The dataset

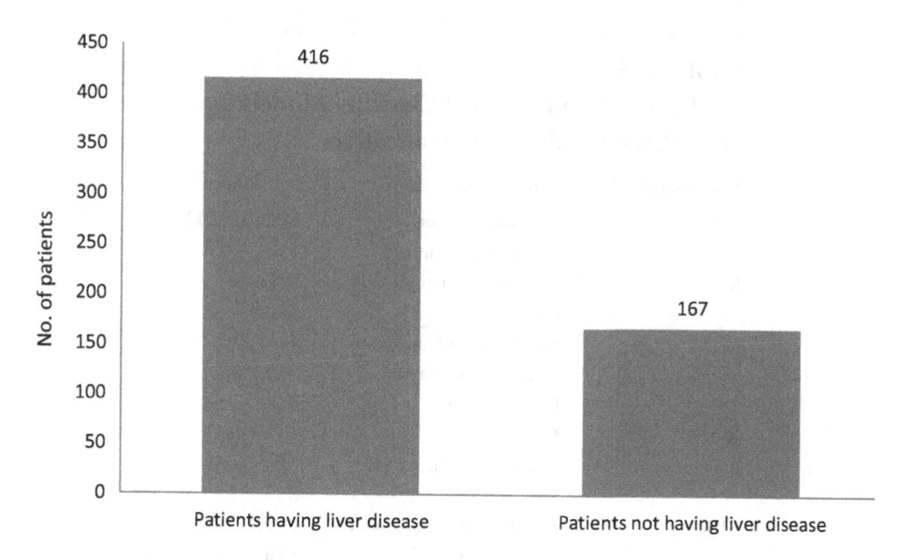

FIGURE 11.3 Distribution of output class for liver disease probability.

consists of 4 missing values for albumin/globulin ratio attribute, and those values are replaced by the mean value of the corresponding attribute. This step is followed by the attribute scaling process. Relevant numeric attributes are scaled into a range to be fitted into a classifier. Preprocessing techniques will assist in obtaining the transformed dataset. It is segregated into the training dataset and the testing dataset with a ratio of 7:3. Input to the classifier model is the training dataset, and the testing dataset is used for prediction. This fit and prediction process to the classifier is accompanied by adjusting the necessary parameters for these classifiers. The summary of these parameter adjustments is given in Table 11.6.

11.5 EXPERIMENTAL RESULTS

This section illustrates the utility of ML algorithms in the disease classification task. A comparative analysis is drawn among the existing well-known classification techniques. Considering three diseases, the application of numerous classification techniques such as k-NN, DT, NB, MLP, SVM, GB, AdaBoost, and RF is implemented.

11.5.1 Analysis for CKD Detection

For detecting CKD at an early stage, the classifier models are implemented, and their prediction efficiencies are compared based on accuracy, F1-score, and MSE. Analytical study, as mentioned in Table 11.7, shows that ensemble-based AdaBoost classifier model can detect CKD with the highest prediction accuracy and the lowest error rate.

11.5.2 Analysis for CVD Detection

Analyzing the input parameters for CVD, all the aforementioned classifier models are implemented. After comparing the predictive models, it can be realized that two

TABLE 11.6
Implementation Details of Classifier Models for Liver Patients' Disease Classification

Classifier Models	Parameters Used	Values
NB	Type of classifier	Multinomial NB
	Smoothing parameter	1.0
MLP	Activation function	ReLu
	Optimizer	Adam
	Number of hidden layers	4
	Size of hidden layers	64,32,16,8
	Learning rate	0.001
K-NN	K	15
	Distance metric	Minkowski
	Leaf size	30
SVM	Regularization parameter (C)	C=1
	Kernel used	RBF
DT	Criterion	Gini
	Splitter	Best
	Number of leaves	169
	Depth of the tree	21
RF	Criterion	Gini
	Base estimator	DT
	Number of base estimators	500
GB	Criterion	Friedman MSE
	Loss	Deviance
	Learning rate	1.0
	Number of estimators	500
AdaBoost	Algorithm	SAMME.R
	Base estimator	DT
	Number of base estimators	500
	Learning rate	1.0

TABLE 11.7
Prediction Efficiency Results for CKD Detection

Performance Measure Metrics	Accuracy (%)	F1-Score	MSE
K-NN	94.7	0.95	0.053
DT	94.7	0.95	0.053
NB	96.11	0.961	0.04
MLP classifier	97.73	0.98	0.023
SVM	96.21	0.962	0.0379
GB	97.73	0.977	0.0227
AdaBoost	99.01	0.99	0.01
RF	98.48	0.98	0.02

TABLE 11.8
Prediction Efficiency Results for CVD Detection

Performance Measure Metrics	Accuracy (%)	F1-Score	MSE
k-NN	89.09	0.89	0.109
DT	98.23	0.982	0.018
NB	81.12	0.81	0.189
MLP classifier	99.12	0.991	0.009
SVM	97.05	0.97	0.03
GB	99.41	0.994	0.006
AdaBoost	99.41	0.994	0.006
RF	99.12	0.991	0.009

TABLE 11.9
Prediction Efficiency Results for Liver Disease Detection

Performance Measure Metrics	Accuracy (%)	F1-Score	MSE
k-NN	75.65	0.76	0.24
DT	67.36	0.67	0.33
NB	74.09	0.74	0.26
MLP classifier	75.13	0.75	0.25
SVM	74.98	0.75	0.25
GB	70.98	0.71	0.29
AdaBoost	72.54	0.73	0.27
RF	72.84	0.73	0.27

ensemble-based models, namely, GB and AdaBoost, show the best results. Hence, for CVD disease classification task, these two models can be inferred as the top predictive models. Comparative study is summarized in Table 11.8.

11.5.3 Analysis for Liver Disease Detection

Based on the comparative analysis as given in Table 11.9, it can be easily observed that k-NN is the best technique for identifying the patients having liver disease. In conclusion, it can be inferred that distance-based k-NN classifier attains the highest efficiency and the lowest error rate with respect to other implemented models. This model requires the k value as 15 to reach this accuracy.

11.6 CONCLUSIONS

Healthcare plays an important key in observing the health-related aspects of the humans around the globe. An intense attention toward the aforementioned diseases and their preventive actions is desirable at most urgent to avoid the various deadly side effects. The presented analysis detects the feasibility of utilizing ML-based techniques for disease classification purposes. For CKD, CVD, and liver disease detection, a comprehensive diagnostic tool is favored that assists the experts in interpreting the early diagnosis of patients. Using ML methods, an efficient automated system is constructed for each of the considered diseases. Different well-known classifier models are applied for constructing these disease diagnostic tools. Finally after comparing their performance, the best classifier model is selected for each of the considered diseases. It is to be noted that all ML models will not give the same accuracy for all problem domains. For instance, in CKD detection, the ensemble-based AdaBoost classifier model reaches an accuracy of 99.01% and an MSE of 0.01. A distance-based k-NN classifier exhibits an accuracy of 75.65% and an MSE of 0.24 for liver disease detection. An accuracy of 99.41% is shown by both AdaBoost and GB for CVD detection. This clearly shows that a particular model will not provide the highest efficient results for all disease classification tasks. The comparative analysis results in identifying the best automated model for achieving the target. However, it is to be noted that incorporating more interfering attributes while constructing the model may help in achieving more promising results. This work can even be extended in the future by analyzing the effect of human habits that can lead to such life-threatening diseases.

REFERENCES

1. Hocine, M., N. Balakrishnan, T. Colton, B. Everitt, W. Piegorsch, F. Ruggeri, and J. Teugels. *Wiley Statsref: Statistics Reference Online*. John Wiley & Sons, Ltd., NewYork, 2014.
2. Wiebe, C.B., and E.E. Putnins. "The periodontal disease classification system of the American Academy of Periodontology-an update." *Journal-Canadian Dental Association* 66, no. 11 (2000): 594–599.
3. Anothaisintawee, T., S. Rattanasiri, A. Ingsathit, J. Attia, and A. Thakkinstian. "Prevalence of chronic kidney disease: A systematic review and meta-analysis." *Clinical Nephrology* 71, no. 3 (2009): 244.
4. Feigin, V.L., G.A. Roth, M. Naghavi, P. Parmar, R. Krishnamurthi, S. Chugh, G.A. Mensah et al. "Global burden of stroke and risk factors in 188 countries, during 1990–2013: a systematic analysis for the Global Burden of Disease Study 2013." *The Lancet Neurology* 15, no. 9 (2016): 913–924.
5. Yap, S.C., H. Thomas Lee, and D.S. Warner. "Acute kidney injury and extrarenal organ dysfunction: new concepts and experimental evidence." *The Journal of the American Society of Anesthesiologists* 116, no. 5 (2012): 1139–1148.
6. Byass, P. "The global burden of liver disease: A challenge for methods and for public health." *BMC Medicine* 12, no. 1 (2014): 1–3.
7. Chen, P.-H.C., Y. Liu, and L. Peng. "How to develop machine learning models for healthcare." *Nature Materials* 18, no. 5 (2019): 410.
8. Shailaja, K., B. Seetharamulu, and M. A. Jabbar. "Machine learning in healthcare: A review." *In 2018 Second International Conference on Electronics, Communication and Aerospace Technology (ICECA)*, pp. 910–914. IEEE, Coimbatore, India, 29–31 March, 2018.
9. Pisner, D.A., and D.M. Schnyer. "Support vector machine." In *Machine Learning*, pp. 101–121. Academic Press, Cambridge, MA, 2020.

10. Safavian, S.R., and D. Landgrebe. "A survey of decision tree classifier methodology." *IEEE Transactions on Systems, Man, and Cybernetics* 21, no. 3 (1991): 660–674.
11. Ali, N., D. Neagu, and P. Trundle. "Evaluation of k-nearest neighbour classifier performance for heterogeneous data sets." *SN Applied Sciences* 1, no. 12 (2019): 1559.
12. Rish, I. "An empirical study of the naive Bayes classifier." In *IJCAI 2001 Workshop on Empirical Methods in Artificial Intelligence*, vol. 3, no. 22, pp. 41–46, IBM, New York, 2001.
13. Murtagh, F. "Multilayer perceptrons for classification and regression." *Neurocomputing* 2, no. 5–6 (1991): 183–197.
14. Breiman, L. "Random forests." *Machine Learning* 45, no. 1 (2001): 5–32.
15. Friedman, J.H. "Stochastic gradient boosting." *Computational Statistics & Data Analysis* 38, no. 4 (2002): 367–378.
16. Schapire, R.E. "Explaining adaboost." In B. Schölkopf, V. Vovk, and Z. Luo (eds.) *Empirical Inference*, pp. 37–52. Springer, Berlin, 2013.
17. Aljaaf, A.J., D. Al-Jumeily, H.M. Haglan, M. Alloghani, T. Baker, A.J. Hussain, and J. Mustafina. "Early prediction of chronic kidney disease using machine learning supported by predictive analytics." In *2018 IEEE Congress on Evolutionary Computation (CEC)*, pp. 1–9. IEEE, Rio de Janeiro, Brazil, 2018.
18. Rady, E.-H.A., and A.S. Anwar. "Prediction of kidney disease stages using data mining algorithms." *Informatics in Medicine Unlocked* 15 (2019): 100178.
19. Vijayarani, S., S. Dhayanand, and M. Phil. "Kidney disease prediction using SVM and ANN algorithms." *International Journal of Computing and Business Research (IJCBR)* 6, no. 2 (2015): 1–12.
20. Kumar, K., and B. Abhishek. *Artificial Neural Networks for Diagnosis of Kidney Stones Disease*. GRIN Verlag, Munich, 2012.
21. De Falco, I. "Differential Evolution for automatic rule extraction from medical databases." *Applied Soft Computing* 13, no. 2 (2013): 1265–1283.
22. Luukka, P. "Fuzzy beans in classification." *Expert Systems with Applications* 38, no. 5 (2011): 4798–4801.
23. Elizondo, D.A., R. Birkenhead, M. Gamez, N. Garcia, and E. Alfaro. "Linear separability and classification complexity." *Expert Systems with Applications* 39, no. 9 (2012): 7796–7807.
24. Ramana, B.V., M. Surendra Prasad Babu, and N. B. Venkateswarlu. "A critical study of selected classification algorithms for liver disease diagnosis." *International Journal of Database Management Systems* 3, no. 2 (2011): 101–114.
25. El-Shafeiy, E.A., A.I. El-Desouky, and S.M. Elghamrawy. "Prediction of liver diseases based on machine learning technique for big data." In *International Conference on Advanced Machine Learning Technologies and Applications*, pp. 362–374. Springer, Cham, 2018.
26. Khan, B., P.K. Shukla, M.K. Ahirwar, and M. Mishra. "Strategic analysis in prediction of liver disease using different classification algorithms." In G. Rani, P. K. Tiwari (eds.) *Handbook of Research on Disease Prediction Through Data Analytics and Machine Learning*, pp. 437–449. IGI Global, Hershey, PA, 2019.
27. Jin, H., S. Kim, and J. Kim. "Decision factors on effective liver patient data prediction." *International Journal of Bio-science and Bio-Technology* 6, no. 4 (2014): 167–178.
28. Chauhan, A., A. Jain, P. Sharma, and V. Deep. "Heart disease prediction using evolutionary rule learning." In *2018 4th International Conference on Computational Intelligence & Communication Technology (CICT)*, pp. 1–4. IEEE, Ghaziabad, India, 2018.
29. Gonsalves, A.H., F. Thabtah, R.M.A. Mohammad, and G. Singh. "Prediction of coronary heart disease using machine learning: An experimental analysis." In *Proceedings of the 2019 3rd International Conference on Deep Learning Technologies*, pp. 51–56, Xiamen, China, 2019.

30. Austin, P.C., J.V. Tu, J.E. Ho, D. Levy, and D.S. Lee. "Using methods from the data-mining and machine-learning literature for disease classification and prediction: A case study examining classification of heart failure subtypes." *Journal of Clinical Epidemiology* 66, no. 4 (2013): 398–407.
31. Kirmani, M.M. "Cardiovascular disease prediction using data mining techniques: A review." *Oriental Journal of Computer Science & Technology* 10, no. 2 (2017): 520–528.
32. Reddy, P.S.C., P. Palagi, and S. Jaya. "Heart disease prediction using ANN algorithm in data mining." *International Journal of Computer Science and Mobile Computing* 6, no. 4 (2017): 168–172.
33. Bahrami, B., and M.H. Shirvani. "Prediction and diagnosis of heart disease by data mining techniques." *Journal of Multidisciplinary Engineering Science and Technology (JMEST)* 2, no. 2 (2015): 164–168.
34. Mohan, S., C. Thirumalai, and G. Srivastava. "Effective heart disease prediction using hybrid machine learning techniques." *IEEE Access* 7 (2019): 81542–81554.
35. Alpaydin, E. *Introduction to Machine Learning*. MIT press, Cambridge, MA, 2020.
36. Zhang, H., T.-W. Weng, P.-Y. Chen, C.-J. Hsieh, and L. Daniel. "Efficient neural network robustness certification with general activation functions." In *Advances in Neural Information Processing* Systems, pp. 4939–4948, 32nd Conference on Neural Information Processing Systems (NeurIPS 2018), Montréal, Canada, 2018.
37. Zhang, C., and Y. Ma, eds. *Ensemble Machine Learning: Methods and Applications*. Springer Science & Business Media, Berlin, 2012.
38. Handelman, G.S., H.K. Kok, R.V. Chandra, A.H. Razavi, S. Huang, M. Brooks, M.J. Lee, and H. Asadi. "Peering into the black box of artificial intelligence: Evaluation metrics of machine learning methods." *American Journal of Roentgenology* 212, no. 1 (2019): 38–43.
39. Anupama, Y. J., and G. Uma. "Prevalence of chronic kidney disease among adults in a rural community in South India: Results from the kidney disease screening (KIDS) project." *Indian Journal of Nephrology* 24, no. 4 (2014): 214.
40. Dua, D. and Graff, C. (2019). "UCI repository of machine learning databases" [http://archive.ics.uci.edu/ml]. Department of Information and Computer Science, University of California, Irvine, CA, 1998.
41. Wessels, A., M.W.M. Markman, J.L.M. Vermeulen, R.H. Anderson, A.F.M. Moorman, and W.H. Lamers. "The development of the atrioventricular junction in the human heart." *Circulation Research* 78, no. 1 (1996): 110–117.
42. C. Blake, E. Keogh, and C.J. Merz, "UCI repository of machine learning databases" [http://www.ics.uci.edu/~mlearn/MLRepository.html], Department of Information and Computer Science, University of California, Irvine, CA, 1998.
43. Rinella, M.E. "Nonalcoholic fatty liver disease: A systematic review." *JAMA* 313, no. 22 (2015): 2263–2273.
44. M. Kahn, St. Louis. "UCI repository of machine learning databases" [http://archive.ics.uci.edu/ml]. Department of Information and Computer Science, University of California, Irvine, CA, 1998.

12 Nursing Care System Based on Internet of Medical Things (IoMT) through Integrating Non-Invasive Blood Sugar (BS) and Blood Pressure (BP) Combined Monitoring

Patrali Pradhan
Haldia Institute of Technology

Subham Ghosh and Biswarup Neogi
JIS College of Engineering

CONTENTS

12.1 INTRODUCTION

Abnormal blood sugar (BS) level or diabetes is a major health issue in the society worldwide because billions of people are suffering from it [1,2]. As it is an incurable disease, life can be prolonged by a proper monitoring and therapy for maintaining a normal glucose level. Typical procedures include the blood sample collection and blood analysis from time to time. For those persons suffering from diabetes mellitus, blood has been often withdrawn many times a day [3]. For the most of diabetic patients in the world, it is essential to externally apply insulin in order to keep the blood glucose level in a balanced way. Conventional treatment includes the form of injection of insulin into subcutaneous tissues of the arms, legs, abdomen, or buttocks. Except this painful treatment, if patients were alert about their daily food habits and other habits with continuous noninvasive monitoring by the proper diet/nutrient chart, then mass people will be facilitative [4–8]. All the conventional ways of measuring and maintaining the acceptance level of glucose in blood are very painful, and all are invasive methods. Imbalance level of BS or glucose creates the metabolism disorder, and several other organs are affected by an imbalance in blood pressure (BP) due to abnormal BS. Also, an invasive method is outmoded to measure the glucose level in the era of smart society. In this chapter, we explain how BS and BP can be controlled in a smarter way with some noninvasive methods as the measurement mode.

Several survey data show that nonfunctional adrenal incidentaloma (NFAI) individuals may have a problem of undetectable autonomous cortisol secretion and exhibit a higher incidence of impaired glucose tolerance and insulin resistance (IR) than controls [9–11]. Some recent study observed that the analysis of glucose monitoring indicated glycometabolism in patients with adrenal diseases compared with that of healthy controls with general blood glucose, within-day and day-to-day glucose variability, and glucose-target-rate levels [12–14]. A real-time monitoring of glucose level makes blood glucose levels in healthy controls which were observed earlier at postprandial periods in the Cushing syndrome and primary aldosterone's groups; at nocturnal, fasting, and postprandial periods in the pheochromocytoma group. Significant IR and abnormal β-cell function were observed in the Cushing syndrome group compared with those in healthy controls [15–17].

In addition, it has been shown in a paper that a man aged 30 years presented with a major head injury, his brain CT scan exhibited joint frontal contusion and subarachnoid hemorrhage, and his BP was 100/60 mmHg at a temperature of 100°F and BS level was 70 mg/dL with head elevation at 45° [14–18]. Moreover, in 2002, a patented device was introduced by an inventor for measuring a user's BS level. In particular, the method and device are noninvasive and are capable of measuring the user's BS level continuously. Furthermore, the measurement of BS level traditionally involves both capillary blood and venous blood. The present inventors have recognized that the source of BS that will adversely affect a person's organs and cause organ damage and tissue perfusion is the blood at the capillary end of arterial blood vessels. That is, the region before glucose in the blood is released to the tissue [19–22]. Some other studies revealed that bioimpedance spectroscopy, microwave/RF sensing [23], fluorescence equipment, mid-infrared spectroscopy, near-infrared spectroscopy, optical coherence tomography, optical polarimetry, Raman spectroscopy, reverse iontophoresis, and ultrasound technology are useful in measuring BS levels. But remarkably, none of these techniques were commercially available and had a clinically consistent device; therefore, much work is needed to be done [24].

This chapter introduces the conceptual design with an objective of the real-time glucose monitoring (cloud-based) system, which includes miniaturization device as a wearable device for the patient's well-being in mobility and accuracy modes. This intelligent system analyzes data for providing the good and healthy diet chart to patients in order to sustain their life smartly with a better understanding of the complex system. Another focus of this chapter is continuous observation and care by connecting physicians to the patients for the clinical advice at anytime from anywhere.

12.2 REVIEW OF EXISTING LITERATURE

Diabetes is often called a "silent killer" as no early-stage symptoms are visible to the subjects. Researcher at IIS, Bangalore [25], has invented the two new methods used to diagnose diabetes. One method uses a device called "field-effect transistor," which is based on electrical signals, and the other method uses "Bragg grating" [26], which is a device used for a wide range of applications like measuring pulse in humans. The Bragg grating [26] is based on graphene and water, which creates APBA (aminophenylboronic acid) molecules. Thus, when the device is in contact with blood, the glucose molecules in the blood get attached to the APBA molecules, which changes the reflected wavelength in the grating procedure. This change in reflected wavelength is measured, which determines the exact concentration of glucose in the blood.

India's first diabetes app Diabeto [27], launched on World Diabetes Day in 2015, is the first application developed that helps the patient to track their blood glucose data, upload it, and store securely onto the cloud. Diabeto is a startup project, which is now a full-mode company. This application allows the patients to choose a doctor of their choice and schedule a teleconsultation from a pool of diabetologists available on the app. Diabeto is a cost-effective application as it is free to download and there is no charge for the cloud. The only cost one would need to pay is for consultation [7]. Effective diabetes management can reduce the risk of the long-term complications associated with the disease, which include heart disease, blindness, stroke, kidney disease etc. [25].

12.2.1 The Conventional Way of Glucose Monitoring

The conventional way of measuring blood glucose level is to prick a finger using lancet to take a small drop of blood. This is a painful process for the patients. There are over 65 blood glucose monitoring techniques [28–30]. In conventional continuous glucose monitoring technique, a disposable glucose sensor is placed just under the skin, and the sensor is linked to a nonimplanted transmitter that communicates with a radio receiver. A reader/receiver records the values and displays them in it.

12.2.2 Minimally Invasive Glucose Monitoring

In minimally invasive glucose monitoring technologies, there is no need to hurt on the skin barrier and puncture any blood vessels. Such systems lack the accuracy. In this technique, the patient still experiences discomfort and pain.

12.2.3 Noninvasive Way of Glucose Monitoring

In noninvasive method, blood glucose is measured without penetrating the skin wall; rather, some painless methods are used to collect a continuous measurement value. Three general categories of techniques for measuring glucose levels are as follows:

- Optical techniques
- Transdermal techniques
- Electrochemical techniques

Photoacoustic method [31] is one of the optical techniques. In this method, laser pulse is applied for a certain period to excite glucose in the blood. Light creates a hit with the volumetric expansion, and in the absence of light, it returns to the normal state. Continuous periodic light energy application creates stress and strain in the medium, thus generating pressure wave. This wave travels outward and is collected by transducer. The amplitude of the pressure wave determines the level of glucose. Digital storage oscilloscope collects the PA waveform and transforms it into a digital signal in order to send to the output device.

12.3 IMPORTANCE OF CONTINUOUS MONITORING BLOOD SUGAR (BS) AND BLOOD PRESSURE (BP)

Diabetes is a common noncontagious disease in the present-day period. The insulin disorder affects kidney and results in heart diseases. The flowchart representation shown in Figure 12.1 lucidly determines the entire presence and function of blood glucose in the human body in Figure 12.1 [32]. From this diagram, it is observed that how blood glucose level is fluctuated. There are various medical procedures to test the blood in daily routine. In every procedure, the collection of actual blood sample from the patients is made, followed by blood analysis. The total PA method is depicted in Figure 12.2. In this method, blood glucose is continuously measured, and the data are collected using the digital device. If any patient is aware of their blood glucose level with zero pain and using some smart digital devices, then that patient can be benefited to keep themselves fit and healthy instead of BS [33]. Continuously data are uploaded to cloud-based environment for further analysis. Computational

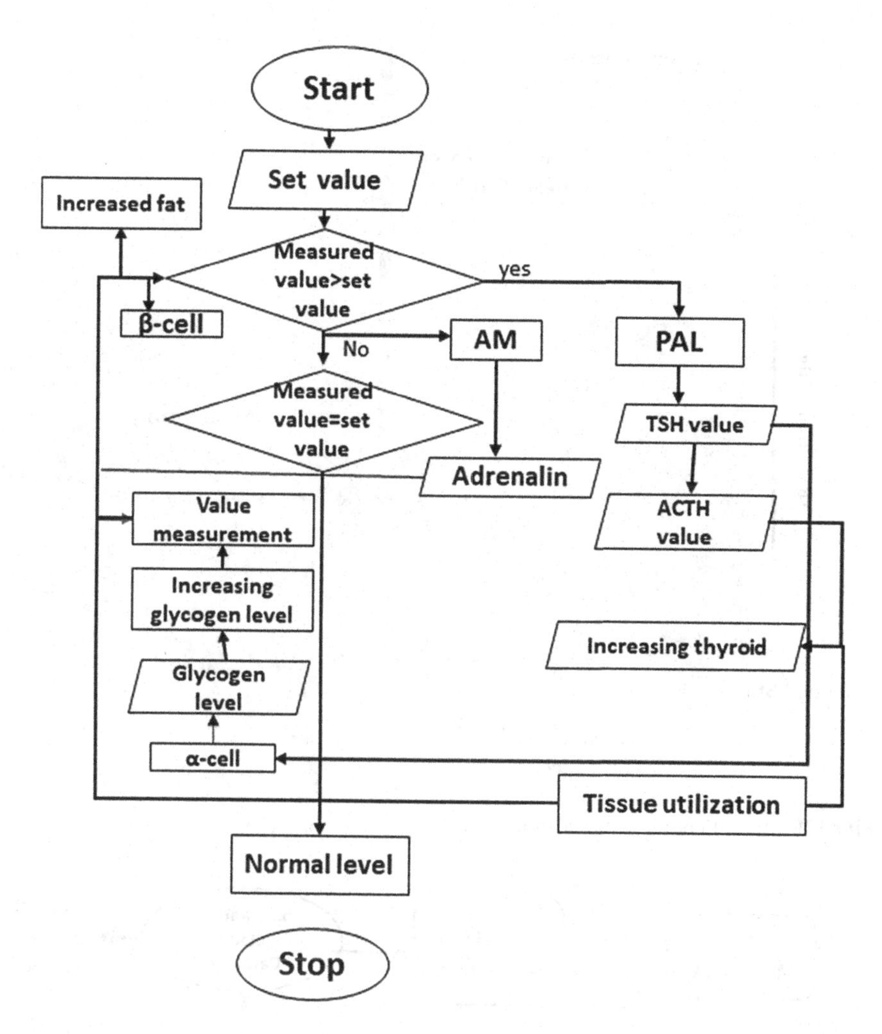

FIGURE 12.1 Functions of all the organs to affect glucose level [32].

cloud-based module is attached to the PA module (Figure 12.3) to make this process a smart process of measuring glucose levels in the human blood. Thus, BS detection is essential to be done at frequent intervals to know if, when, and how much insulin is needed to control the glucose level in the blood, and know what food habits need to be changed. In the early research work done by P. Pradhan et al. [32,33], a preliminary simulation has been done, and it is necessary to detect how the glucose level can be controlled by stimulating pancreas.

Diabetic patient's life can be prolonged by a proper therapy and a perfect time consultation. The proposed approach is associated with therapy, daily alert, and consultation of the qualified physician in a nominal cost. As smartphones, wearable devices, and other mobile health devices continue to be adopted throughout the

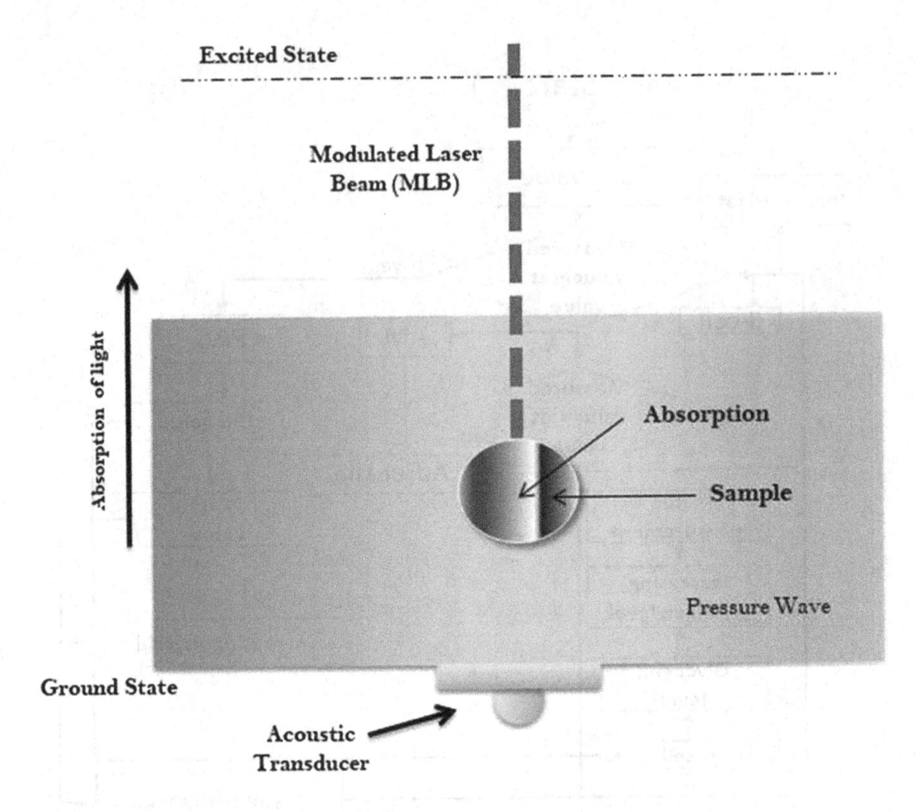

FIGURE 12.2 Photoacoustic method.

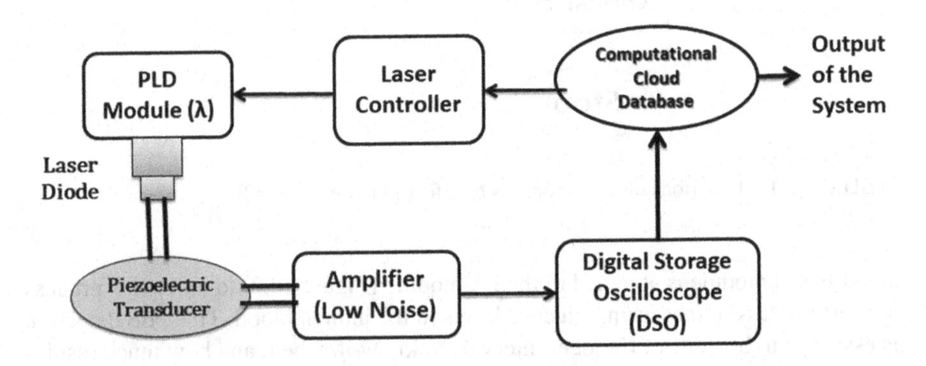

FIGURE 12.3 New approach of cloud-based computing module with the PA method.

healthcare industry, the need for wearable devices and smart sensors is driving the adoption of IoT in healthcare. These wearable devices and sensors will enable patients to get any kind of push notification to monitor and be alert about the day-to-day habits. Smart sensor device using PA noninvasive method will measure the glucose level on a real-time basis and send it to the cloud-based database. Neuro-fuzzy system will analyze that data to provide the actual level and guide a patient with a proper diet.

12.4 MEASUREMENT OF BLOOD PRESSURE (BP) AND BLOOD SUGAR (BS)

12.4.1 Mean of the Blood Pressure Measurement (MBP)

The pulse pressure is the difference between the measured systolic and diastolic pressures (Figures 12.4–12.7)

$$P_{\text{pulse}} = P_{\text{systolic pressure}} - P_{\text{diastolic pressure}}$$

Some measurements of MATLAB plot provide the information plotted in Figures 12.4 through 12.7.

12.5 METHODOLOGY DETAILING STEPWISE ACTIVITIES AND SUBACTIVITIES

Here, an approach to produce a wearable intelligent and smart device is explained. Device consists of cloud storage to store the real-time biometric data and an artificial intelligent diagnostic system to analyze BS and BP of a patient using PA spectroscopy

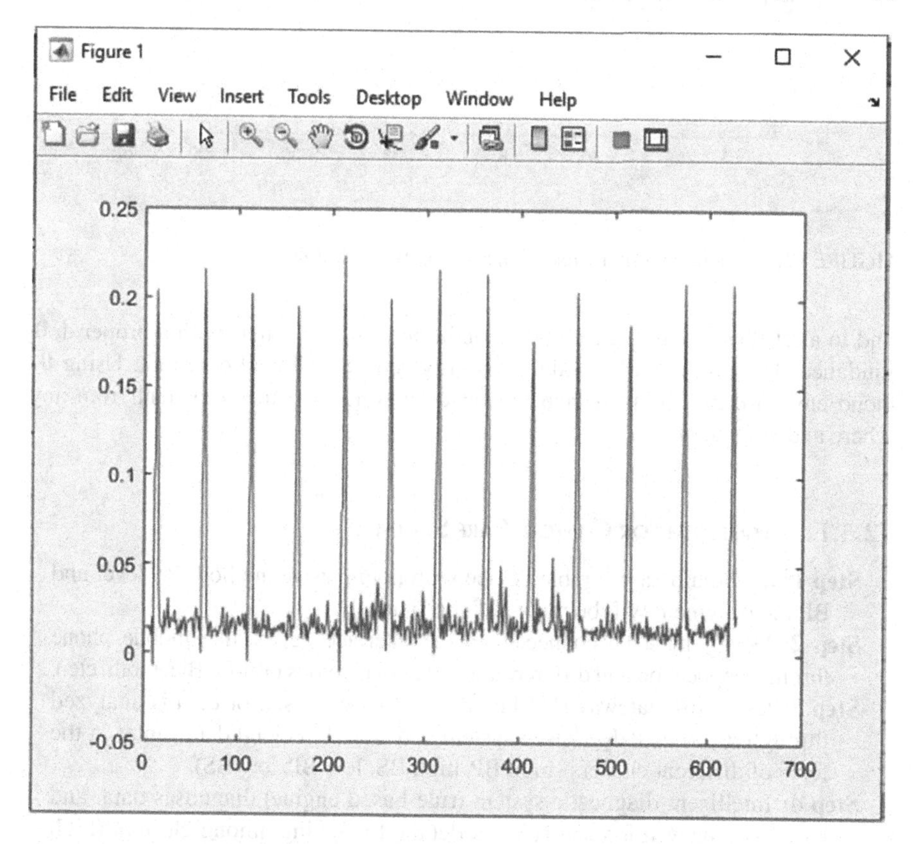

FIGURE 12.4 Plotted human pulse of measuring BP without noise.

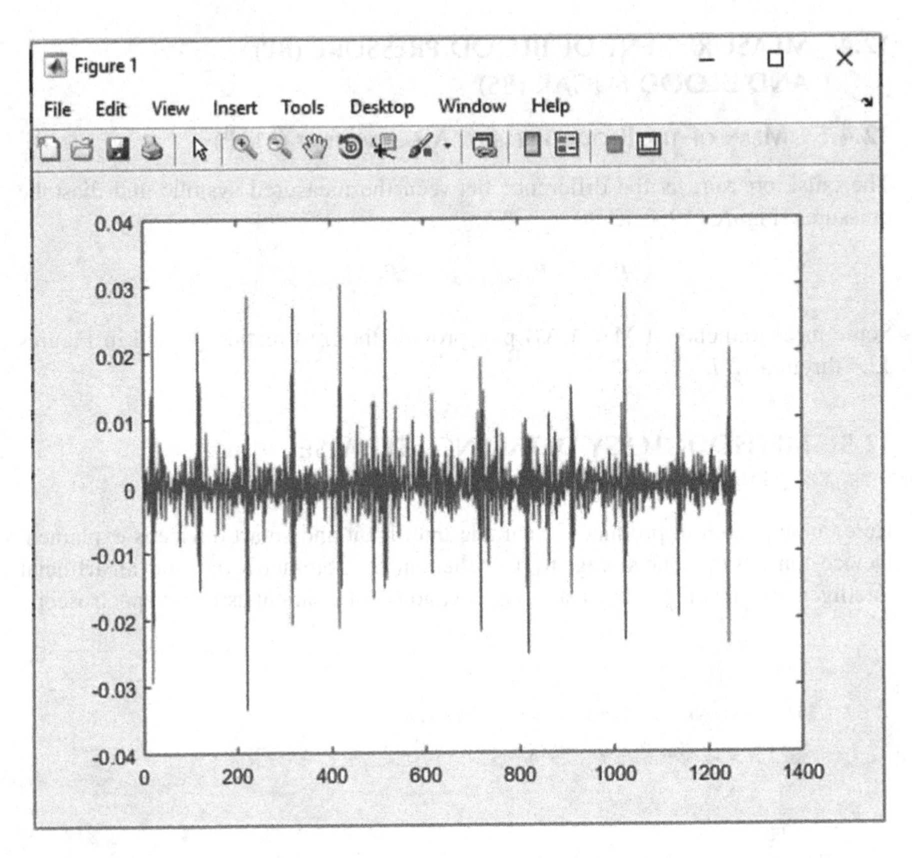

FIGURE 12.5 Plotted human pulse of measuring BP with noise.

and to alert them about their clinical condition or to live smart with a proper daily guidance. The proper daily guidance is provided as a clinical care unit. Using the cloud environment, the physician will also be connected to the patient from anywhere and at anytime.

12.5.1 Algorithm for Clinical Care System

Step 1: It would be a wearable device with noninvasive method. BS level and BP measurement will be recorded continuously.

Step 2: Device must be connected to the interface device like mobile phone through application and different connectivity methods (Wi-Fi, Bluetooth, etc.).

Step 3: Using IoT gateway (HTTP, MQTP [34] etc.), sensor data is analyzed through the knowledge-based system and stored in cloud data center in the form of different clusters (high BP, high BS, low BP, low BS).

Step 4: Intelligent diagnostic system (rule-based engine) diagnoses data, and based on fuzzy inference rules, a detailed mapping among clusters (high

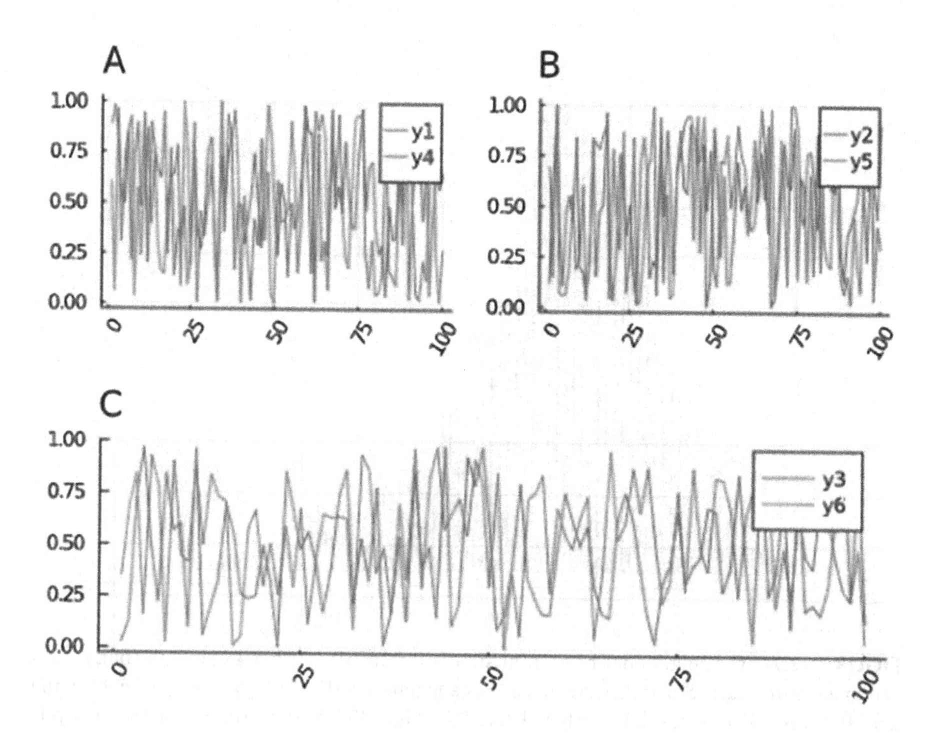

FIGURE 12.6 Computational simulation without noise in BP and BS measurements using Julia Scientific Language Package integrated with Jupyter interface; (a) plotted BP for time in *Y*-axis against pulse in *X*-axis at high frequency where the systolic pressure is in focus; (b) plotted BP for time in *Y*-axis against pulse in *X*-axis at high frequency where the diastolic pressure is in focus; (c) plotted BS for time in *Y*-axis against pulse in *X*-axis at high frequency where noise is eliminated at the maximum range.

BP-high BS, high BP-low BS, low BP-high BS, low BP-low BS) will be performed. As BP and BS are very much related, it claims a proper analysis; otherwise, only monitoring of glucose level would not be effective to reduce risks happening from high BS.

Step 5: Decision support system then takes a decision after the entire data processing by producing an alert in day-to-day food habits or activities.

Step 6: Alert will be shown to interface device as patient can prevent the immediate risks easily.

Step 7: Connected physicians also get an alert about risks of the undertaken patient. So, the physicians can also start an immediate recovery process.

12.5.2 Flowchart to Show Relationship between BS and BP

Different log records on BS and BP have been published, which show the direct or indirect relation between BS and BP. It shows that continuous imbalanced BS can damage kidney's capillaries that are the main components for filtering. Fructose

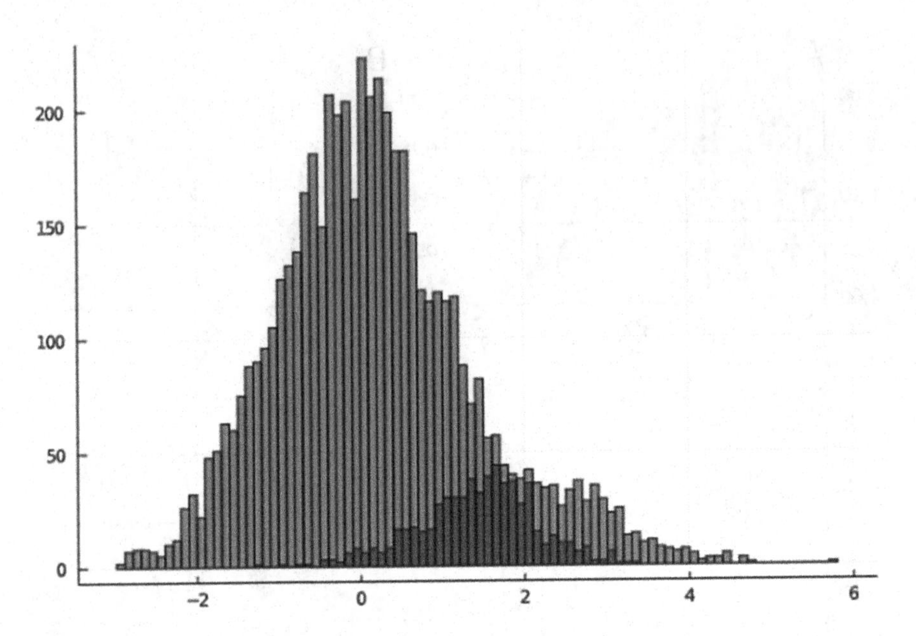

FIGURE 12.7 Computational histogram simulation in BP (off black) and BS (blue) measurements using Julia Scientific Language Package integrated with Jupyter interface, showing high BP pulse (*Y*-axis) result directly bolstered the high BS level according to complete cycle gapes (*X*-axis).

thickens the wall of capillaries. BP is gradually increased to maintain the normal blood flow through capillaries [35]. For this reason, less blood is flown through the muscles, thus decreasing the size of the muscle. Similarly, the sugar level is decreased throughout the muscle cells, thus resulting in an increase in the free sugar in blood vessels. The level of free sugar damages glomeruli, and altered blood is flown through the pancreas. How alpha and beta cells are affected is shown in Figure 12.1. Based on the observed data [36], it is noticed that alpha and beta cells of pancreas play an important role in insulin imbalance. Insulin level is decreased and BS is in abnormal level. Abnormal BS level creates an abnormal BP level. This is true when fructose of BS is broken and indirectly causes high BP. So, it is proved that BS and BP are related to other.

As BP and BS are related, each or both cause many other chronic diseases (Figure 12.10). To reduce the risk of other chronic disease, we should have a proper and transparent knowledge. Our system is for diagnosis based on BP and BS monitoring. High BS for more than three months causes diabetes, and one of the symptoms is high BP. Figure 12.8 shows that BS contains glucose and fructose. Fructose is broken down by the liver into uric acid, low-density cholesterol, fat globules, and triglycerides, thus causing fatty liver and increasing BP that results in kidney disease. So, high BP and high BS can both be affected by the excessive consumption of sugar (Figure 12.9).

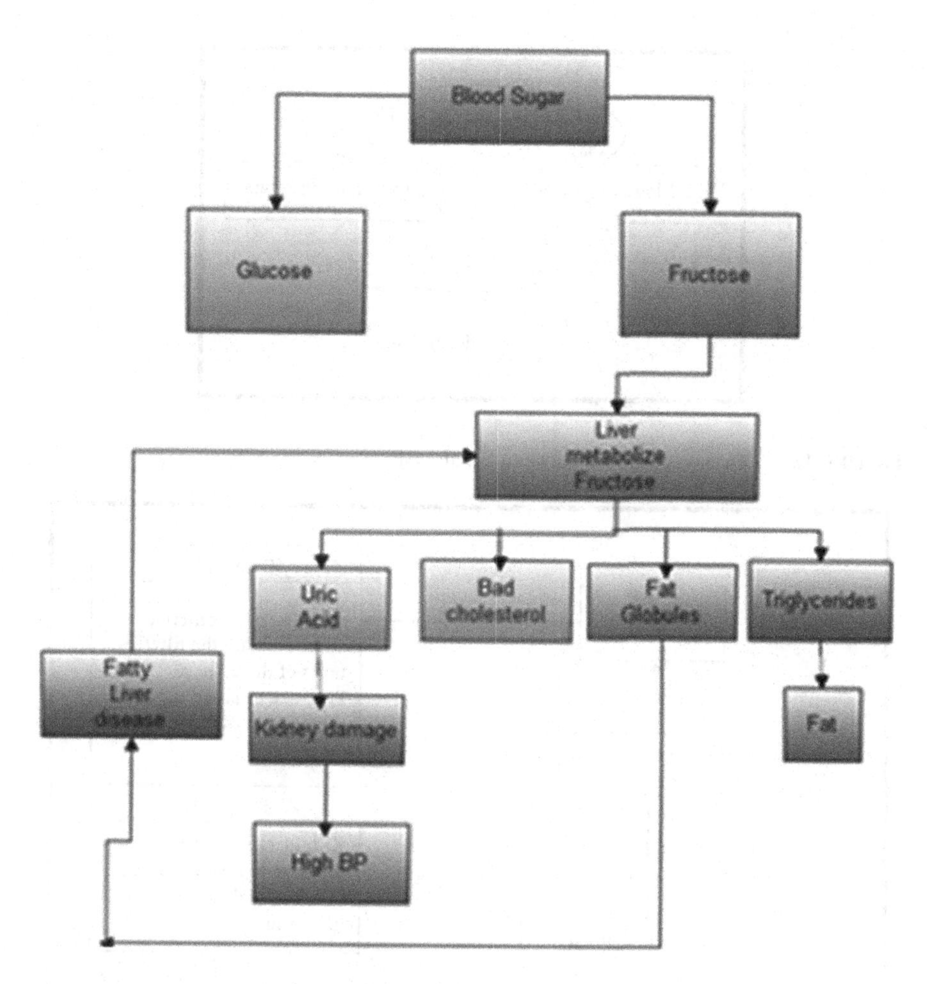

FIGURE 12.8 How BS affects different organs.

12.6 ARCHITECTURE OF THE PROPOSED DESIGN

12.6.1 Device-Level Architecture in Application of Internet of Medical Things (IoMT)

Here, in nursing care system based on Internet of Medical Things (IoMT), the following three types of devices have been developed:

I. **Wearable device:** This could be any type of wearable device but should be able to measure BP and BS. So, this device would have the four major units, namely, BP measuring unit, BS measuring unit, interactive display unit, and other microcontroller processing unit like wireless connection with smartphone or intelligent system. BP measuring unit contains a pressure sensor. BP is created in the arteries when blood is pumped around the body by the heart.

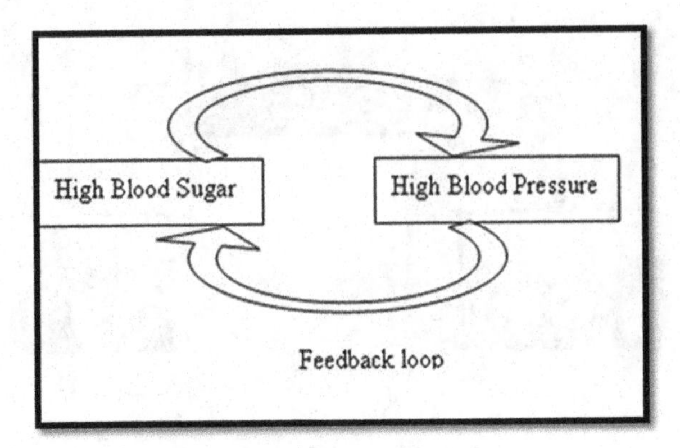

FIGURE 12.9 Two-way relation between BS and BP.

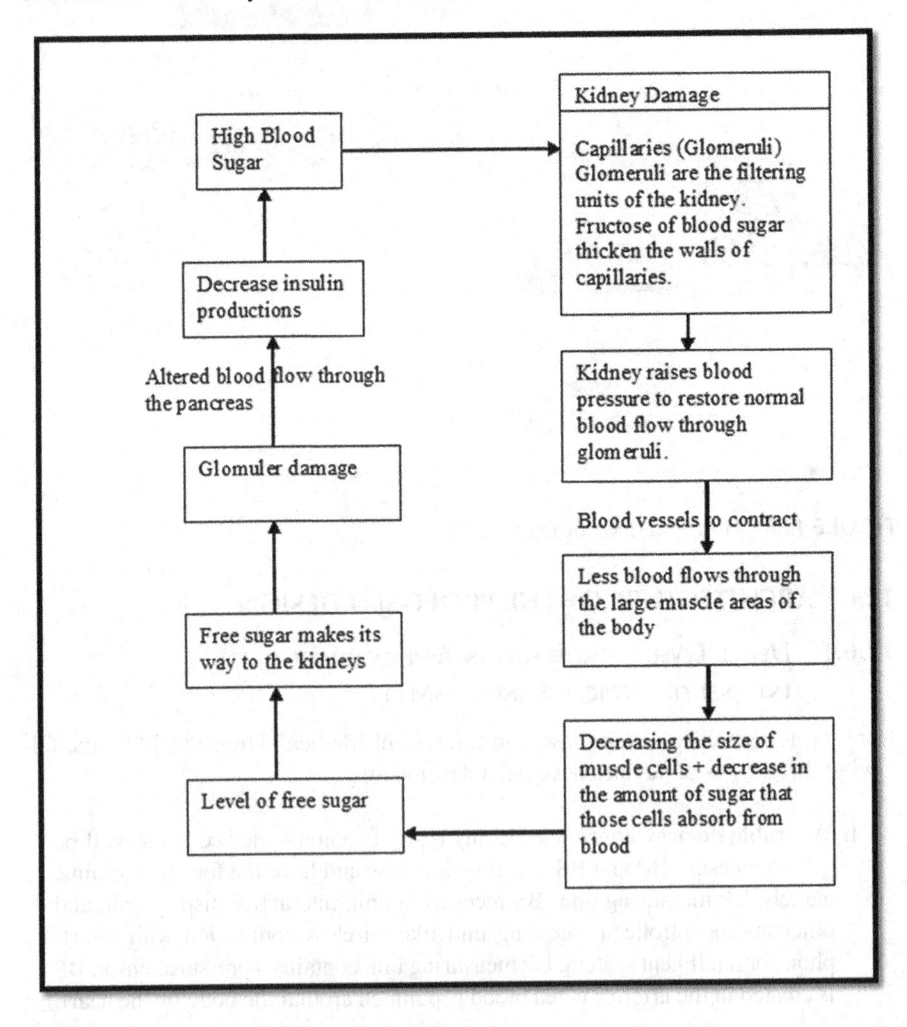

FIGURE 12.10 Relation between BP and BS.

BP is presented with two components, namely, the systolic pressure (as the heart beats) and the diastolic pressure (as the heart relaxes between beats).

II. **Intelligent diagnostic system:** It is a rule-based system. Based on BP and BS data, there are six rules (normal BP, low BP, high BP, normal BS, low BS, and high BS) that are applied to diagnose the monitored data before storing, and there are 8 rules (if normal BP & normal BS, If low BP & normal BS, low BP & high BS, If low BP & low BS, If high BP & normal BS, If high BP & low BS, and If high BP & high BS) that are required after retrieving the analyzed data to make people aware about their health condition and to alert them. In Tables 12.1 and 12.2, it is shown that how BP and BS vary in human beings in respect to age and different situations (Figure 12.11).

III. **Cloud environment:** It is mainly required to store the real-time data as the real-time monitoring would be huge. Cloud architecture is shown in Figure 12.12.

12.6.2 Intelligent Rule-Based System

In this section, fuzzy rule-based system and solution approach have been produced in different tables based on various BP and BS levels. Fuzzy IF-THEN rule-based system is applied for various levels of BS and BP. Actual values are fuzzified by the fuzzy engine and then processed. Tables 12.1 and 12.2 [37] shows different levels of BP and BS for different age groups.

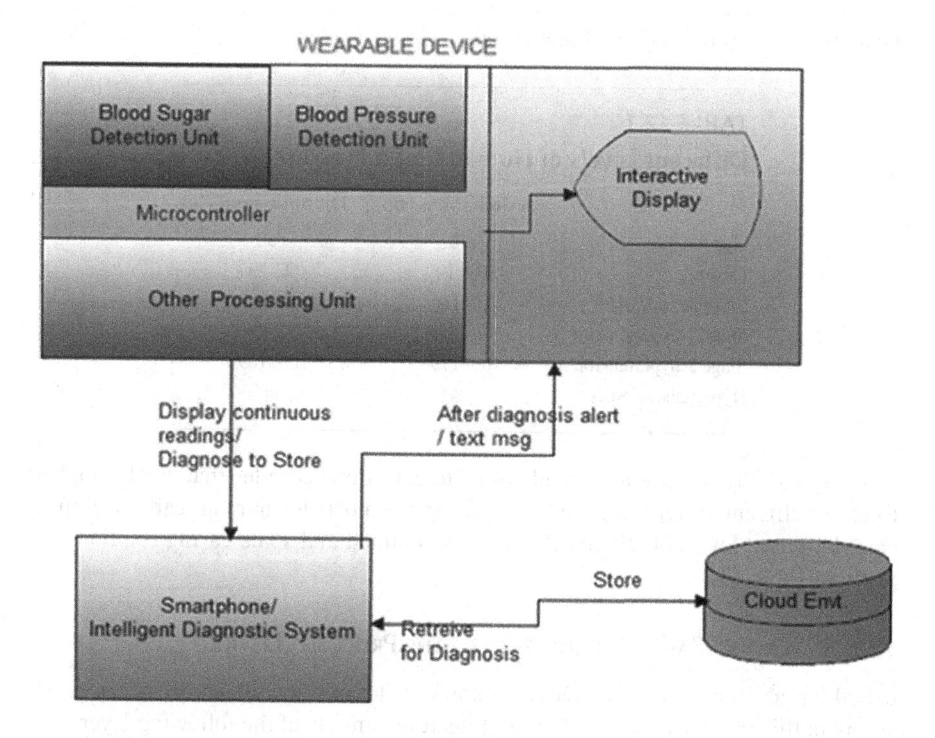

FIGURE 12.11 System-level diagram.

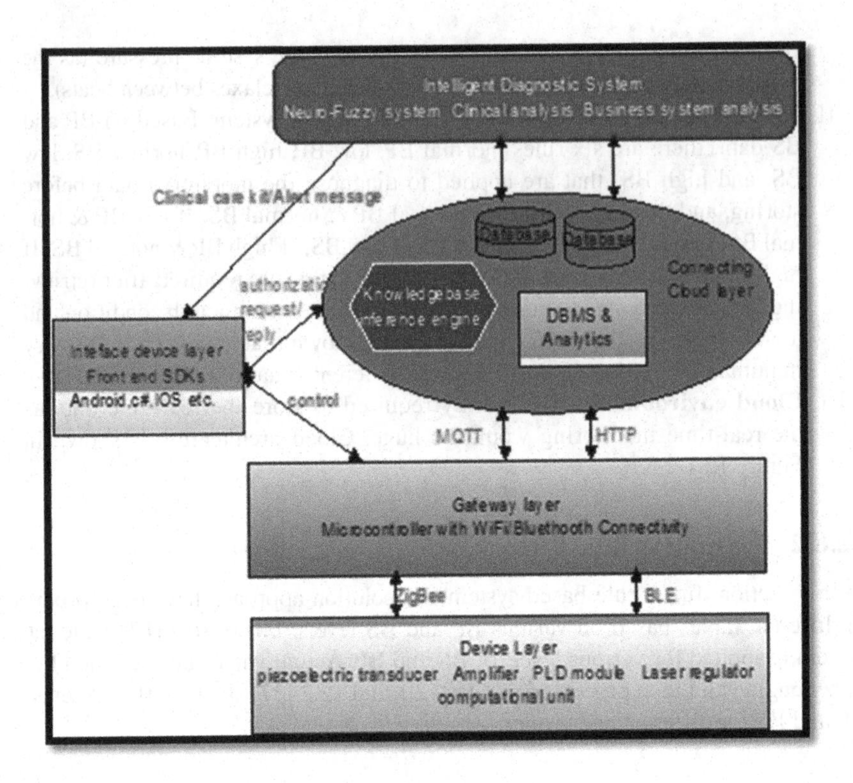

FIGURE 12.12 Cloud-based IoT architecture.

TABLE 12.1
Different Levels of Human Blood Pressure

	Systolic (mm Hg)	Diastolic (mm Hg)
Hypotension	<90	<60
Desired	90–119	60–79
Prehypertension	120–139	80–89
Stage 1 hypertension	140–159	90–99
Stage 2 hypertension	160–179	100–109
Hypertensive crisis	≥180	≥110

Rule-based fuzzy engine is made of different inference rules that can be applied to the intelligent system to generate a proper diagnosis for nursing care or clinical care. Different levels of BP and BS rules are defined and some caring solutions are given in Table 12.3.

12.6.3 Cloud-Based Architecture of the Proposed Device

Cloud-based architecture is needed to know that cloud infrastructure services are acting in this proposed device. This architecture consists of the following layers:

TABLE 12.2
Levels of Glucose in Human Blood Based on Age

Suggested Time	Age (Yrs)	mg/dl	mmol/l	Status
Fasting (a.m) or no food for 2 hrs	Below 5	80–200	4.5–11.1	Fine
Fasting (a.m) or no food for 2 hrs	5–11	70–180	3.9–10.0	Fine
Fasting (a.m) or no food for 2 hrs	12 or above 12	70–150	3.9–8.3	Fine
Bedtime (before bedtime snack or during the night)	Below 5	Above 150	8.3	Fine
Bedtime (before bedtime snack or during the night)	5–11	Above 130	7.3	Fine
Bedtime (before bedtime snack or during the night)	12 and above	Above 130	7.3	Fine

Application interface layer: It acts as an interface between user or patient and intelligent system layer. With this interface, patients can enter the system to see the glucose level, pressure level, and alert messages and precautionary measure into the android platform. This interface is mainly based on the android platform interface.

Intelligent layer: This layer is responsible for the clinical analysis based on the real-time data with neuro-fuzzy system. Best utility of the system depends on activities of this layer. Neuro-fuzzy system is used to minimize the response time and cost. Rule-based methods are used in this layer to establish the relationship between BP and BS. This layer is directly connected to cloud server or used as a local storage for the data.

Gateway layer: It is a gateway interface between the intelligent layer and the device layer. Edge device or the proposed device is connected to the intelligent layer through this gateway interface. Device is connected to the server using HTTP, MQTT [34] server with Wi-Fi, or Bluetooth connectivity. Real-time data from device is uploaded to the server through this layer.

Device layer: It is the most important layer that contains necessary portable chips to read data from human body as it is attached to the human body. It consists of PLD unit, computational unit, piezoelectric transducer etc. Reading data of the device is uploaded through the gateway layer with ZigBee connection.

12.6.4 Output-Based Design of Proposed Approach

Output-based design shows how the total system is working. Mobile edge device contains android application interface through which patients can read their BS and BP levels, which can be altered by the system. Data coming from the device goes to the intelligent system, and after necessary diagnosis is made, alert message is shown in the mobile display unit. Wearable device sends data to mobile application and to

TABLE 12.3
Set of Rules for Fuzzy Analysis

Rules	Diet Type	Example Diet	Instruction to follow
If BP and BS are normal	Normal diet	Morning at 6: 1/2 teaspoon fenugreek powder + water. Morning at 7: I cup sugar free tea + 1–2 sugar free biscuits. Morning at 8.30: 1 plate oatmeal+ half bowl sprouted grains + 100 ml cream-free milk without sugar. Morning at 10.30: 1 small fruit or lemon water. Lunch at 1: 2 roti of mixed flour, 1 bowl rice, 1 bowl pulse, 1 bowl yogurt, half cup soybean or cheese vegetable, half bowl green vegetable, one plate salad	Exercise for 30 mins or walk
If BS high and BP normal	Follow the prescribed diabetic diet	Eliminate milk from the normal diet	Eliminate sugar, sweets, dry fruits containing sugar, honey, sweet potato, pumpkin, etc. and do exercise regularly, consult physician
If BP high and BS normal	Follow high BP diet	Standard sample diet as in Fig	Reduce sodium, potassium, alcohol, eat more vegetables and fresh fruits, fiber. Exercise daily
If BS moderate and BP high	Follow strict high BP diet	Standard sample diet as in Fig	Try to maintain sugar consumption, daily exercise, walk
If BS high and BP low	Strict diabetic diet with physician's concern	—	Daily exercise, strictly eliminate sugar, walk, daily contact with physician.
If BS and BP high	Strict diet	Standard sample diet as in Fig	Consult physician immediately

the intelligent system. As the BP and BS levels must be visible to the patients, the mobile application is needed to install. On the other hand, after analyzing the data, the intelligent system provides necessary actions, which are also visible through mobile application to the patients. Diet chart or any alert message is shown in the mobile screen, so that patients can do further actions (Figure 12.13).

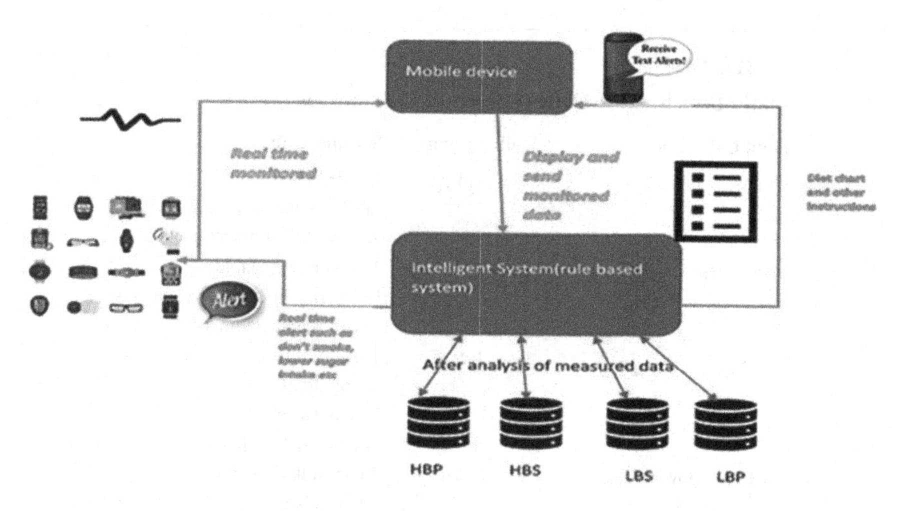

FIGURE 12.13 Output-based proposed design.

12.7 OUTPUT-BASED SAMPLE STANDARD DIET ANALYSIS

From Table 12.4 and data shown in Figure 12.1, daily serving of food should be analyzed. This analysis is done by considering the required food intake structure people either are diabetic or suffering from Hypertension.

It is necessary to maintain a sensitive diet every day for diabetic and hypertensive people. This analysis with diet is provided by the nursing care unit (Table 12.4).

12.8 LIKELY IMPACTS OF THE PROPOSED DEVICE

The main impact of the device will be on society in a wider way with IoT, cloud computing services, and android platform technology. Diabetic patients or people are forced to be panic about food, daily activities, and other effects on body organs. So, they usually go through malnutrition and meanwhile welcome other disease too. This device is unique in alerting about food habits, and in providing daily diet chart and physician consultation.

Mostly, it is about the application of noninvasive method of diabetes monitoring without taking insulin or that can avoid taking insulin. This proposed idea can reach in the following aspects of socio-health zone:

On prediabetic people: Everyday diet chart and real-time monitoring of this proposed device will make large amount of people more sensible from occurring diabetes.

On diabetic people: Number of diabetic people is increasing day by day. Daily lifestyle that has led to a decreased physical activity and increased consumption

TABLE 12.4
Daily Servings of Different Food Categories

Food Categories	Daily Servings	Serving Unit
Grains	6–8	1 slice bread
		½ –1 ¼ cups of dry cereal
		½ cup cooked rice or pasta
Vegetables	4--5	1 cup raw vegetables
		½ cup raw or cooked vegetables
		½ cup vegetable juice
Fruits	4–5	1 medium fruit
		¼ cup dried fruit
		½ cup cut-up fruits
		½ cup any fruit juice
Fat-free or low-fat milk	2–3	1 cup milk or yogurt
		1 ½ oz cheese
Fish, meat	6 or less (based on nutrition value)	1 oz cooked meat, fish
		1 egg
Nuts, seeds, legumes	4–5 per week	1/3 cup nuts
		2 tbsp peanut butter
		2 tbsp seeds
		½ cup cooked legumes
Fats and oils	2–3	1tsp margarine
		1tsp vegetable oil
		1tsp mayonnaise
		2 tbsp salad dressing
Sweets and added sugar	5 or less per week	1 tbsp sugar
		1 tbsp jelly or jam
		½ cup gelatin
		1 cup lemonade

of fat and sugar levels, affects insulin sensitivity and results in obesity. Only continuous awareness makes people to learn what should do, what should eat, and how to live healthy life having diabetes. This chapter shows with natural diet how diabetic people can maintain a normal life with low risk.

On cost: Our device will be available in a minimal cost; as it will be wearable device, it will be convenient to use. This cost-effective device is especially useful for those who needed at low cost as it is portable to use.

On other risks: As it is seen that diabetic patients often suffer with other physical risks, the main component of this device is intelligent diagnosis system, which provides a pure analysis on the real-time data generated from patient's body. Any people knowing diabetic level and continuous monitoring data could get rescue from other risks with the real-time awareness and correct physician consultation.

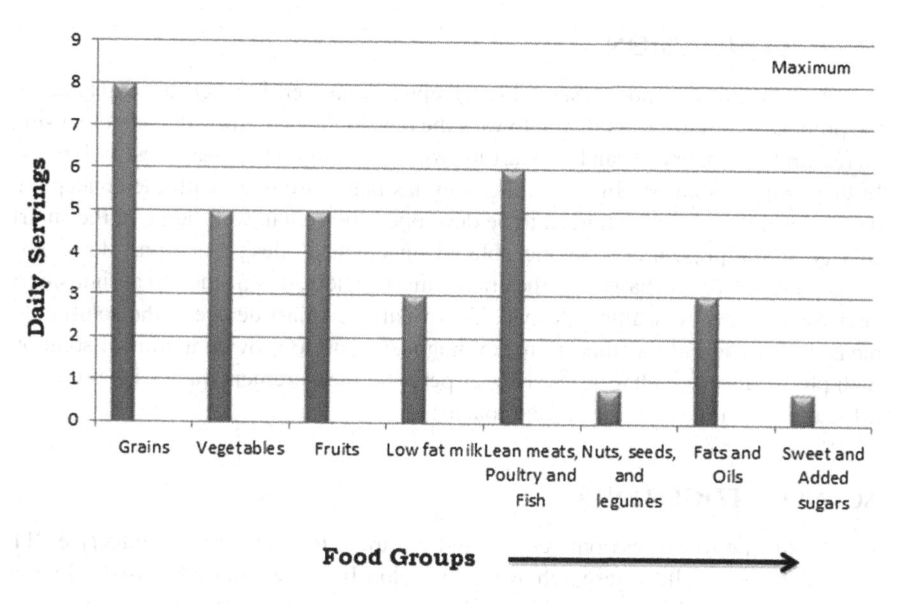

FIGURE 12.14 Daily food serving analysis for high BS and high BP patients.

12.9 PARAMETERS EFFECTING THE RESEARCH

The usefulness of this idea must be measured with respect to the below parameters:

Cost: Costly device or costly treatment is expectable in diabetic disease. Determination of perfect cost is the challenging concern in country like India. So, it is a big issue that how to minimize the cost for the proposed device.

Wearable device design: The miniature design is a major parameter to measure the effectiveness of the proposed device. Various kinds of wearable devices are already available in the market, but this device would be more useful if it is cost-effective, portable, and risk-free. In this chapter, for a continuous monitoring of blood glucose and pressure, individual must be worn this device all the time so that it can damage physical body in other way. It is a concern that it should be ensured that it is risk-free and all-time wearable.

Intelligent diagnostic system design: Diagnosis is the main key component in this device. Here in this intelligent diagnostic system, assembled intelligent program does the necessary analysis based on the real-time data. If diagnosis is not perfect—being available huge continuous data—then the total system would be error-prone or failed. Some rule-based engines are applied to examine the data, store the time-sensitive data, and detect the problems for providing prerisk preventive measures.

12.10 CONCLUSION

Post-project activities are presented in a stepwise manner. Further this explanation, the proposed system-oriented aim toward the development manner depicted focusing on research periphery. It can be a startup project with more necessary research work. In this chapter, some preliminary research has been discussed with the conceptual device-level designs, which need to be developed for human well-being in the smart society. In the present era, a noticeable advancement in design of smart devices is the key factor of this chapter. In the era of smart society, it is needed to design smart devices in everyday healthy lifestyle. This wearable smart device is the solution to measure BS and BP together, to make diagnosis, and to provide a clinical solution with physician's consultation. Storing of periodic measurement values is no more a difficult task with a cloud-based approach.

ACKNOWLEDGEMENTS

We would like to express our respect and gratitude to Prof. Swapna Banerjee, IIT KGP, for her excellent research work on "Non-Invasive Photo-Acoustic Method of Blood Glucose Measurement," which is our main motivating area to write this chapter. Also, we are thankful for the researchers who have done an extraordinary research in this field.

REFERENCES

1. The Diabetes Control and Complications Trial Research Group, 1993. The effect of intensive treatment of diabetes on the development and progression of long-term complications in insulin-dependent diabetes mellitus. *The New England Journal of Medicine*, 329(14):977–986.
2. D.R. Whiting, L. Guariguata, C. Weil, and J. Shaw, 2011. IDF diabetes atlas: Global estimates of the prevalence of diabetes for 2011 and 2030, *Diabetes Research and Clinical Practice*, 94(3):311–321.
3. D.D. Cunningham, and J.A. Stenken, 2010. *In Vivo Glucose Sensing*, John Wiley & Sons, Inc., Hoboken, NJ.
4. V. Tuchin, 2008. *Handbook of Optical Sensing of Glucose in Biological Fluids and Tissues*, CRC Press, Boca Raton, FL.
5. N. Bashkatov, E.A. Genina, V.I. Kochubey, and V.V. Tuchin, 2005. Optical properties of human skin, subcutaneous and mucous tissues in the wavelength range from 400 to 2000 nm. *Journal of Physics D: Applied Physics*, 38(15):2543–2555.
6. M. Ivović, L.V. Marina, S. Vujović, M. Tančić, M. Stojanović, N.V. Radonjić, et al. 2013. Nondiabetic patients with either subclinical Cushing's or nonfunctional adrenal incidentalomas have lower insulin sensitivity than healthy controls: clinical implications. *Metabolism: Clinical and Experimental*, 62(6):786–92.
7. A. Tabarin, 2018. Do the diagnostic criteria for subclinical hypercortisolism exist? *Annales d'Endocrinologie (Paris)*, 79(3):146–8. doi:10.1016/j.ando.2018.03.013
8. L. Warren, and P. Hixenbaugh, 2020. Adherence and diabetes. In L. Myers, and K. Midence (eds.) *Adherance to Treatment in Medical Conditions* (pp. 423–453). CRC Press, Boca Raton, FL.
9. D. Donizetti-Trevisan, R. Nazário-Aoki, M.M. Wopereis-Groot, M. Aurélio-Boes, and A.R. de Souza Oliveira-Kumakura, 2020. Validation and applicability of instrument

for documenting the nursing process in intensive care. *Enfermería Clínica (English Edition)*, 30(1):4–15.
10. G. Parati, and J.E. Ochoa, 2019. Blood pressure variability. In G. Mancia, S. Julius, and R. Zimlichman (eds.) *Prehypertension and Cardiometabolic Syndrome* (pp. 395–417). Springer, Cham.
11. V. Puri, R. Kumar, D.N. Le, S.S. Jagdev, and N. Sachdeva, 2020. BioSenHealth 2.0—a low-cost, energy-efficient Internet of Things–based blood glucose monitoring system. In V.E. Balas, V.K. Solanki, and R. Kumar (eds.) *Emergence of Pharmaceutical Industry Growth with Industrial IoT Approach* (pp. 305–324). Academic Press, Cambridge, MA.
12. V.S. Patil, and N.A. Khatib, 2020. Triterpene saponins from Barringtonia acutangula (L.) Gaertn as a potent inhibitor of 11β-HSD1 for type 2 diabetes mellitus, obesity, and metabolic syndrome. *Clinical Phytoscience*, 6(1):1–5.
13. S. Abokyi, P.A. Ayerakwah, S.L. Abu, and E.K. Abu, 2020. Controlled blood sugar improves the eye's accommodative ability in type-1 diabetes. Eye, pp. 1–7.
14. R. Chawla, R. Senthilkumar, and N. Ramakrishnan, 2020. Intracranial pressure monitoring and management. In R. Chawla, and S. Todi (eds.) *ICU Protocols* (pp. 327–338). Springer, Singapore.
15. J.G.S. Latorre, and D.M. Greer, 2009. Management of acute intracranial hypertension: A review. *The Neurologist*, 15(4):193–207.
16. G. Citerio, and P.J. Andrews, 2009. Intracranial pressure part two: Clinical applications and technology. In G. Hedenstierna, J. Mancebo, L. Brochard, M. Pinsky (eds.) *Applied Physiology in Intensive Care Medicine* (pp. 109–112). Springer, Berlin.
17. P.J. Andrews, and G. Citerio, 2004. Intracranial pressure. *Intensive Care Medicine*, 30(9):1730–1733.
18. A. Bhatia, and A.K. Gupta, 2007. Neuromonitoring in the intensive care unit. I. Intracranial pressure and cerebral blood flow monitoring. *Intensive Care Medicine*, 33(7):1263–1271.
19. J.A. Ronen, M. Gavin, M.D. Ruppert, and A.N. Peiris, 2019. Glycemic disturbances in pheochromocytoma and paraganglioma. *Cureus*, 11(4):e4551. doi:10.7759/cureus.4551
20. E.S. Kilpatrick, A.S. Rigby, and S.L. Atkin, 2006. The effect of glucose variability on the risk of microvascular co mplications in type 1 diabetes. *Diabetes Care*, 29(7):1486–1490. doi:10.2337/dc06-0293.
21. M.T. Corwin, S.M. Navarro, D.G. Malik, T.W. Loehfelm, G. Fananapazir, M. Wilson, et al., 2019. Differences in growth rate on CT of adrenal adenomas and malignant adrenal nodules. *American Journal of Roentgenology*, 213(3):632–6. doi:10.2214/AJR.19.21342.
22. M. Han, X. Cao, C. Zhao, L. Yang, N. Yin, P. Shen, J. Zhang, F. Gao, Y. Ren, D. Liang, J. Yang, Y. Zhang and Y. Liu, 2020. Assessment of glycometabolism impairment and glucose variability using flash glucose monitoring system in patients with adrenal diseases. *Frontiers in Endocrinology*, 11:544752. doi:10.3389/fendo.2020.544752.
23. C.M. Ting, 2002. Method and device for measuring blood sugar level, US 2002/0198443A1.
24. W. Yu, and S.Y. Huang, 2018. "T-shaped patterned microstrip line for noninvasive continuous glucose sensing". *IEEE Microwave and Wireless Components Letters*, 28 (10):942–944. doi:10.1109/LMWC.2018.2861565.
25. Researcher in IISC, Bangalore have done research work which is published as article in https://epaper.livemint.com/Home/ArticleView.
26. N. Mohammad, W. Szyszkowski, W. Zhang, E. Haddad, J. Zou, W. Jamroz, and R. Kruzelecky, 2004. Analysis and development of a tunable fiber Bragg grating filter based on axial tension/compression. *Journal of Lightwave Technology*, 22:2001–2013. doi:10.1109/JLT.2004.832439.
27. Diabeto is a remote patient monitoring, chronic disease management, and wellness solution for people with diabetes and their care teams. http://www.diabe.to

28. H. Teymourian, A. Barfidokht, and J. Wang, 2020. Electrochemical glucose sensors in diabetes management: An updated review (2010–2020). *Chemical Society Reviews*, 49:7671–7709.
29. NON, G.C.B.A.A., Available Online through Research Article.
30. A. Sola-Gazagnes, P. Faucher, S. Jacqueminet, C. Ciangura, D. Dubois-Laforgue, H. Mosnier-Pudar, R. Roussel, and E. Larger, 2020. Disagreement between capillary blood glucose and flash glucose monitoring sensor can lead to inadequate treatment adjustments during pregnancy. *Diabetes & Metabolism*, 46(2):158–163.
31. P. Pai, P. Sanki, and S. Banerjee, 2015. A photoacoustics based continuous non-invasive blood glucose monitoring system. *2015 IEEE International Symposium on Medical Measurements and Applications, MeMeA 2015 - Proceedings*. doi:10.1109/MeMeA.2015.7145181.
32. A. Das, B. Neogi and P. Pradhan, 2007. Diabetic control by pancreatic stimulation and its process control realization. *Calcutta Medical Journal*, 104(6):25–31.
33. P. Pradhan, A. Das, and B. Neogi, 2007. Controlling glucose level using computerized method in human blood. *International Journal HIT Transaction on ECCN*, 2(8):443–449. ISSN: 0973-6875
34. MQTT is an OASIS standard for IoT connectivity. 1999. https://mqtt.org/getting-started/.
35. G.M. Grassi, and P.M. Nilsson, 2016. Specific blood pressure targets for patients with diabetic nephropathy? *Diabetes Care*, 39 (Supplement 2):S228–S233.
36. Blood Sugar Blood Pressure Log Book: Diabetes Journal and Blood Pressure Log Book, Monitor Blood Sugar and Blood Pressure levels for Your Health, Daily, Frances Walker (Author), CreateSpace Independent Publishing Platform (July 12, 2018). ISBN-10: 1723010057, ISBN-13:978-1723010057.
37. S. Roy, 2014. Design approaches on Auto Computational Guidance for maintained Sugar level with Proposed IDPC unit model.

13 Eye Disease Detection from Retinal Fundus Image Using CNN

Padma Selvaraj
Madanapalle Institute of Technology and Science

Pugazendi Rajagopal
Government Arts College

CONTENTS

13.1 INTRODUCTION

Medical field is retrieving different types of data from patients for the diagnosis of disease. The image is playing a vital role in this field. X-ray images, different types of scan images, and ultrasound images are few of them. Signals are also retrieved from ECG and EEG. Images can be of different format, size, and color. Previous researches have paved the way for medical diagnosis at the earlier stage with the images [1]. Handling of gray-scale images is different from executing color images [2]. Human body consists of several parts, with unique importance. Eyes are considered to be the most important organ in the human body. It is to sense the picturization of the environment, and thereby, the brain stores in it. Eyes are made of several parts, including iris, pupil, and retina. Perfect vision of a human is described as 20/20 vision. The rods and cones existing in the eyes are enabling us to see the light.

Surveys released by the World Health Organization (WHO) for the year 2020 represent that globally one billion people have problems in their vision. People greater than 50 years of age are normally affected by several eye diseases, which may cause blindness if not diagnosed at the initial stage. Persons affected from diabetes are rapidly increasing year by year. The major organs affected for a diabetic patient are eyes, kidneys, and heart. Cardiovascular disease, cancer, chronic respiratory disease, and diabetes are the major life-threatening diseases.

Many diseases affect retina, and if it's not diagnosed at the initial stage, then chances for vision loss will become increased [3]. The medical field has been improved with several technologies for the identification of diseases. The time taken by the physician for analyzing the test is comparatively more, as the number of patients is also increased. Screening of fundus images and diagnosing with the support of additional computer-aided tools prevent the people from the sufferings. Existing tools for medical diagnosis may not suit to diagnose the retinal images taken.

13.1.1 Retinal Fundus Images

Retinal fundus images are those taken from the back part of the eyes. It is a thin layer that gets affected for a diabetic patient easily and may lead to mild retinopathy, observable retinopathy, referable retinopathy, proliferative retinopathy, etc. Diabetic retinopathy (DR) is observed in the young people. Persons affected from these retinal diseases are predicted to be 288 million by 2040. Identification of disease from the fundus images is better compared to that of the other ophthalmic images. These retinal fundus images help to identify several eye disorders. The use of raw retinal images is difficult for the methodology framed. Retrieved images may be of different size, intensity, and color. Before utilizing the computer-aided tools, few preprocessing steps are to be executed.

Retinal fundus images help to diagnose various eye diseases, which may lead to visionless. These eye diseases are common and affect persons at different age groups. People affected from other major diseases will be easily affected by the eye diseases. Being a vital organ in the human body, earlier diagnosis flourishes light in many lives. Table 13.1 lists few eye diseases that can be identified by the retinal fundus image. This image specifies the abnormality change in the eyes and the symptoms for it.

Some of the important eye diseases that could be identified from the retinal fundus image are shown in Figure 13.1. Figure 13.1 shows the image of normal eyes along with images of eyes with several diseases. The box portion is the infected part of the eyes. Identification of these diseases at early stages prevents the vision loss for many people at different age groups.

13.1.2 Machine Learning

Artificial intelligence (AI) concepts are incorporated in various applications as it is well known for its effective execution. Traditional machine learning (ML) has established its power in different domains of today's modern society. Few applications that can be listed are searching the web using filtering on social media and recommendations on e-commerce websites, and its necessity is increased and required by the customers. ML applications are also extended in identifying images, language processing, time-series data handling, and video analytics.

TABLE 13.1
Eye Diseases Identified through Retinal Fundus Images

Eye Disease	Leads To	Symptoms
Tessellated fundus [4]	Reduced pigmentation	Blurry vision, rainbow-colored haloes
Optic cups [5]	Danger due to change in the size of optic cups	Pale disk, imaging
Retinal vein occlusion [6]	Blockage of central retinal vein, painless vision loss	Distorted vision
Glaucoma [7]	Visual disturbance due to optic cup and nerve degeneration	Severe headache, eye pain, blurred vision
Optic atrophy [8]	Death of the retinal ganglion	Blurred vision, difficulties with side, color vision
Hypertensive retinopathy [9]	Due to high blood pressure or hypertension	Reduced vision, eye swelling, risk of stroke
Disk swelling [10]	Build pressure in and around brain, symptom of brain tumor or hemorrhage	Blurred vision, fever
Dragged disk [11]	Retinopathy due to prematurity, detachment of retina may occur	Scar-like appearance in retinopathy
Congenital abnormalities [12]	Impair visual function	Morning glory syndrome
Retinitis pigmentosa [13]	Breakdown of cells due to generic disorders	Vision problem at the night and also loss of side vision
Crystalline dystrophy [14]	Vision loss due to deposition of a large number of small white or yellow fatty compounds	Night blindness
Lattice degeneration [15]	Retina will be thin, which leads to affect the near-sight of the person	Blurred vision, flashing lights
Branch retinal vein occlusion (BRVO) [16]	Blockage in one or more retinal veins	Peripheral vision loss, blurred central vision

Traditional ML algorithms have proved their efficiency in various aspects. ML performs better for classification, clustering, and regression. In this chapter, it is much focused towards the classification of the images. The important techniques of data mining are compressed to the three types of learning, namely, supervised learning, unsupervised learning, and reinforcement learning. Supervised learning classifies the data based on the class labels; in other words, it maps perfectly an input feature to an output feature of class labels [17]. Imagine there are images of 1000 cars; the aim of the problem is to classify similar model cars and also to predict the test image. The model for the execution will be built on the two separate sets, namely, training and testing. Training is to train the model with its features and its relevant classes. After continuous training, the model gains the capacity of learning the features of the dataset. Test the ML model with the test image, and the classifiers' performance is evaluated based on the measures. The studies on different classifiers

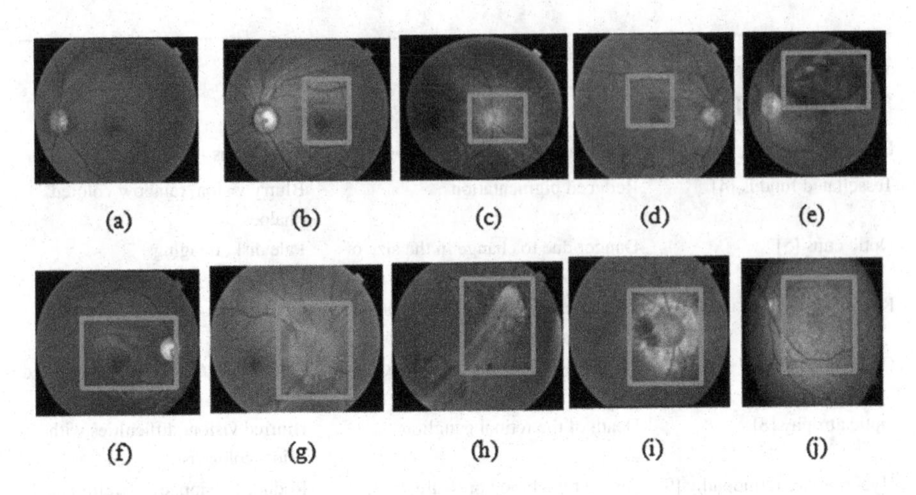

FIGURE 13.1 Retinal fundus image sample. (a) Normal image. (b) Tessellated fundus. (c) Optic cup. (d) Glaucoma. (e) Retinal vein occlusion. (f) Optic atrophy. (g) Disk swelling. (h) Dragged disk. (i) Congenital abnormalities. (j) Crystalline dystrophy.

are described below. Researches are executed to approximate the complex nonlinear problems efficiently. ML can be extensively used for classification, which is used to solve the real-world problems.

The above-mentioned classification can be done either through sequential learning or through batch learning. In batch learning, the entire dataset is divided into several batches and made the model to learn. These methods require the entire data specified for training to be executed more number of times to reduce the approximation errors. It requires more time and space as it executes with the entire training data every time.

Single-layer feed-forward network (SLFN) is a three-layer network comprising the input layer, the hidden layer, and the output layer, as shown in Figure 13.2. The input layer comprises the input neurons that are the input features. The input values are moved to the next layer, the hidden layer with additional weights and bias. The hidden layer holds the activation function that determines the neuron firing for the execution. The output of the activation function will be updated by necessary weights and bias to identify the class labels correctly [18].

Through the study on various algorithms, the weights are considerably playing an important role in the entire execution. Initially, the weights are assigned randomly; these weights can also be learned by orthogonal least squares (OLS), extended Kalman filter (EKF), and mean square error (MSE) [19]. Update in weights reduces the error, which ultimately reduces the overfitting and improves the generalization of the classifier. Projection-based learning–radial basis function (PBL-RBF) is a method to update the weight using the least mean square errors. It works on the principle of minimizing error by finding the optimal weight for the execution [20].

An addition to the simple three-layer neural network is the inclusion of self-regulatory principles within the network. Learning strategies like sample deletion avoid overtraining, control neuron growth, and update parameters using EKF [17].

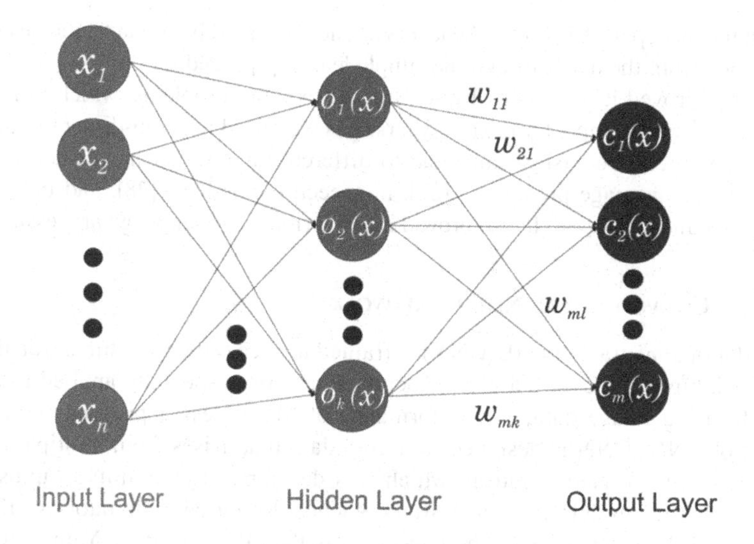

FIGURE 13.2 Three-layer neural network.

Nelson and Naren defined a model for cognition [21]. This model comprises two components, namely, cognitive and meta-cognitive. These components control and monitor the flow of information. The three-layer RBF was incorporated with the cognitive principles to produce meta-cognitive neural network (McNN) [22]. The weight of the network is updated using the PBL along with fuzzy concepts, thus framing a new way to PBLF-McNN [23].

Batch learning is efficiently done in the extreme learning machine (ELM), in which the weights are randomly assigned [24]. It is a fast learning algorithm, which has proved its efficiency in various applications. The weight update using PBL along with the cognitive concepts performs well when compared to the other existing algorithms [25]. Conventional ML methods face their difficulty in processing the real data, where the transformation has to be done.

13.1.3 Deep Learning

Representation-based learning breaks over the above-said difficulty. Automatic discovery of patterns and detection with the raw data is said to be as a representation learning. Deep learning (DL) is the one that executes the images automatically and helps to detect the correct classes [26]. DL is a method with multiple levels of representation, which converts the nonlinear method into the abstract level. It starts with the raw input and transforms the input into the expected one. Exclusively for classification, it identifies the important feature for identifying the class labels and suppresses the other features that are unimportant. For example, an image is the array form of its pixel values, and the first layer represents the features of the images. The second layer identifies the values with some variations, and the third layer focuses on the important features that are required for classification. The remaining layers form a combination of these layers to detect the objects and their class labels. The important concept of DL is that the layers are not designed by humans; the layers can be learned from the data through the simple learning procedure.

DL has proved its efficiency by solving the existing problems, which were done through several attempts for the past years. It is well used for high-dimensional data, and hence, it can be easily applicable to different domains. It has beaten the ML performance in image processing [27], in speech recognition [28], and in working with genes and DNA [29]. It also proved its performance in language processing [30].

13.1.4 Convolutional Neural Network

Convolutional neural network (CNN) is framed to access the two-dimensional data. CNN is a type of DL with a greater depth of network especially applied to image data. In using image data, the performance of ML is less appropriate compared to that of CNN. CNN is designed to access data that arises from multiple arrays. CNN has a name Neocognitron, which was developed by Kunihiko Fukushima, a researcher from NHK Broadcasting Science Research Laboratories, Kinuta, Setagaya, Tokyo, Japan [31]. The concept was then developed by Yann LeCun, a researcher from AT & T Bell Laboratories in Holmdel, New Jersey, United States. LeNet LeCun applied this concept in his research on numerical and handwriting recognition [32].

The working of CNN is similar to that of a common multilayer perceptron (MLP). But in CNN, each neuron is represented in two dimensions, whereas in MLP, neuron is represented in a single dimension. The operations of CNN are different in calculating the weights of the network. CNN contains numerous layers and many neurons in each layer. For a CNN, it is difficult to set the rules and its applications. It has proved its applications in image processing, video recognition, and natural language processing. The architecture of CNN is shown in Figure 13.3.

The architecture is continuous of different stages. In these few layers, an image is a collection of pixels, which are framed in a matrix format. Flattening of the image matrix to a vector for the easy execution is considered to be as an important feature of CNN. The convolutional layer and the pooling layer are the major layers available in the architecture. Each unit of the convolutional layer is connected to local patches in the feature maps of the previous layer through a set of weights

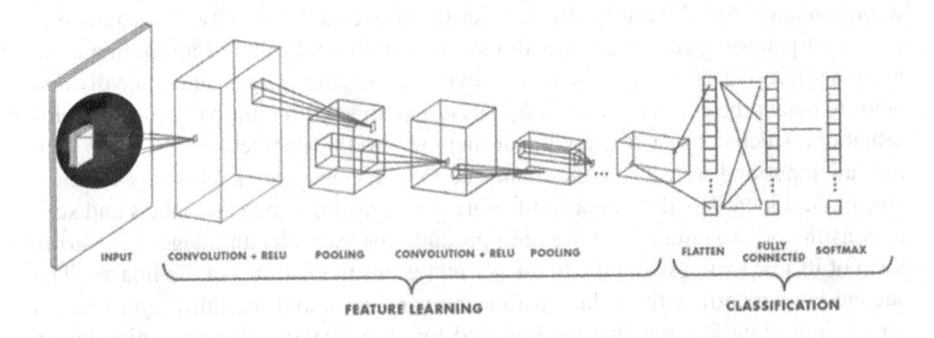

FIGURE 13.3 CNN architecture.

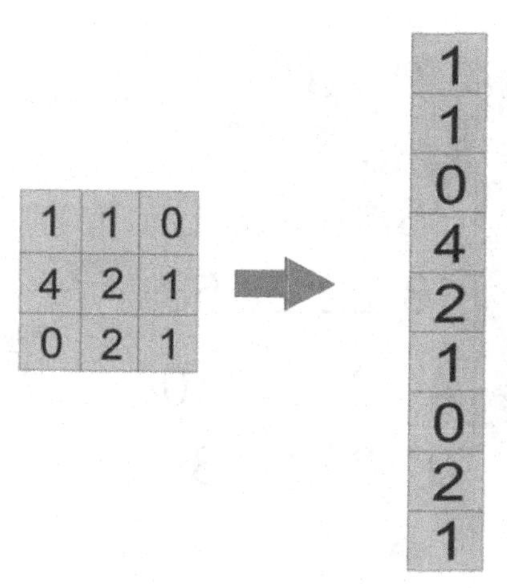

FIGURE 13.4 Flattening 3×3 matrix into a vector.

called filter bank. The activation function used is ReLU. The processed data is now ready for classification, which was forwarded into the fully connected layer. The fully connected layer processes the input neurons, which are activated by the hidden neurons through ReLU function. The output neurons are activated by the softmax function.

Normally, working with images becomes complicate because of the usage of matrices and high-dimensional data. CNN reduces the complexity by flattening the matrices into a simple vector, which can be easily computed as in Figure 13.4. The CNN simplifies the working complexity and is successful in capturing the spatial and temporal values in the image through filters. It performs better fitting due to the parameter reduction and reusability of weights.

The input image taken can be of either gray scale or of RGB, HSV, CMYK etc. The dimensions of these images complicate the computation. The CNN reduces the dimensions without affecting the features or quality of the images. Figure 13.5 represents the three dimensions of the image clearly.

The operation that happens in the convolutional layer is the filtering, which is represented in Figure 13.6. The image pixel values are filtered by a 3×3 matrix where it is convolved. The filtering is done throughout the image matrix, and the output is stored in a separate image with a reduced matrix size. The filters are working without any deviation in the features.

The objective of CNN is to reduce the complexity and not in the quality of the image. By means of padding, the size of the matrices needs to be reduced without losing their original features.

Similar to the convolved layer, the pooling layer tends to reduce the dimensionality of the image. The pooling layer is represented in Figure 13.7. The reduction decreases the complexity of work. It helps to extract the dominant features that are essential. Two types of pooling can be used. Maximum pooling extracts the maximum feature value from the image. Average pooling extracts the average feature value from the image.

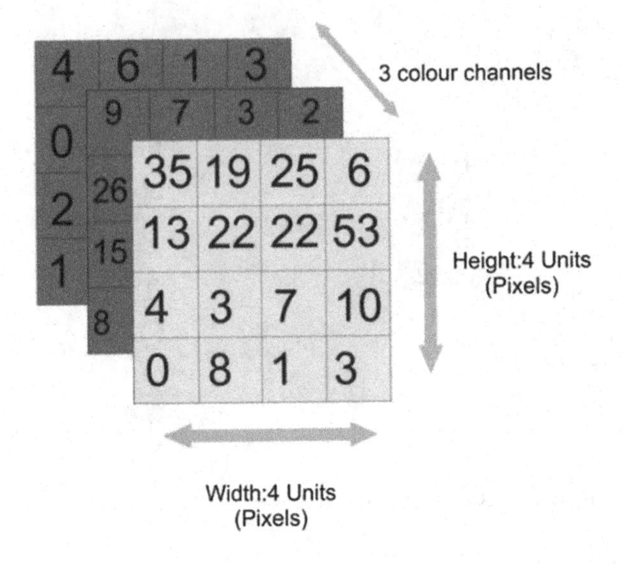

FIGURE 13.5 Multidimensional representation of an image.

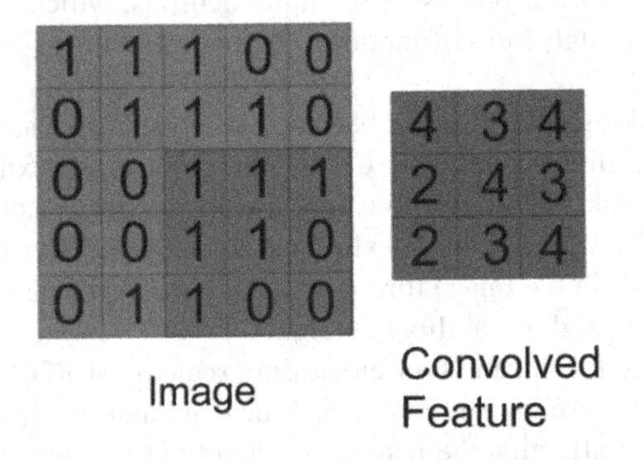

FIGURE 13.6 Sample convolved feature and its original representation.

FIGURE 13.7 Sample pooling matrix with the convolved feature matrix.

13.2 DATASET DESCRIPTION

The datasets were retrieved from kaggle. All these 1000 fundus images that belong to 39 classes are come from the Joint Shantou International Eye Centre (JSIEC), Shantou City, Guangdong Province, China. The class description is listed in Table 13.2. Table 13.2 represents the class names along with the samples available in each class for execution. The data retrieved is highly imbalanced.

TABLE 13.2
Retinal Fundus Image Dataset Description

Class	Class Name	No. of Images per Class
1	Normal	38
2	Tessellated fundus	13
3	Large optic cup	50
4	DR1	18
5	DR2	49
6	DR3	39
7	BRVO	44
8	CRVO	22
9	RAO	16
10	Rhegmatogenous RD	57
11	CSCR	14
12	VKH disease	14
13	Maculopathy	74
14	ERM	26
15	MH	23
16	Pathological myopia	54
17	Possible glaucoma	13
18	Optic atrophy	12
19	Severe hypertensive retinopathy	15
20	Disk swelling and elevation	13
21	Dragged disk	10
22	Congenital disk abnormality	10
23	Retinitis pigmentosa	22
24	Bietti crystalline dystrophy	8
25	Peripheral retinal degeneration and break	14
26	Myelinated nerve fiber	11
27	Vitreous particles	14
28	Fundus neoplasm	8
29	Massive hard exudates	13
30	Yellow-white spot-flecks	29
31	Cotton-wool spots	10
32	Vessel tortuosity	14
33	Chorioretinal atrophy—coloboma	15
34	Preretinal hemorrhage	10

(*Continued*)

TABLE 13.2 (*Continued*)
Retinal Fundus Image Dataset Description

Class	Class Name	No. of Images per Class
35	Fibrosis	10
36	Laser spots	20
37	Silicon oil in eye	19
38	Blur fundus without PDR	114
39	Blur fundus with suspected PDR	45

13.3 EXPERIMENTAL RESULTS AND DISCUSSIONS

The data samples get executed in python 3.8 with the support of Google Colab. The dataset contains color images with an unequal size. Preprocessing of data is required to convert the image sizes into equal. The target size is fixed as 28,28,3. Using the python code, the images are retrieved from the dataset and converted into the target size. The total dataset is divided into 80% for training data and 20% for testing data. Model is built with pooling layer as 2×2 size, and the activation function ReLU is used in the hidden layers. The softmax activation function is used in the output layer.

The dropout is mentioned as 0.25 and 0.5 wherever required. After building the model, compilation started. The total number of parameters used is 1,200,458, which is comparatively too high. After analyzing the model summary, it is identified that a dropout of 0.5 can be included before the ReLU activation function. Once it is included, there is a sudden decrease in the number of parameters used. After executing the model, the training loss and validation loss as well as training accuracy and validation accuracy are plotted in Figure 13.8.

The result of the model is not satisfied. The test accuracy obtained is 0.368750005960464, which is poor. It is made to increase the epochs from 50 to 100 in order to observe the change, which is represented in Figure 13.9.

The results observed from Figures13.8 and 13.9 clearly represent that the model is suffered from overfitting. It is trained much that memorizes the content provided, and hence, it is not able to validate the new image. There are measures to overcome this overfitting but before that, it is tried with batch normalization instead of using dropout before the dense. It is observed that there is an increase in the number of total parameters. Also from the observation while using dropout, the value of the nontrainable parameter is 0, but using the batch normalization, the value of the nontrainable parameter is 18,042, which reflects in the total parameters used by the model. The model is made to execute with an epoch value of 50 and the observed results are plotted in Figure 13.10.

From Figure 13.10, it is observed that there is a slight variation in the validation part and there is a nominal increase in the training part compared to that shown in Figures 13.8 and 13.9. To make the process fine, the number of epochs is increased to 100. The observations are shown in Figure 13.11.

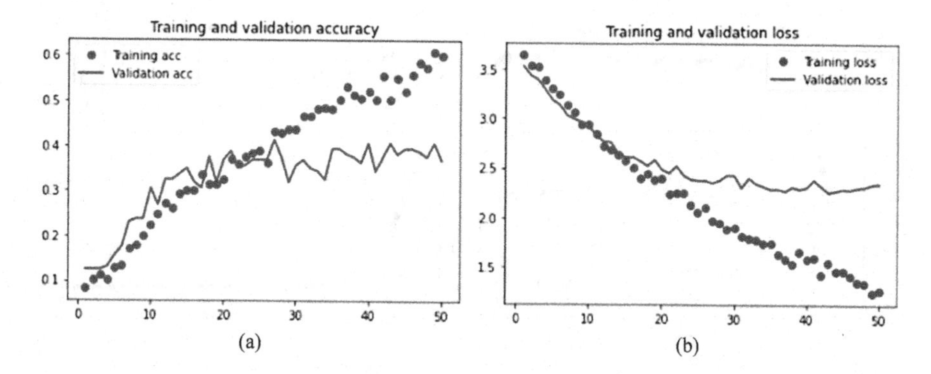

FIGURE 13.8 Plots for dropout 0.5 with 50 epochs. (a) Training and validation accuracy. (b) Training and validation loss.

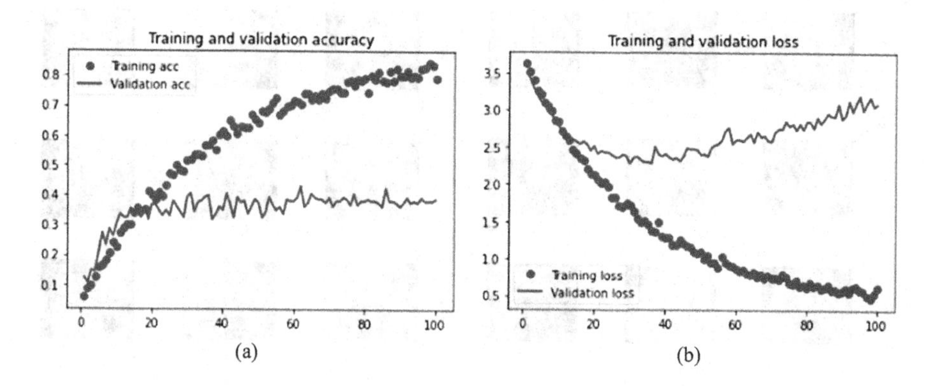

FIGURE 13.9 Plots for dropout 0.5 with 100 epochs. (a) Training and validation accuracy. (b) Training and validation loss.

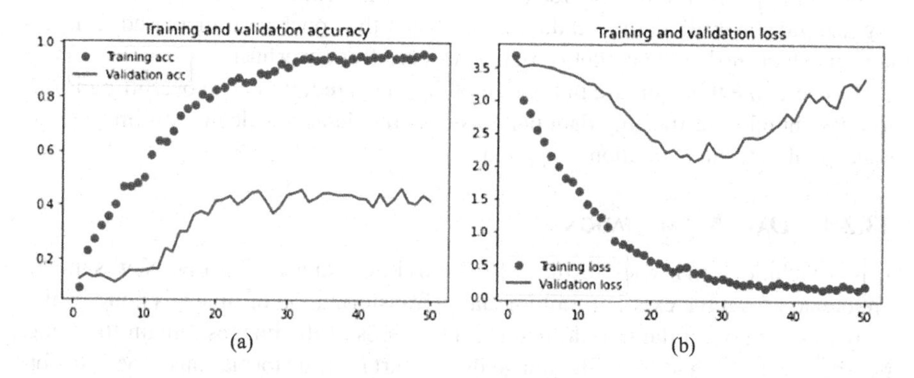

FIGURE 13.10 Plots for batch normalization with 50 epochs. (a) Training and validation accuracy. (b) Training and validation loss.

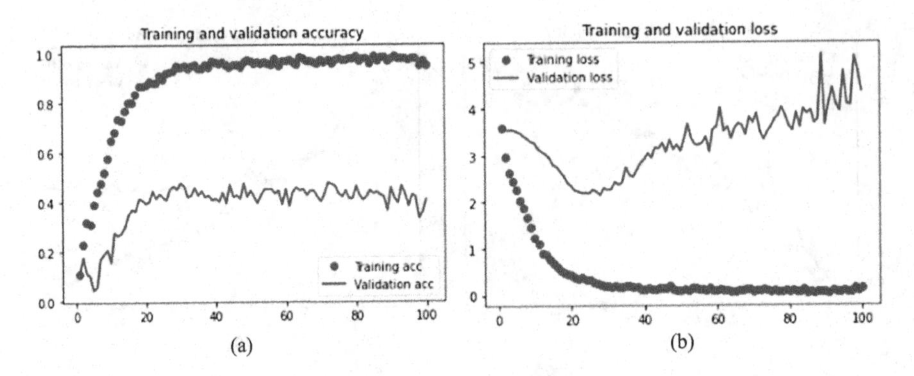

FIGURE 13.11 Plots for batch normalization with 100 epochs. (a) Training and validation accuracy. (b) Training and validation loss.

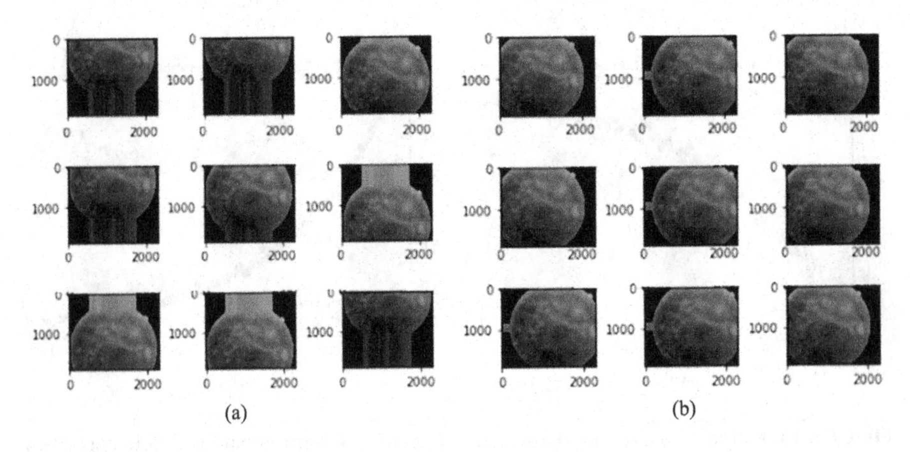

FIGURE 13.12 Data augmentation (a) Horizontal shift. (b) Vertical shift.

From Figure13.11, it is observed that there is some remarkable change in the training accuracy as well as the validation loss when the epochs are increased. But it is very much clear that the model is highly suffered from overfitting.

To overcome this increase in the size of dataset is required. The overfitting is due to a less number of training data per class. As the dataset is dealt with images, the concept of data augmentation is applied.

13.3.1 Data Augmentation

It is a technique that tries to increase the training data artificially. New samples are created from the existing training data. Transformation of image is done, which increases the size of dataset ultimately. The classes of the images remain the same, but there will be changes in the image due to certain transformations. The transformation includes shifts, flips, and zooms both vertically and horizontally. Shifting the image either horizontally or vertically shifts the image pixels in one direction without changing the image dimensions. Some clipping activities are performed here. The horizontal and vertical image shifts are represented in Figure 13.12.

Horizontal and vertical flipping of images reverses the rows and columns of the pixels as per the requirement. To increase the image data as well as different positions of the same data results in best training to the model. The flipping is represented in Figure 13.13. It shows the flipped image in the horizontal view.

Another method of augmentation is random rotation. The image gets rotated clockwise based on a random degree from 0 to 360. The image may leave the frame to no pixel data also, which is shown in Figure 13.14.

The next method of data augmentation used in this chapter is random brightness. The brightness of the image may be increased or decreased randomly or both. It tries to increase the combinations of image at different light levels. The image of the existing training data is augmented using the random brightness method, which is shown in Figure 13.15.

From Figure 13.15, the random brightness is observed; both an increase and a decrease in light is randomly shown.

Zoom augmentation can also be done randomly. It tends to add new pixel values around the image or interpolates the pixel values. A sample of zoom augmentation of retina image is shown in Figure 13.16. The zoom-in and zoom-out are clearly observed from the figure.

After performing the above-explained augmentation, the size of data is made to increase from N to 5N. The increase in data with different representations is fed into the already-designed CNN.

Previously, the model suffered from overfitting, which is overcome by increasing the data. It is observed that DL CNN accuracy increases for the dataset of huge size.

The model is executed with a dropout of 0.5 for the activation of ReLU. The results observed are quiet considerable, which are represented in Figure 13.17.

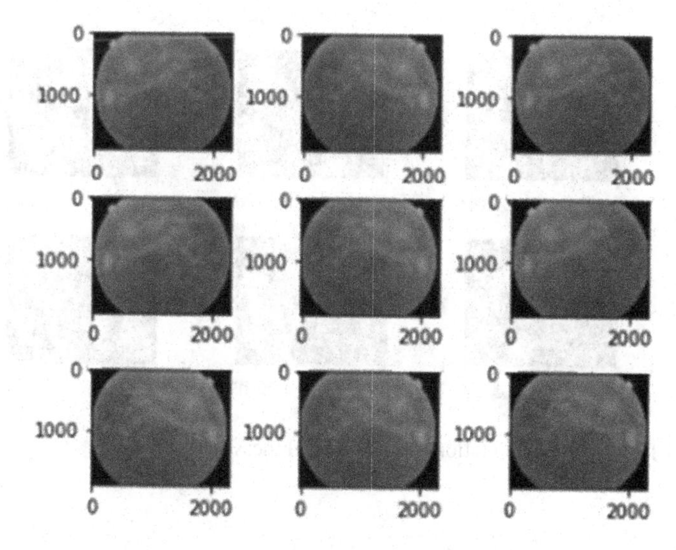

FIGURE 13.13 Data augmentation—horizontal flip.

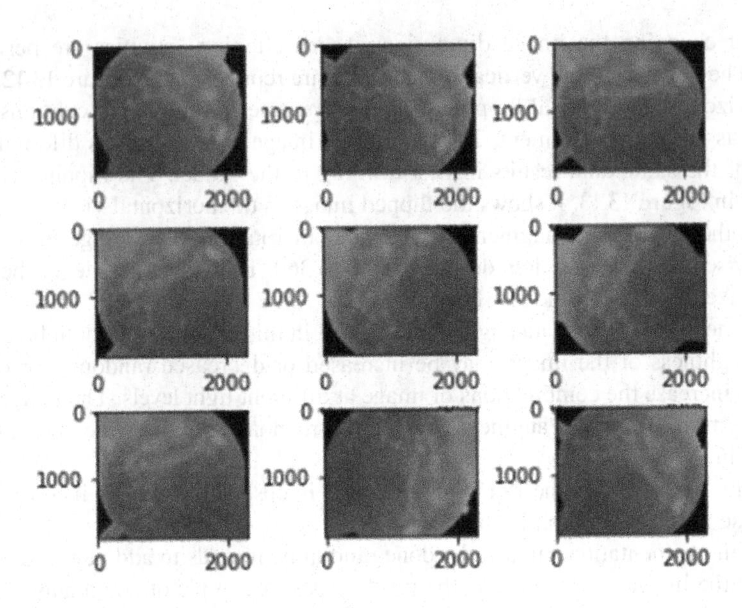

FIGURE 13.14 Data augmentation—random rotation.

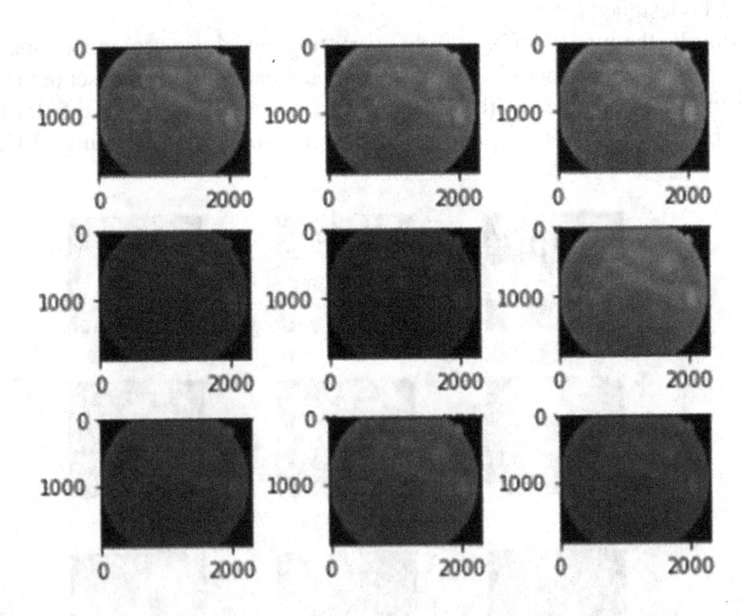

FIGURE 13.15 Data augmentation—random brightness.

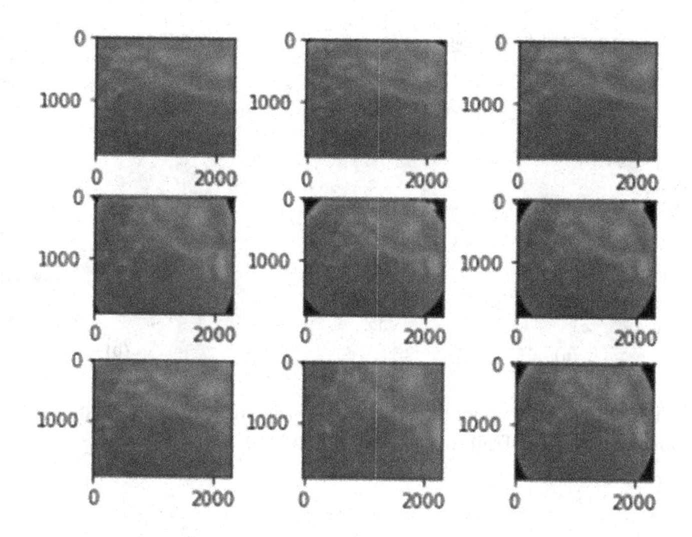

FIGURE 13.16 Data augmentation—random zoom.

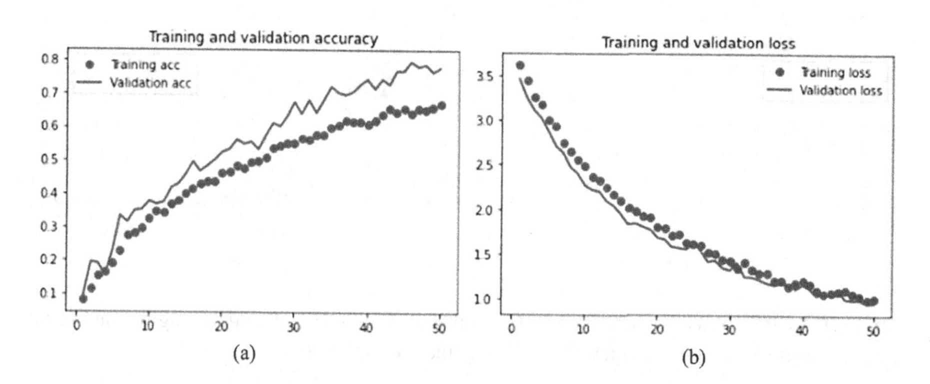

FIGURE 13.17 Plots for dropout 0.5 with 50 epochs after data augmentation. (a) Training and validation accuracy. (b) Training and validation loss.

Figure 13.17 shows that the model is well trained and it is free from overfitting. The results are average, which tends to increase the epochs to 100. The results are shown in Figure 13.18.

Increase in the number of epochs increases the validation accuracy and reduces its loss. The model is now trained to access the data after augmentation using the batch normalization. From the previous results, it is identified that even for the small data size, it performs well compared to dropout. To make sure of it, the model is executed with 50 epochs, and the results are represented in Figure 13.19.

The results are much better, and the accuracy of both training and validation reaches the expected level. Once the epochs are increased, the variations in the results are observed, which are shown in Figure 13.20. The accuracy of both training and validation is achieved.

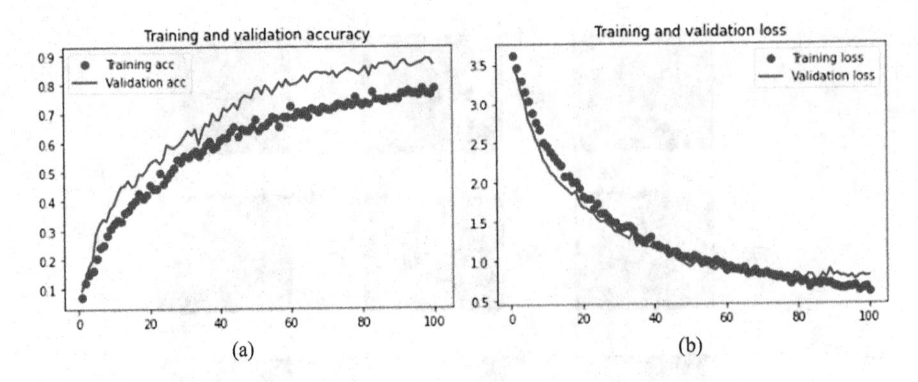

FIGURE 13.18 Plots for dropout 0.5 with 100 epochs after data augmentation (a) Training and validation accuracy. (b) Training and validation loss.

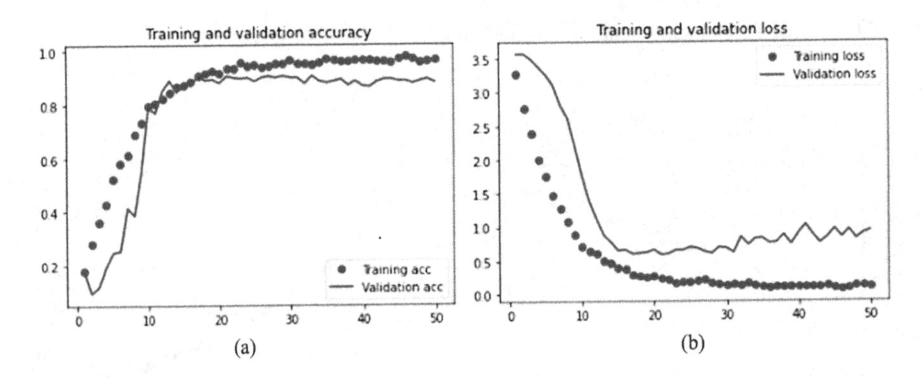

FIGURE 13.19 Plots for batch normalization with 50 epochs after data augmentation. (a) Training and validation accuracy. (b) Training and validation loss.

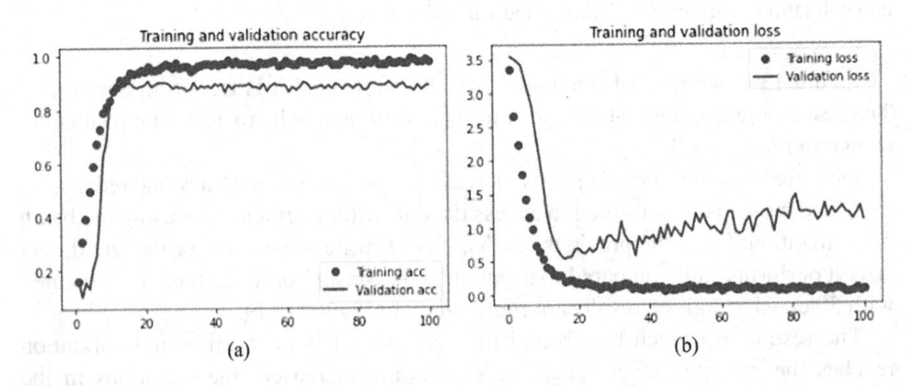

FIGURE 13.20 Plots for batch normalization with 100 epochs after data augmentation (a) Training and validation accuracy. (b) Training and validation loss.

The above result helps to diagnose different diseases that can be identified through the retinal fundus images.

13.4 CONCLUSION

The model developed for the execution of the dataset is important. CNN performs well for huge data. This chapter clearly represents how to increase the dataset size without including the replicated images. Data augmentation transforms the original image into different aspects so that the model can be trained for it. For a single image, the samples at different views can be provided while training the model. Training the model in this way makes it much comfortable while validating the image. This chapter also tries to represent that dropout can be avoided, and instead of it, the batch normalization trains the model well. With these results, the CNN performs well with 96% of accuracy in diagnosing the eye disease. The result can be fine-tuned with different regularization methods if necessary.

ACKNOWLEDGMENTS

The sample images are retrieved from kaggle dataset. All of these 1000 fundus images that belong to 39 classes come from the Joint Shantou International Eye Centre (JSIEC), Shantou City, Guangdong Province, China.

REFERENCES

1. S. Padma and R. Pugazendi. 2020. Combined fuzzy and projection based learning in META-cognitive neural network for MAMMOGRAM classification. *J. Comput. Int. Syst.*, 4, 93–98
2. B. K. Singh, G.R. Sinha and B. Mazumdar. 2010. *ICTACT Journal on Image and Video Processing*, 22–26.
3. B. K. Triwijoyoa, B.S. Sabargunaa, W. Budihartoa and E. Abdurachmana. 2020. Deep Learning approach for classification of eye diseases based on color fundus images in Diabetes and Fundus OCT. In A.S. El-Baz and J.S. Suri (eds.), *Diabetes and Fundus OCT*, pp. 25–57. Elsevier, Amsterdam.
4. D.J. BOptom, O.K.P. BOptom, T.J. Naduvilath, C. Fedtke, M.J. BOptom, H. Zou, P. S. BOptom. 2018. Tessellated fundus appearance and its association with myopic refractive error in Clinical and experimental optometry. *Clin. Exper. Optometry*, 102, 378–384.
5. A. Almazroa, R. Burman, K. Raahemifar, and V. Lakshminarayanan. 2015. Optic disc and optic cup segmentation methodologies for glaucoma image detection: A Survey. *J. Opthalmol.*, 2015, 28.
6. S.S. Hayreh. 1994. Retinal vein occlusion. *Indian J. Ophthalmol.*, 42, 109–132.
7. R.N. Weinreb, T. Aung, and F.A. Medeiros. 2015. The pathophysiology and treatment of glaucoma a review. *JAMA Netw.*, 311, 1901–1911.
8. M.R. Chaddah, K.K. Khanna, and G.D. Chawla. 1971. Optic atrophy (Review of 100 cases). *Indian J. Ophthalmol.*, 19, 172–176.
9. A.D. Henderson, B.B. Bruce, N.J. Newman, and V. Biousse. 2012. Hypertension-related eye abnormalities and the risk of stroke. *PMC*, 2012, 1–9.
10. J.J. Jung, S.-H. Baek, and U.S. Kim. 2011. Analysis of the causes of optic disc swelling. *Korean J. Ophthalmol.*, 25(1), 33–36.

11. S.H. Narnaware, and P.K. Bawankule. 2019. Disc drag: Sequelae of spontaneously regressed retinopathy of prematurity. *Int. J. Med. Ophthalmol.*, 1(1), 34–35.
12. M.W. Ansari, and A. Nadeem. 2016. Congenital anomalies of eye. In: *Atlas of Ocular Anatomy*, pp. 99–101. Springer, Cham.
13. M.A. Musarella, and I.M. MacDonald. 2010. Current Concepts in the Treatment of Retinitis Pigmentosa.
14. G.P. García-García, M. Martínez-Rubio, M.A. Moya-Moya, J.J. Pérez-Santonja, and J. Escribano. 2019. Current perspectives in Bietti crystalline dystrophy. *Clin. Ophthalmol.*, 13, 1379–1399.
15. L.P. Semes. 1992. Lattice degeneration of the retina and retinal detachment. *Optom. Clin.*, 2(3), 71–91. PMID: 1463916.
16. J. Li, Y.M. Paulus, Y. Shuai, W. Fang, Q. Liu, and S. Yuan. 2017. New developments in the classification, pathogenesis, risk factors, natural history, and treatment of branch retinal vein occlusion. *J. Opthalmol.*, PMID: 28386476.
17. S. Padma, and R. Pugazendi. 2015. A survey on study of various machine learning methods for classification. *Int. J. Database Theory Appl.*, 8(5), 265–272.
18. S. Padma and R. Pugazendi. 2018. Solving classification problems using projection-based learning algorithm with fuzzy radial basis function neural network. *Int. J. Comput. Intell. Appl.*, 17(3), 1850013.
19. Y. Wu, H. Wang, B. Zhang, and K.-L. Du. 2012. Using radial basis function networks for function approximation and classification. *Int. Sch. Res. Not.*, 2012, 34.
20. S. Padma, and R. Pugazendi. 2017. Improved radial basis functions using projection based learning algorithm for classification problems. *J. Comput. Intell. Syst.*, 1(1), 22–25.
21. T. Nelson, and L. Narens. 1990. Metamemory: A theoretical framework and new findings. *Psychol. Learn. Motiv.*, 26, 125–173.
22. G.S. Babu and S. Suresh. 2012. Meta-cognitive neural network for classification problems in a sequential learning framework. *Neurocomputing*, 81, 86–96.
23. S. Padma and K.M. Arun. 2014. Classification of Escherichia coli bacteria using meta-cognitive neural network. *Int. J. Comput. Sci. Eng. Technol.*, 5(2), 141–149.
24. G.-B. Huang, Q.-Y. Zhu and C.-K. Siew. 2006. Extreme learning machine: Theory and applications. *Neurocomputing*, 489–501.
25. S. Padma and R. Pugazendi. 2020. Breast cancer detection and classification using fuzzy and projection based learning in meta-cognitive extreme learning. *Compl. Eng. J.*, 11, 265–279.
26. Y. LeCun, Y. Bengio, and G. Hinton. 2015. Deep learning. *Nature* 521(7553), 436–444.
27. J. Tompson, A. Jain, Y. LeCun, and C. Bregler. 2014. Joint training of a convolutional network and a graphical model for human pose estimation. In *Proceedings of the Advances in Neural Information Processing Systems*, 27, pp. 1799–1807.
28. T. Sainath, A.-R. Mohamed, B. Kingsbury, and B. Ramabhadran. 2013. Deep convolutional neural networks for LVCSR. In *Proceedings of the Acoustics, Speech and Signal Processing*, 8614–8618.
29. M.K. Leung, H.Y. Xiong, L.J. Lee, and B.J. Frey. 2014. Deep learning of the tissue-regulated splicing code. *Bioinformatics* 30, i121–i129.
30. S. Jean, K. Cho, R. Memisevic, and Y. Bengio. 2015. On using very large target vocabulary for neural machine translation. In Proc. ACL-IJCNLP http://arxiv.org/abs/1412.2007.
31. E. Grisan. 2005. Automatic Analysis of Retinal Images: Retinopathy Detection and Grading, (PhD dissertation).
32. C.D. Murray. 1926. The physiological principle of minimum work. I. The vascular system and the cost of blood volume. *Proc. Natl. Acad. Sci.* 12(3), 207–214.

Index

Note: **Bold** page numbers refer to tables and *Italic* page numbers refer to figures.

D

E

F

G

H

I

N

R

S

Printed in the United States
by Baker & Taylor Publisher Services